PROCEED WITH CAUTION

Proceed with Caution

Predicting Genetic Risks in the Recombinant DNA Era

Neil A. Holtzman, M.D., M.P.H.

Department of Pediatrics, Johns Hopkins University School
of Medicine, and Departments of Epidemiology and Health Policy
and Management, Johns Hopkins University School of Hygiene
and Public Health

THE JOHNS HOPKINS UNIVERSITY PRESS   BALTIMORE AND LONDON

The Johns Hopkins University Press
701 West 40th Street
Baltimore, Maryland 21211
The Johns Hopkins Press Ltd., London

The paper used in this publication meets the minimum requirements
of American National Standard for Information Sciences—Permanence
of Paper for Printed Library Materials, ANSI Z39.48-1984.

LIBRARY OF CONGRESS CATALOGING-IN-PUBLICATION DATA
Holtzman, Neil A. (Neil Anton), 1934–
    Proceed with caution.
    (The Johns Hopkins series in contemporary medicine and public health)
    Bibliography: p.
    Includes index.
    1. Medical genetics.   2. Genetic counseling.   I. Title.   II. Series. [DNLM:
1. DNA, Recombinant.   2. Genetic Counseling.   3. Hereditary Diseases—
prevention & control.   4. Risk. QZ 50 H758p]
    RB155.H59   1989   616'.042   88-29658
    ISBN 0-8018-3730-8
    ISBN 0-8018-3737-5 (pbk.)

To my father, **Irving N. Holtzman** (1909–1987), who was the first to teach me skepticism, but who knew the price. He concluded his last letter, "Illegitimes non carborundum."

Contents

Acknowledgments

This work grew out of a report commissioned by the Henry J. Kaiser Family Foundation in 1984. Alvin Tarlov, president of the Foundation, originally asked me to consider the policy implications of testing individuals for genetic predispositions to the harmful effects of exposure to environmental agents. Few genetic predispositions had been discovered, but advances in recombinant DNA technology made it inevitable that they would be. As I examined the progress made with this new technology, it became apparent that genetic testing would soon encompass considerably more than susceptibilities to environmental exposures. My earlier studies of genetic screening persuaded me that the expansion of testing posed many difficult questions for society. I am grateful to Dr. Tarlov for permitting me to broaden the scope of the report and for the Foundation's support. Critiques of the report by Dr. Tarlov, and also by Barton Childs, Eric Holtzman, and Anthony Robbins, were very helpful as I set out to explore the topic in greater depth. For many years Barton Childs has encouraged me to pursue unconventional interests in genetics.

With support from the Kaiser Family Foundation, I was able to visit a number of biotechnology companies and to interview several geneticists and molecular biologists, some of whom were affiliated with the companies I visited. Conversations with Norm Arnheim, Jon Beckwith, David Botstein, Henry Erlich, Jim Gusella, Leonard Lerman, Tom Maniatis, and, at Johns Hopkins, Stylianos Antonarakis, Barton Childs, Haig Kazazain, Victor McKusick, and David Valle were very helpful. Special thanks to Dr. Antonarakis for a critical review of the final draft of chapter 4.

The Bureau of Maternal and Child Health and Resources Development (BMCH), Health Resources and Services Administration, U.S. Department of Health and Human Services, and the Health Program, Office of Technology Assessment (OTA), U.S. Congress, provided support for a survey of the interest of American biotechnology companies in genetic testing. Maria Hewitt, an analyst at OTA, played a key role in designing the follow-up questionnaire and in analyzing survey responses. Maria's criticisms of an early draft of the book were very helpful. BMCH and OTA also supported a workshop held at OTA in July 1986 on "Applications of Biotechnology to Tests for Human Genetic Disorders." A number of workshop participants prepared papers for OTA (with the support of BMCH) that gave me a greater insight into recombinant DNA technology and the applications of genetic testing. For these papers I want to thank Lori Andrews, Bob Baumiller, David Blumenthal (with Richard Zeckhauser), Jim Bowman, Henry Erlich, Ruth Faden, Irene Forsman, Charles Hall, David Housman, Abby Lippman, Phil Reilly, and Frank Ruddle (with Kevin Bentley and Anne Ferguson-Smith). Additional invited papers by Rochelle Mayer (with Anna Hamilton and William Rorie), Joe McInerney, and Kay Noel also were helpful, as were materials made available by Jerry Donlon, John Fletcher, and Bob Greenstein.

Maria Hewitt and I prepared a draft of an OTA report on recombinant DNA and genetic testing which was never released. Eighty people reviewed the draft, and the comments of many of them refined and sharpened my writing of this book. In addition to several of those already mentioned, I owe special thanks to Fred Bergmann, Bernard Davis, Clarke Fraser, Philippe Frossard, Victor Fuchs, Susan Gleeson, Kiki Hellman, Mary Sue Henifin, Angela Holder, Larry Jones (who also arranged for input from the Health Insurance Association of America and the American Council of Life Insurance), Sylvia Krekel, Jane Lin-Fu, Joan Marks, Arno Motulsky, Elena Nightingale, Gil Omenn, Barbara Katz Rothman, Mark Rothstein, Charles Scriver, and Nancy Wexler.

BMCH provided additional support to enable me to finish writing the book and to make possible its wide dissemination. I am particularly grateful to Irene Forsman and Vince Hutchins for their continued interest. In December 1987, as I was putting the finishing touches on the manuscript, I was invited by the Harvard Medical School graduate students in genetics to deliver a seminar entitled "A Pandoran View of Genetic Testing." Conversations with the students, and also with Paul Billings, Ruth Hubbard, and Eric Lander, helped me polish the manuscript before I submitted it to the Johns Hopkins University Press. At the Press, I am indebted to Wendy Harris for her encouragement and patience.

The large number of people with whom I consulted forced me to defend to the utmost, and sometimes to modify, my arguments. I take sole responsibility for the content of the book.

It would be surprising if the author of a book on genetics did not mention family members. Genes account for only part of their role, however. My debt to my father is expressed on the book's dedication page. In addition to contributing her genes to our children, Barbara Starfield introduced me to epidemiology. She endured restless nights as I hacked at the word processor. Each of our children had a hand in this project. In 1979, when Robert, our oldest, graduated from Reed College, he and Jon (our second) engaged me in a spirited discussion of prenatal diagnosis and abortion on the side of Mt. Hood. That discussion may well have sowed the seeds for this undertaking. Jon's and Steve's (our third) criticisms of the early chapters of the first draft prompted me to start all over again. Deborah (number four) joined in dinner table discussions in which I sought clarification of my own thoughts. She also prepared some of the book's references. Together, our children inspired me to write about the issues of genetic screening that they and their children will face.

Baltimore, Maryland

PROCEED WITH CAUTION

Introduction: The Shape of Things to Come

Genetics does not matter much to the delivery of medical care. Its meager contribution, except in the detection and management of a few rare, serious diseases, is due not to the absence of genetic factors in many diseases but to an inability to identify them. Until recently, genetic diagnosis relied on inferences from observations far removed from the gene. For only a few diseases were sufficient data available to draw correct inferences.

The coming of the recombinant DNA era has changed all that. The ability to chop up DNA, the stuff of which genes are made, and move the pieces, permits the direct examination of the human genome. As a result, the genetic components in a wide variety of rare and common disorders —cardiovascular, neoplastic, psychiatric, neuromuscular, skeletal, renal, metabolic, hematologic, immune, endocrine—have already been discovered. The data and methods that will permit medical science to go even further are being acquired rapidly.

By pointing the way to effective treatment or prevention, these discoveries may ultimately improve the prospects for the many people who at some point in their lives will manifest a disease with a genetic component. Sometimes recombinant DNA technology will provide the drugs and biologics—as it already has for insulin, growth hormone, and antihemophilic factor—for improving outcome. More immediately, however, genetic tests based on this new technology will be used for diagnosis in those whose health is already impaired and for prediction in those who are still healthy. Tests can predict future disease not only in oneself but also in one's offspring. It is in using genetic tests to predict future disease that caution is needed.

The Scope of the Book

Unfortunately, the congruence of genetics with a few rare diseases has ill prepared many health professionals and the public to appreciate the magnitude of the change made possible by the new technology. The possibility that genes play a role in common diseases, or that genes that increase risk can be identified in time to stop the occurrence of disease or to change its course, will be doubted by many health care providers. The first part of this book is devoted to dispelling this skepticism. In order to do this, I first present some fundamental "axioms" of genetics in chapter 1 and introduce genetic terms that should make reading the chapters that explain the role of genes and of recombinant DNA technology relatively painless.

The role of genetics in common diseases is also finding slow acceptance because of adherence to the doctrine of disease causation that came into vogue with the discovery of microbial pathogens: diseases had single or "specific" etiologies. That an altered gene can cause a few rare diseases (a fact first recognized by Garrod in the early 1900s) fits well with this concept. That several factors—genes at different loci, or genetic plus environmental factors, or several environmental factors—can interact to cause common diseases has gained recognition slowly, even by medical investigators; it is much easier to track down one thing at a time. Further complicating the standard doctrine is the growing evidence for disease heterogeneity; the same clinical entity may be the end result of different combinations of etiologic factors. In chapter 2, I explore these problems further and suggest how diseases whose etiology is complex can be analyzed. Separating causal factors into "discrete" (under which most genetic and environmental factors can be subsumed) and "modulating," I also classify interventions for reducing the burden of disease.

I turn my attention fully to genetics in chapter 3, in which the basis for a genetic role in common diseases is explained by showing that common variants exist for many genes and that some of these variants do increase susceptibility to disease. The apparent contradiction between selection against deleterious genes and the genetic basis of common diseases also is discussed. The chapter summarizes the "classical" and "neoclassical" methods of genetic diagnosis.

The new methods for localizing the genes responsible for many diseases to specific regions of specific chromosomes and for identifying their function are described in chapter 4. This is probably the most difficult chapter to comprehend, but it is essential for an appreciation of the magnitude of the changes made possible by recombinant DNA technology and of some of the pitfalls of using the methods.

The first practical application of human gene identification, and by far the one that will affect the most people, is genetic testing. In the first part of chapter 5, I describe the types of tests that will be developed to determine the presence of the disease-related genes discovered by recombinant DNA technology. Genetic tests will be introduced into health care in one of two ways, depending on the level of scientific knowledge. When the disease-related gene has been localized to a specific region of a chromosome but not yet identified, testing will be limited to families in which the disease has already occurred. Once the gene is identified, tests for the mutation(s) that cause, or increase the risk of, disease will be developed. This will permit genetic *screening*, a population-based search that does not depend on one's having an affected relative. Screening to predict the risk of future disease, therefore, can affect most people.

With population-based predictive tests, the chance for mislabeling is relatively high, even when the tests are based on elegant recombinant DNA technologies. Some people in whom the genetic factor is present (as detected by testing) will not develop clinical disease, because other factors necessary for it to manifest are absent. Some people in whom the test fails to detect an etiologic genetic factor (because it is truly absent) will still develop the disease because of the presence of other etiologic factors. I describe parameters needed to assess the validity (correct labeling ability) of genetic tests.

Another common source of skepticism about the importance of genetics is the belief that little can be done once the presence of a "harmful" gene is detected. Genetic tests can be used to identify asymptomatic individuals at risk for a disease in time to prevent the appearance of the disease. Yet effective interventions have been discovered for relatively few diseases. Until more interventions are discovered, genetic tests will be used to identify individuals, and couples, who are at risk of having affected offspring, so they can take steps to avoid such a conception or birth. Moreover, recombinant DNA technology makes possible the development and application of such tests for any disease in which one or a few genes have been implicated. The uses and sequelae of genetic tests are described in greater detail in the second part of chapter 5.

Having the ability to develop tests is not synonymous with their actual development. A good deal of basic research remains to be done, and then tests suitable for use in routine medical care must be developed. The transfer of knowledge from the research laboratory to organizations that will develop genetic tests for use by health care providers is considered in chapter 6. This transfer involves primarily universities, which have conducted most of the research with public support, and private corporations, which will develop the tests. I consider first the recent changes that have facilitated this transfer and their implications for future research. Then I examine the current interest of biotechnology companies in genetic testing. Much of this work is based on a mailed survey of companies and on personal interviews with executives and scientists at a few companies. There is little doubt that the transfer is taking place.

In chapter 7 I discuss the transmittance of genetic tests from the companies developing them, through the health care providers who will perform them, to the public, which is the ultimate recipient. I consider whether current procedures for regulating medical devices—the category defined by amendments to the Food, Drug, and Cosmetic Act, under which genetic tests fall—are adequate to ensure that tests approved for marketing have been adequately validated. The problem of ensuring reliable test performance in the laboratories that will perform the tests (including physicians' office laboratories as the technology becomes simplified) also is addressed. In the remainder of the chapter, I deal with the knowledge and attitudes of physicians and consumers toward genetic testing. I present evidence that most physicians have been inadequately trained and are inadequately prepared to administer and interpret genetic tests. Nor is the base of public knowledge sufficient to ensure that people coming for testing will necessarily understand the implications of the test. However, a lack of knowledge on the part of either health care providers or consumers will probably not deter the wide use of genetic tests.

The results of predictive genetic tests have such significant consequences that it is important to ensure that people are tested only when they understand the implications of the test and have the opportunity to refuse. Yet a number of situations arise in which people are not given this opportunity. Some of these are paternalistic. Physicians or communities often pressure people to be tested (or may test them without obtaining their informed consent) because they believe they are acting in the people's best interest.

Some testing will be performed to benefit persons other than those being tested. Testing performed in adoption procedures or to obtain insurance or employment may be in the best interest, respectively, of the couple doing the adopting or of the insurance company or employer. I examine these uses of genetic testing in chapter 8. I also consider the possible emergence of a new eugenics. Some geneticists, ethicists, and legal experts argue for the abortion of fetuses destined to suffer severe disease, regardless of the pregnant woman's wishes. They base their argument on the concern that no infant should be allowed to suffer unnecessarily (abortion provides the means of avoiding such suffering) and on economic considerations (abortion usually costs much less than keeping such infants alive).

The continued expansion of genetic testing to more diseases and to more people, however, could increase the threat to personal autonomy. It could also interfere with the ability of people with positive test results to obtain adequate health care. In chapter 8 I also examine some of the legal barriers to the coercive use of genetic tests. By and large these are inadequate to protect individual autonomy.

Finally, in chapter 9 I summarize how genetic tests are likely to be used in the near future and I offer some prescriptions for ensuring that they will be performed safely and effectively while preserving the opportunity of each individual to decide whether to be tested.

Why Proceed with Caution?

In order to persuade the reader of the need for caution—in a sense, to justify the book—I present here in capsule form three reasons why genetic testing may be perilous: (1) the past use of genetics in public and corporate policy; (2) the current trend toward commercialization in biotechnology; (3) and the disparity between diagnosis and effective intervention to reduce the burden of genetic diseases in those born with them.

Genetics in public and corporate policy

Despite its small contribution to personal medical care, genetics has played a role in shaping public policies in the United States. The scientific claims of some early geneticists, or, more properly, eugenicists, were used to justify sterilization and immigration policies in the early part of this century.[1] 1 Although it has been thoroughly repudiated, this inglorious occurrence should keep us alert to the possibility that the identification of specific genetic traits could be used to interfere with individuals' reproductive rights, employment opportunities, or access to adequate health care.

Genetic testing has already been used as an instrument of public policy. When it became possible to detect phenylketonuria (PKU) in apparently healthy newborns, the National Association for Retarded Children and its allies secured the passage of laws in most states that compelled the screening of newborns for increased concentrations of phenylalanine in the blood, an indicator of the possible presence of PKU.[2] At the time, the ability of a low-phenylalanine diet to prevent the appearance of retardation had not been established.[3] Although it is now clear that most infants with persistent, large elevations of blood phenylalanine will benefit from the special diet, a few of them will not; nonresponsive forms of the disorder are now known.[4] Had those forms predominated, screening for PKU would have proved a waste of public funds. PKU screening has also confirmed a point I made earlier. The test is not a perfect predictor of PKU; some infants with the disorder are missed by screening while others who have positive test results do not have PKU.[5]

In the early 1970s, screening for sickle cell anemia and the sickle cell trait rapidly proliferated, frequently with the use of public funds and sometimes as a result of compulsory legislation.[6] Neither treatment nor prenatal diagnosis was available, and just what young adults who were identified as being carriers did with the information was never determined. A study in Orchomenos, Greece—a village in which the sickle cell gene is present in high frequency—indicated that some carriers who were detected by screening hid their status and that probably no reduction in matings between carriers resulted from screening.[7]

Genetic testing has also been adopted by a few corporations to identify workers with genetic susceptibilities who might suffer harm from workplace exposures. There is little evidence to justify the use of current tests for this purpose,[8] but many more tests will be possible in the future. Screening out workers discovered to be at risk by genetic tests may still leave other workers susceptible.

Thus, there is ample precedent for embarking on genetic screening without adequate evidence of the benefits and without adequate consideration of the harmful effects. In the case of PKU, some infants were falsely labeled as having the disease and suffered irreparable damage.[9] In sickle cell screening, some individuals found to have the trait suffered severe psychological reactions because its benign nature was never explained.[10] In the workplace, genetic screening can be used as an alternative to improving working conditions.

Until now, genetic testing has been undertaken for relatively rare disorders. With the advent of recombinant DNA technology, the detection of those at risk for many more conditions, some of them quite common, will be possible. Thus, the opportunity for reducing the burden of disease becomes much greater. But if the mistakes of past genetic testing programs are repeated, the dangers also will become much greater.

Commercialization in biotechnology

When genetic tests for rare disorders were developed—usually as a result of publicly supported research—they were usually provided under research budgets at little cost to the patient. When newborn screening became possible, and later, carrier screening for sickle cell, thalassemia, and Tay-Sachs, the tests were subsidized by states or community groups in many parts of the country. Chromosome analysis (karyotyping) in older pregnant women for the prenatal diagnosis of Down syndrome was provided primarily by university laboratories that were part of genetic service centers. Until the early 1980s many of these centers received federal support. Cutbacks in federal support for genetic services,[11] together with a growing recognition of the market for genetic and chromosome tests, led commercial laboratories to expand their testing. A few biotechnology companies perceive a market in DNA-based genetic testing and have invested in test development.

Commercial involvement will accelerate the development of genetic tests and their dissemination to the public, but it is not clear that the tests will be applied appropriately. Once again, the historical record is instructive. In the 1970s, a few American pharmaceutical companies asked the Food and Drug Administration (FDA) to approve the marketing of diagnostic kits for the detection of neural tube defects (anencephaly, spina bifida) in the fetus. Obstetricians, pediatricians, and geneticists feared that despite the test's reliability it could easily be misused, misinterpreted, or not appropriately followed up. As a consequence, unaffected fetuses could be aborted.[12] They called for restrictions on the marketing of the test. The manufacturers, together with the American Medical Association and clinical pathologists, maintained that as long as the test was accurate, restricting its use would infringe excessively on physicians' abilities to practice medicine. Under the Carter administration, the FDA sided with the obstetricians.[13] The proposed rule was reversed by the Reagan administration and the kits are now being marketed with virtually no restrictions.[14]

The use, interpretation, and follow-up of recombinant DNA tests for genetic diseases, particularly the common ones, will be at least as difficult as those of the tests for neural tube defects. It is by no means clear that the FDA will deal with DNA-based tests any differently than it has dealt with tests for neural tube defects. Without much greater understanding of tests and their implications, neither physicians nor prospective recipients will appreciate when to use the tests or how to interpret the results. Physicians tend to underestimate the occurrence of false positive and false negative test results. And even when the results of the test are correct, they still may not provide adequate information.

Companies make no secret of the importance of profit in motivating their interests in specific areas. When tests are costly and the number of people likely to use them is small, companies lose interest. Tests may be aggressively marketed for common diseases but not, therefore, for rare ones. It is not clear that university laboratories will retain an interest in these rare disorders. Consequently tests for them might not be available to people who could benefit from them.

Uneven development: Detection precedes correction

Although recombinant DNA research may eventually lead to the development of effective treatments for genetic disorders, it will lead to the development of genetic tests much sooner. In the interim, controversial and sometimes novel means of avoidance will be the primary consequences of detecting those at risk. Biotechnology companies developing genetic tests are not deterred by this time lag. Predictive tests will be on the market before treatments for the disorders they predict are developed or their efficacy is demonstrated.

Recombinant DNA technology will greatly increase the number of disorders for which prenatal diagnosis is possible. By the relatively new technique of chorionic villi sampling (CVS), fetal cells can be obtained as early as the ninth week of pregnancy (compared to the sixteenth to twentieth weeks for amniocentesis). If proven as safe as amniocentesis, CVS will probably make prenatal diagnosis acceptable to more pregnant women.

With DNA-based tests, many more disorders will be detectable in the fetus. In the quest for perfect babies and lower health expenditures, prenatal diagnosis and abortion could be used for many of them. (In this book, questions will be raised as to where the line should be drawn in determining the appropriateness of a condition for prenatal diagnosis and abortion, and who should draw it.) Genetic tests could foster a new eugenics in which pressure is exerted on women whose offspring would be at risk to avoid their conception or birth.

And what about the living who harbor genes for serious diseases in themselves? Over a decade ago Lewis Thomas pointed out that the costs of medical care are highest when we are only "halfway along" in our understanding of underlying disease mechanisms.[15] That is the stage we will be at for quite some time after the genetic factors in diseases are elucidated. Until the costs go down, private insurance companies and employers, who pay a large portion of our health care bills, could use genetic tests to foster a new form of discrimination in which they deny coverage or jobs to those who are at greater risk, thereby reducing the costs to insurance companies and employers respectively.

Gene detection is likely to touch the lives of many people, and soon! How this will happen, what implications it will have, and what can be done to avoid misuse are the subjects of this book.

Chapter 1

The Structural Basis of Genetic Differences

Exposure to a specified dose of some environmental agent—be it a germ, chemical, or dietary constituent—will result in illness in some, but not all, individuals, even if all other environmental events could be kept constant. Among those who do become sick, the interval between exposure and the onset of symptoms, the extent of the illness, and the response to it will vary. Genetic differences account for most of these variations. The mechanisms accounting for genetic variation will be considered further in chapters 2 and 3. In this chapter I present the structural basis of genetic differences. The statements that follow are presented as axioms, but they all have proofs. Presentation of the evidence would fill several volumes. I refer back to specific axioms at several points in subsequent chapters. Those who have studied or read about genetics *recently* may want to skip this chapter.

Axiom 1. Genes are segments of DNA arranged in tandem along chromosomes. The position occupied by a gene is called its locus. The chromosomes reside inside the cell's nucleus.

Axiom 2. One set of chromosomes is inherited from the mother and one from the father (figure 1), via the egg and sperm, respectively. Each of these germ cells contains one set of twenty-three chromosomes. Twenty-two of them are autosomes; the twenty-third (the sex chromosome) is either an X or a Y chromosome. Normally, all the other nucleated cells in the body—called somatic cells—have a pair of each autosome and either two X chromosomes (for a female) or an X and a Y chromosome (for a male), for a total of forty-six chromosomes. The two members of a pair of autosomes (one from the mother, one from the father) are called homologous chromosomes.

Since each somatic cell has two sets of chromosomes, each also has two sets of genes. The genes occupying identical loci on homologous

---

FIGURE 1.1

Nucleus of a somatic cell (or germ cell precursor).
Segments of only 2 of the pairs of autosomes
are shown. The member of each pair derived
from the ovum of the previous generation is
designated **M** (maternal). The other member,
derived from the sperm that fertilized the
ovum, is designated **P** (paternal). Specific gene
loci are designated by number. Alleles at a
locus (see axiom 9) are indicated by locus
number with and without primes (') following
the number—e.g., 4 and 4' are two different
alleles at locus 4. Each chromosome has started to
replicate; the individual strands are called chromatids.

---

chromosomes also are homologous. A female has two X chromosomes,
so she has two sets of genes for the X chromosome, although in any cell
only one set functions. A male, however, has only one X and one Y chromosome, so he has only one set of genes for each.

Axiom 3. The precursor cells of an egg and a sperm also have two sets of
chromosomes, for a total of forty-six. During meiosis this number is reduced to twenty-three. Early in meiosis, homologous chromosomes pair
with each other and line up in the middle of the cell. The members of
each pair are on opposite sides of an imaginary plane that divides the cell.
The different autosomes line up independently of one another, so a random combination of maternally *and* paternally derived autosomes is on
each side of the plane (figure 1.2). Thus each ovum or sperm that results

---

FIGURE 1.2

Early meiosis. In meiosis, homologous chromosomes in precursor cells of the germ cells pair
with each other. A random combination of
maternally and paternally derived autosomes
will be on each side of the cell. "Synapsing" (attachment) of maternal and paternal members of a pair occurs as a result of
breakage at points along the chromatids;
an **M** chromatid at one side of the break
point joins to the **P** chromatid at the other,
forming "chiasmata." The result is known as
"crossing over" or "recombination." (The recombined chromosomes are shown in figure 1.3.)

Synapse
(crossing over)

FIGURE 1.3

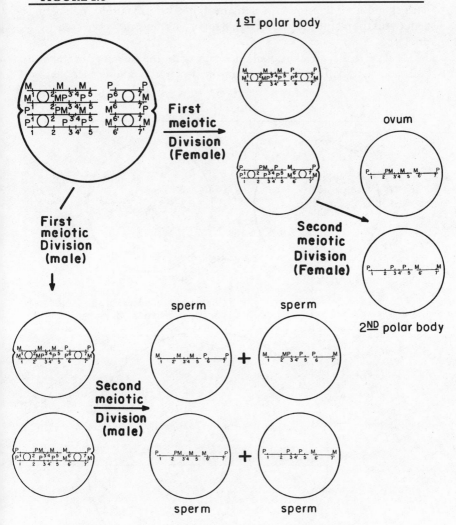

First and second meiotic divisions. In the first meiotic division, the homologous pairs separate, one member going to each "daughter" cell. As a result of crossing over, each member of a chromosome pair now contains alleles derived from the mother and the father of the previous generation. In females one of the daughter cells is discarded as the "first polar body."

In the second meiotic division, the chromatids separate, one going to each germ cell. In females, only one of the two cells becomes an ovum; the other is discarded as the "second polar body." In males, all four of the cells derived from one precursor become sperm.

from the division of these cells will carry chromosomes derived from both the mother and the father (figure 1.3). At fertilization, the sperm penetrates the ovum and a new double set of chromosomes is created (figure 1.4).

During meiosis, an additional opportunity for the exchange of maternally and paternally derived chromosomal material, and consequently

FIGURE 1.4

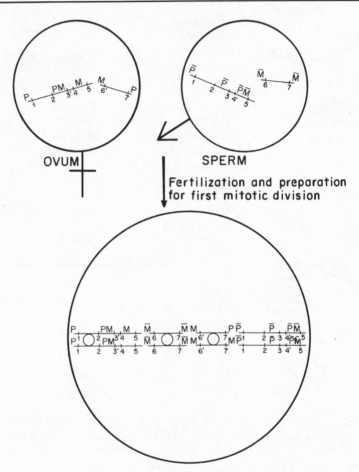

Pronucleus of the ovum in figure 1.3 following fertilization. The maternal and paternal origins of the gene loci on the sperm are designated $\overline{M}$ and $\overline{P}$, respectively. Note that crossing over in the chromosome from the sperm has occurred at a different point than that in the ovum.

genes, presents itself. When homologous chromosomes pair, the homologous genes face each other and are in close proximity. This allows an exchange of genetic material, or crossing over (see figure 1.2) to take place. A chromosome that came entirely from one parent before meiosis will have segments from the other parent interspersed along it after meiosis. Crossing over is often reciprocal; the segments lost from one chromosome are gained by the other. The closer two genes are to each other on a chromosome, the less likely it is that crossing over will occur between them; the two are said to be linked.

Axiom 4. DNA (deoxyribonucleic acid) consists of two long strands of polynucleotide entwined around each other in the shape of a double helix. Each polynucleotide consists of long sequences of deoxyribonucleotides. Each of these consists of a purine or pyrimidine base attached to a sugar (deoxyribose). The deoxyribonucleotides are covalently bound to each other by phosphates attached to the fifth (5') carbon of one sugar and the third (3') carbon of the next. There are four different bases: adenine, guanine, cytosine, and thymine. Through hydrogen bonding, each base on one strand pairs with a specific complementary base on the other strand: adenine with thymine, and guanine with cytosine. In DNA replication, the strands separate. With the help of enzymes, each strand serves as the template for synthesis of the complementary strand. Complementary strands of DNA are bound to each other by the pairing of their complementary bases (figure 1.5). The pairing of complementary strands is also called hybridization.

FIGURE 1.5

DNA replication. Both strands serve as templates. Synthesis always proceeds by adding deoxyribonucleotides to the free 3' end. A cytosine deoxyribonucleotide forms a hydrogen bond with guanine on the upper template. The phosphate on the fifth carbon of the cytosine's deoxyribose backbone is about to be linked to the third carbon of the thymine deoxyribose to its right.

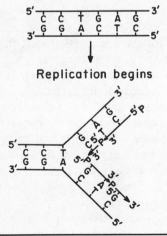

Axiom 5. The sequence of nucleotides of a gene determines its *unique* function. Genes that are directly responsible for the synthesis of polypeptide chains, of which proteins are comprised, are called structural genes.

a. Because of the presence of sequences that are recognized by the appropriate enzymes, some genes are transcribed into RNA (ribonucleic acid) (figure 1.6). This process is similar to DNA replication, but in this case, instead of serving as a template for pairing with complementary deoxyribonucleotide bases, one strand serves as a template for pairing with complementary ribonucleotide bases. (Ribose, rather than deoxyribose, is the sugar of ribonucleotides.) Adenine pairs with uracil ribonucleotides (there are no thymine ribonucleotides), but thymine, guanine, and cytosine deoxyribonucleotides of DNA pair with adenine, cytosine, and guanine ribonucleotides, respectively, in a manner similar to DNA replication. Transcription occurs at different times in the cell cycle than DNA replication and is catalyzed by different enzymes.

b. The transcribed RNA of structural genes contains sequences of nucleotides that encode for the synthesis of polypeptide chains. Each polypeptide chain consists of a sequence of amino acids, of which there are twenty. The sequence of nucleotides—taken in groups of three, called codons—determines the specific order of amino acids in the chain (figure 1.7, top), as well as the termination of chain synthesis. This sequence is contained in messenger RNA (mRNA) molecules, the products of the transcription process. Each molecule in another class of RNA, transfer RNA, contains one triplet (anticodon), whose bases are complementary to one codon in mRNA. (A molecule of mRNA carries a string of codons arranged sequentially; a molecule of transfer RNA carries only one anticodon.) Each transfer RNA molecule is also capable of binding one of the twenty different amino acids. In polypeptide synthesis, the transfer RNAs, with their respective amino acids attached, find their way, one after the other, to the complementary codons of the mRNA molecule. With enzymatic assistance, the peptide bonds are formed between the amino acids, which by this process are brought close to each other. This process is called translation (figure 1.6, bottom).

Portions of the nucleotide sequences of structural genes do not code for amino acids. Some of these noncoding sequences, called introns, are interspersed between the encoding sequences, or exons, while others precede the first exon and others succeed the last. Intron sequences are transcribed, but they are then excised from putative mRNA; the exons are then spliced together. Portions of the preceding and succeeding sequences influence the initiation and termination of transcription and play a role in initiating translation, but the function, if any, of other noncoding sequences is unknown.

c. Long nucleotide sequences of each chromosome are not transcribed

FIGURE 1.6

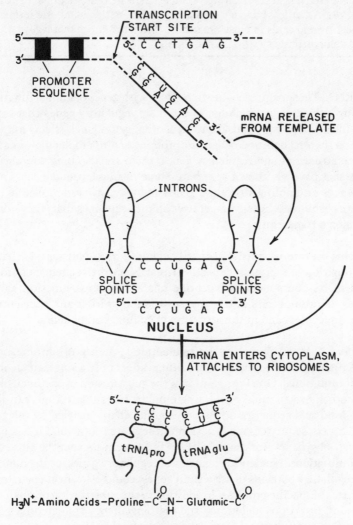

DNA transcription. RNA polymerase (not shown) recognizes two promoter sequences that are almost identical for all structural genes. The enzyme then initiates transcription at a fixed "start" site, using only the 3'-to-5' strand of the DNA molecule that permits synthesis of mRNA to proceed in the 5'-to-3' direction. Note that in mRNA the base uracil replaces thymine in complementary pairing. The sequences that "tell" RNA polymerase to stop transcribing are not shown. Intron regions are "spliced out" before the finished mRNA molecule enters the cytoplasm. In translation, shown in the bottom part of the figure, codons on mRNA are recognized in turn by complementary anticodons on tRNA molecules to which specific amino acids are attached at their carboxyl ends. There are more than twenty different tRNAs, at least one for each amino acid. Peptide bonds are formed between amino acids in close proximity. When the entire message is "read," polypeptide synthesis is complete.

---

into RNA. These sequences are in tandem with genes of known function, bearing a fixed position. Some of them are regulatory genes that influence the activity (e.g., transcription) of other genes. Such effects may depend on their recognition of specific proteins or other molecules. In addition to structural and regulatory genes, there are also long stretches of DNA that have no known function. Some of these, pseudogenes, have sequences resembling structural genes and may have functioned in progenitors of humans but no longer have all the sequences that enable them to undergo transcription.

Axiom 6. Proteins consist primarily of one or more polypeptide chains. The function of a protein depends primarily on the sequence of amino acids in its component polypeptide chains. Proteins function as enzymes, hormones, and antibodies; in the recognition and transport of other molecules; and in the structure of cellular components.

Axiom 7. Mutations alter the nucleotide sequence of chromosomal DNA (figure 1.7). The smallest mutations affect only a single nucleotide (point mutations). One type results in the substitution of one nucleotide for another. In structural genes, single-nucleotide substitutions can alter the amino acid sequence of the polypeptide chain encoded by the gene and, as a consequence, the function of the protein of which it is a part. The rate of synthesis or the stability of the protein also may be altered by point mutations. Nucleotide changes in regulatory genes, or the noncoding, regulatory portions of structural genes, could also affect the rates of synthesis of specific proteins. In addition to the substitution of single nucleotides, insertions, deletions, and rearrangements of nucleotides also occur. Some mutations do not have any detectable effect.

Large insertions may result in the introduction of a repeat sequence of an entire gene (gene duplication). They may arise as a result of crossing over when the two strands of DNA do not match perfectly (unequal crossing over). Sometimes these sequences will not be transcribed (pseudogenes), or if they are, they will not lead to the presence of a functional polypeptide because the complete sequence is not present. At other times the duplicate gene will undergo further mutation that will give it a new function.

FIGURE 1.7

```
                    -C C U G A G G A G-    "wild type" nucleotide sequence
                    -P r o-G L u-G L u-    "wild type" amino acid sequence
```

Types of mutation (⇩ indicates site of mutation, <u>amino acid</u> changes are <u>underlined</u>)

I Single nucleotide substitution

```
                              ⇩
            a) -C C U G A G G A G-    "wild type"
               -C C U G U G G A C-    substitution
               -P r o-Va L-G L u-
                            ⇩
            b) -C C U G A G G A G-    "wild type"
               -C C U U A G G A G-    substitution
               -P r o  Stop
```

II Deletion

```
                          ⇩
            -C C U G A G G A G-    "wild type"
            -C C U A G G A G -     deletion (frameshift)
            -P r o-Arg-Arg-
                        Ser
```

III Insertion

```
                      ⇩
            -C C U G A G G A G-    "wild type"
            -C C U U G A G G A G-  insertion (frameshift)
            -P r o  Stop
```

IV Inversion

```
              ⇩           ⇩
            -C C U G A G G A G-    "wild type"
            -G A G U C C G A G-    inversion
            -G L u-Se r-G L u-
```

Types of mutation. Mutation occurs on DNA, but if the segment is transcribed, it is reflected in the nucleotide sequence on the mRNA, as shown in the figure. The arrows indicate the site or sites of mutation. The original or "wild type" mRNA sequence and the segment of the polypeptide for which it encodes are shown at the top of the diagram. I(a): The substitution of uracil for adenine in the second position of the second codon results in the substitution of valine (val) for glutamic acid (glu) on the polypeptide. This is, in fact, the mutation of sickle cell anemia. I(b): The substitution of a uracil for guanine in the first position of the second codon introduces a "stop" codon, UAG. This codon is not recognized by any tRNA, and peptide synthesis terminates prematurely. II: The deletion of the guanine in the first position of the second codon, without any substitution, shifts the "reading" frame for translation. The codon GAG is gone and all subsequent nucleotides are now out of frame by one nucleotide. The second codon is now AGG, which is recognized by the tRNA for arginine. The large number of differences in amino acid sequence, as well as a possible premature termination of polypeptide synthesis, will drastically alter the function of the polypeptide. **III:** The insertion of a U after the first codon also shifts the reading frame so that a stop codon, UGA, is read. **IV:** The first and second codons are inverted, resulting in a sequence that codes for glu and serine (ser). If the inversion does not involve multiples of three nucleotides, frame shift will occur.

Axiom 8. For mutations to be transmitted to the next generation, they must occur in the germ cells or their precursors. Mutations in somatic cells that continue to divide after the mutation occurs will be transmitted only to "daughter" cells that contain the DNA on which the mutation occurred.

Axiom 9. In any individual, the two members of a gene pair—one inherited from the mother, the other from the father—do not necessarily have identical DNA sequences. A mutation in one gene could have been received from the germ cell of one parent but not the other. Genes at a locus on a chromosome that differ in their DNA sequences are called alleles. Although an individual can never have more than two alleles—one from each parent—at a locus, within the population there may well be many alleles at the locus, each arising from a different mutation. Individuals with two different alleles at a locus are heterozygotes. Individuals who have inherited the same allele from both parents are homozygotes. Males are hemizygotes for alleles on the X chromosome. The alleles present at a locus define the genotype at that locus.

Axiom 10. The presence of more than one allele at a locus can be inferred by experimental matings in animals and plants, and sometimes by analysis of pedigrees in humans. If two alleles, A and a, exist at a locus, then six matings of the genotypes listed below are possible. A parent can pass only one allele to any one child. The genotypes of the offspring are shown after the colon. If more than one genotype is possible from the mating, the ratio of their respective probabilities of occurrence is shown in parentheses. (In contrast to the book's illustrations, in which numbers represent genes and primes represent different alleles, upper- and lowercase letters are used here in keeping with standard genetic nomenclature.)

1. AA × AA: AA
2. AA × aa: Aa
3. AA × Aa: AA (1), Aa (1)

4. Aa × Aa: AA (1), Aa (2), aa (1)
5. Aa × aa: Aa (1), aa (1)
6. aa × aa: aa

The phenotype, or the observed characteristic, does not always distinguish different genotypes. Thus, genotypes *AA* and *Aa* may have identical characteristics—that is, the same phenotype. The phenotype due to *A* is then said to be dominant over the phenotype due to *a*. Only when present in the *aa* homozygote is the characteristic due to *a* expressed. The *aa* phenotype is then said to be recessive. If that is the case, then in cross (3) only one phenotype is observed, and in cross (4) two phenotypes are observed with probabilities in the ratio of 3:1. In the heterozygote, when both alleles are expressed they are said to be codominant.

(In the above example, the locus was assumed not be on an X or a Y chromosome. Unless a woman is homozygous for an allele on the X chromosome, the trait for which the allele is responsible will be manifested more strongly in males with the allele. This is because in some cells of the heterozygous female the allele carrying the trait will be active, while in others the other allele will be the active one (only one X chromosome remains active in each cell in the female (axiom 2). This attenuates the expression of the allele. Half of the male offspring of a woman heterozygous for an allele on the X chromosome will, on average, inherit the allele.)

Genes that are located on different chromosomes are passed to the next generation independently of each other. This follows from the arrangements of the chromosomes at meiosis. In addition, because of the likelihood of crossing over, genes at widely distant loci on the same chromosome also will be inherited independently of each other.

The basic rules of inheritance described in axiom 10 were first proposed by the monk Gregor Mendel in the latter half of the nineteenth century as a result of his crosses of different varieties of garden peas.[1] Mendel did not have the benefit of axioms 1–9 to guide him, however; neither genes nor chromosomes had yet been discovered. By hybridizing plants that differed in one characteristic (e.g., white or gray seed coat color), he observed that the hybrids inherited one or the other alternative (e.g., they were *either* gray *or* white), in a ratio of 3:1. We now know that such segregation, as Mendel put it, is due to the segregation of alleles. Mendel himself coined the terms *dominant* and *recessive* to explain the ratios. To this day, traits due to alleles at single loci are said to be Mendelian. Mendel also recognized that the inheritance of one characteristic (e.g., seed coat color) did not depend on the inheritance of another (e.g., pod texture). This he described as independent assortment. These independent characteristics were determined by genes that were on different chromosomes or far apart (unlinked) on the same chromosome.

Many of the traits of the garden peas that Mendel worked with produced continuous variation and consequently did not demonstrate clear-cut segregation. Two possible explanations can account for this. The first is that there are multiple (more than two) alleles at a single locus, and each combination of two (genotype) has a different expression (phenotype). As demonstrated in axiom 10, when two alleles are present, three genotypes are possible. If three alleles are present, six genotypes are possible, and with four alleles, ten are possible. The second explanation is that the trait is determined by alleles at more than one gene locus, each of the loci is unlinked to the others, and each genotype has a different phenotype. If there were two separate loci A and B and two alleles at each of them (A,a;B,b), then nine genotypes would be possible: aabb, aabB, aaBB, aAbb, aAbB, aABB, AAbb, AAbB, and AABB. It will be very difficult to distinguish between these two possibilities.

The British physician Sir Archibald Garrod was the first to recognize that certain rare disorders are inherited as Mendelian traits.[2] Some twenty years later he suggested the possibility of genetic predispositions to a much wider range of disorders even though Mendelian inheritance could not be established.[3] Recombinant DNA technology opens up the possibility—to a much greater degree than ever before—of finding the specific gene loci, and the alleles at them, that account for these predispositions.

Chapter 2

The Complexity of Diseases: No More Magic Bullets

Death rates at every age have plummeted since 1900 in the United States and other developed countries. Will the strategies that have been responsible for this decline continue to be effective, or will new approaches be needed? How important a part could genetic testing play? To begin to answer these questions, I examine the changes in the prevalence of disease during this century, and the interventions that have been responsible for increased survival. On the basis of this analysis, I present a classification of the determinants of disease that provides a systematic approach to discovering causal factors. The classification is also useful in categorizing interventions for reducing the burden of disease and disability.

Changes in Disease Prevalence

In 1900, the leading causes of death were pneumonia, tuberculosis, and diarrhea. The great success of Pasteur, Koch, and other microbe hunters in showing that these and other common diseases of the time were caused by microorganisms set the tone of biomedical research until the present day: "They imposed upon medical thought; they transfixed its theoretical and philosophical corpus with the vivid concept of the specific etiological factor, and by necessity also with its corollary, the specific antidotal, curative agent, 'the magic bullet,' now so dear to the science romancer."[1]

Their search and their success were facilitated by the congruence between the clinical and pathologic features of a disease on the one hand and its etiology on the other. This congruence is supported by the observation that many of the names of the common diseases of the time, which were descriptive of the clinical picture or the pathology (e.g., pneumonia, tuberculosis, pertussis, tetanus, diphtheria), were given to the bacteria that were proved to cause them. The congruence was so great that even in the absence of laboratory tests demonstrating the presence of the infectious agent, one could be certain of the diagnosis most of the time. Only later—after laboratory tests became an adjunct in diagnosis—did medical practitioners recognize that not everyone who harbors a pathogenic microorganism actually develops the disease.

Despite the correctness of the germ theory, and the effectiveness of the "magic bullets" that followed, the decline in the occurrence of infectious diseases started long before the introduction of vaccines and antibiotics.[2] Public health measures such as water purification, sewage treatment, milk processing (Pasteurization), and less crowded housing reduced the likelihood of infection. Better nutrition and clothing undoubtedly raised resistance. Without this rise in living standards, "modulating" factors, in ways that were poorly understood, enhanced the infectious qualities of the specific etiologic agents.

With the decline in infectious diseases, a greater proportion of infants survived to older ages. Concomitantly, the leading causes of death at all ages changed. Heart disease, cancer, stroke, accidents, and chronic obstructive lung disease now outrank pneumonia, influenza, and tuberculosis as causes of death among adults.[3] In contrast to 1910, when diarrhea was the leading cause of death in infancy,[4] congenital abnormalities are today.[5]

There is less congruence between the symptom complex and etiology of the diseases prevalent today than there was for the common infectious diseases. There are several explanations for this:

1. Different people with the same pathologic condition may develop it from different causative factors. There is considerable etiologic *heterogeneity*. Although increased risk of coronary artery disease is associated with hypercholesterolemia, most who suffer the disease have moderate cholesterol levels. Cleft palate or spina bifida occurs more frequently than expected in the offspring of women with seizures who take specific anticonvulsants during pregnancy, but most infants who are born with these abnormalities were not exposed to these drugs in utero. Congenital anomalies of all types are due to a variety of causes, but for most the causative factors are unknown.[6]

This etiologic heterogeneity is not observed for some of the diseases that have occurred in epidemic proportions since World War II. A large proportion of lung cancer is associated with cigarette smoking. Characteristic congenital limb deformities, which appeared suddenly about thirty years ago, were almost all due to the use of the sedative thalidomide early in pregnancy. Most cases of the acquired immune deficiency syndrome (AIDS) are due to infection with human immunodeficiency viruses (HIV).

2. The same factor can be incriminated in the etiology of more than one disease. Cigarette smoking contributes to fetal death and premature birth as well as to heart disease and lung cancer. Toxic chemicals may be

teratogens as well as carcinogens. This *pleiotropic* effect was observed for some of the common infectious agents of the past as well. But each of the different entities attributable to an infectious agent, such as the tubercle bacillus, is not also attributable to a large number of other agents.

3. Even though an agent is found to play a role in the causation of a disease, many individuals exposed to that agent, even at high doses, will never suffer the disease. There is variable *expressivity*. Geneticists also use the term *penetrance* to describe this phenomenon; throughout this book I will use *expressivity* to cover the entire spectrum of variation associated with the presence of an etiologic agent. The spectrum runs from full-blown clinical picture, through intermediate and different clinical manifestations, to the complete absence of manifestations. The classic study on the link between lung cancer and smoking projected that fewer than 2 percent of men over the age of 35 who were heavy smokers would die of lung cancer over the ensuing ten years. The risk of dying from lung cancer is highest in long-time smokers aged 65 to 75, but among them, fewer than 5 percent will die of lung cancer within ten years.[7] Fewer than 3 percent of men aged 40 to 54 who are free of coronary heart disease but are in the highest decile of smoking, plasma cholesterol, and blood pressure will suffer a myocardial infarction or die from coronary heart disease in the ensuing twelve years.[8] Nor is the volume of alcohol imbibed or the duration of high intake a good predictor of who develops cirrhosis.[9] Anticonvulsants taken in pregnancy do not always cause birth defects.

Classifying Etiologic Factors

The doctrine of specific etiology is no longer sufficient to explain disease. Many different factors are potentially capable of causing at least one disease. As seen in the accompanying list, these factors can be divided into two categories: discrete and modulating. Moreover, the discrete factors can be subclassified as genetic or environmental.

Discrete factors

ENVIRONMENTAL
Chemicals (pure, including drugs, and constituents of foods and
    other products)
Physical agents (irradiation of various types, heat, cold)
Microorganisms (bacteria, viruses, protozoans)
Deficiencies of specific nutrients (vitamins, trace metals)
Weapons

GENETIC
Alleles at specific loci (about 100,000 loci): disease-causing;
    susceptibility-conferring

Modulating factors
Age (developmental stage: infancy, childhood, adolescence, adulthood,
    pregnancy, senescence)
Sex
Family
Ethnic group, race
Social class
Climate
Occupation
Sanitation
Housing
Clothing
Nutrition
Stressors (physical, emotional)
Complex physiological functions (absorption, excretion)
Resilience
Past experience (immunity)
Social networks
Personal habits (smoking, drinking)
Drugs (pharmacological and recreational)

Discrete factors

To classify a factor as "discrete," one must first establish a *causal* relationship between the factor and the occurrence of disease in at least some individuals. (The methods for doing this will be introduced in the next section.) Discrete genetic factors are alleles at a specified gene locus that are capable, by themselves, of causing a disease. I call such factors *disease-causing alleles.* For recessive diseases, however, a single dose of a disease-causing allele will not cause the disease. I will use the term *disease-causing genotype* when I am referring to only that dosage of a disease-causing allele capable of causing disease. I will use the term *disease-related gene* to refer to a gene locus at which disease-causing or susceptibility-conferring alleles reside. Discrete environmental factors are those chemical and physical agents that have been proven capable of causing disease at least at some dosages.

The "capability" of discrete factors to cause disease is not tantamount to predicting that they will always cause disease, or cause disease of the same severity. The expressivity of disease-causing alleles will vary. This has recently been demonstrated for Gaucher disease, a Mendelian disorder in which the documented presence of a double (homozygous) dosage of a disease-causing allele caused neurologic manifestations and early death (type 2 disease) in some individuals but a later onset and much less severe manifestations (type 3 disease) in others.[10]

Some diseases will be much more likely to manifest when more than one genetic factor, more than one environmental factor, or one or more of both factors are present. In such cases, the diseases are *multifactorial* in origin. When interaction between genes and environmental factors is needed, I call the genetic factors *susceptibility-conferring alleles*. The presence of certain alleles of a gene on one chromosome 13 greatly increases the risk of retinoblastoma or osteosarcoma,[11] but a mutation at the homologous locus on the second chromosome 13 in retinal cells— occurring either spontaneously or in response to a mutagen in the environment—is needed before cancer appears. An allele or alleles at a locus on chromosome 5 causes familial adenomatous polyposis (FAP).[12] The presence of disease-causing mutations at this locus on both homologous chromosomes in cells of the colon or rectum results in cancer.[13] In patients with FAP, the inherited defect serves as a susceptibility-conferring allele.

Among individuals with a well-defined clinical-pathologic disease, different discrete causal factors will operate from one to another (heterogeneity). A proportion will have the disease because of the presence of disease-causing alleles; different alleles at the same locus, or alleles at different loci, may be capable of causing the same disease in different individuals. Others will manifest the disease because of the presence of susceptibility-conferring alleles and environmental exposures. In others the disease will be multifactorial or purely environmental in origin.

There is strong evidence that about 5 percent of patients with coronary artery disease before the age of 60 have the disease on a single-gene basis.[14] People who are homozygous for an allele that confers deficiency of alpha-1-antitrypsin constitute about 3 percent of all patients with chronic obstructive pulmonary disease.[15] About 10 percent of patients with Alzheimer disease and a small proportion of those with bipolar affective (manic-depressive) disorder have family histories of the disease which suggest Mendelian (single-gene) inheritance.[16] Two different gene loci have already been discovered in families with Mendelian inheritance patterns of bipolar affective disorder; alleles at one are found to account for the disorder in some families, alleles at the second in others. It remains unknown, however, whether the disease-causing alleles that account for diseases when they are inherited in a Mendelian fashion play any role in those in which the inherited pattern is not evident. Other etiologic factors play a role in the majority of patients.

The same discrete factor may cause more than one disease, depending on which other discrete factors are present as well as on modulating factors (see below). For instance, the enzyme product of a gene may catalyze the detoxification of more than one chemical. If that enzyme is defective in an individual—because of the presence of a susceptibility-conferring allele (or pair of alleles)—then the disease manifestation will depend on the properties of the particular chemical to which the individual is exposed. For reasons that are poorly understood, disease-causing alleles for Tourette syndrome, which are present in over 1 percent of the population, are associated with attention-deficit disorders (with or without hyperactivity) in some people, and motor or vocal (coprolalia) tics (with or without the deficit disorder and/or hyperactivity) in others.[17]

Modulating factors

Even when all of the necessary discrete factors are present, the clinical expressivity of some diseases will depend on modulating factors. Rather than *causal* relationships, *associations* between the modulating factors and one or more diseases have been described. In some cases, the association with a particular disease may be spurious; in others, it may be real (a confounding factor). Factors with "real" associations are of two types. The first type enhances or reduces the effect of discrete agents, but is neither necessary nor sufficient to cause disease. Consider the developmental stage, for instance. A pregnant woman exposed to a chemical may have an infant with a birth defect. A young, nonpregnant adult exposed to the same chemical may develop cancer several years later. Exposure in an older adult may have no effect because the latency period exceeds the normal life span. The second type contains a causal element, but one that has not yet been dissected out from the noncausal components. Most diseases occur with greater frequency in lower than in upper social classes, but the mechanisms responsible have not yet been fully elucidated.[18]

As discrete causal factors are discovered, they will at least partially replace the "modulating" factor of which they were components. (The modulating factor may continue to have some effect even after a discrete component is excluded.) For instance, an association may be observed between an occupation and a disease. When it is discovered that exposure to a specific chemical used in that occupation explains the association and is causally related to the disease, then the *modulating* factor of occupation for that disease is replaced by the chemical as a *discrete* environmental agent. Similarly, when specific alleles are found to account for familial effects in causing certain diseases, the discrete genetic factors replace the modulating family factors for those diseases. In these examples, occupation and familial factors remain as modulating factors for other diseases until the causal elements of those diseases are discovered.

A positive family history has long been known to increase the risk of lung cancer.[19] More recently, a discrete genetic factor has been reported that begins to explain this observation, as I will discuss in chapter 3. A family history of coronary heart disease before the age of 55 is a stronger risk factor for heart disease than any other.[20] Discrete genetic factors are being discovered to explain this aggregation.[21] Differences in genetic susceptibility help explain the observations mentioned earlier that only a fraction of men who smoke or have high levels of cholesterol develop lung cancer or coronary artery disease, respectively. The feeding of cow's milk to infants with alpha-1-antitrypsin deficiency increases the risk of early liver disease by an unknown mechanism.[22] The 80–90 percent of these infants who survive to adulthood are more likely to develop chronic obstructive pulmonary disease in early adulthood if they smoke.[23] Although still poorly understood, genetic differences also play a role in alcoholism.[24]

As the causal factors contained within some of the modulating factors are dissected out, knowledge of the etiology of many diseases will increase, but we will never have complete understanding. The total milieu in which humans live is constantly changing. As René Dubos put it, "Men will develop new urges, and these will give rise to new problems, which will require ever new solutions. . . . Disease will remain an inescapable manifestation of [their] struggles."[25] The challenge to unravel the mysteries of disease will be unending.

Searching for Causal Factors

The complex etiology of many modern diseases makes it difficult to use the same criteria that were used to establish the infectious origin of many of the epidemic diseases of the past. To prove that a microorganism caused a disease, Koch postulated that it had to (1) be seen in all cases of the disease, (2) be isolated in culture in material obtained from patients, (3) cause the disease in experimental animals, and (4) be recoverable from those animals. Obviously, postulate (2) is hard to satisfy for noninfectious agents, but one can substitute simple isolation of the substance or a metabolite from patients. With this modification, toxic environmental agents could fulfill the postulates. The postulates could also be fulfilled by a disease-causing allele that caused a unique ("pathognomonic") disease; the mutation or a deficiency or defect of gene product would be found in all cases, satisfying postulates (1) and (2). An animal model with a defect at the analogous locus would satisfy postulates (3) and (4).

Among diseases prevalent today, few satisfy all of these criteria. As I have mentioned, a clinical disease entity can result from different causes, and few agents—either environmental or genetic—are capable by themselves of causing a disease in most people.[26] Occasionally, small differences between patients with a disease entity—such as a family history that suggests Mendelian inheritance, the age of onset,[27] exacerbating events, the symptoms and signs, and laboratory test results—will help distinguish "purer" subtypes in which factors that meet the postulates can be found. More often, however, such divisions will not be possible. The factors that are associated with disease in some patients will not be present in all cases, and will be present in many people who never manifest the disease. They are referred to as *risk factors* rather than etiologic agents.

We can use a different set of "postulates" to determine whether risk factors contribute to the causation of disease. (1) The factor should be present in a higher proportion of those with the disease than those without it (relative risk), controlling for confounding factors. (2) Its presence should precede the appearance of disease. Although an allele responsible for a disease will always be present before the manifestations of the disease, evidence of its presence may not be available early on. Establishing antecedent exposure to an environmental agent also may be difficult. (3) A dose-response relationship, whereby the probability of disease increases with the amount of the agent to which the person was exposed, or when disease occurs only above a threshold dose, also strengthens the association. This will often be the case for environmental agents and in genetically determined enzyme deficiencies in which the intolerance increases with the dose of the offending substance. A different relationship can be observed depending on the dosage of disease-related alleles; the disease that occurs in the presence of two doses of a single allele will often be more severe and different in its manifestations from the disease —if any—that occurs in the presence of one dose. (4) There should be a biologically plausible explanation for the relationship, and evidence to support it, such as histopathologic or biochemical changes. (5) The findings should be reproducible.

Given the multitude of factors that can contribute to the etiology of a specific disease, how are these postulates to be tested for any one of the factors? For environmental factors, it is often possible to begin with a discrete agent. For genetic factors, the investigation usually begins with the analysis of more complex factors. Two general approaches can be used for both environmental and genetic factors. The first begins with persons with the disease in whom a contributory role of the factor is suspected. The second begins with the agent and searches for disease.

Environmental factors

In a "case-control study," evidence of antecedent exposure is sought in patients with a disease and in suitable "controls" in whom the disease is not under investigation. Disease registers, such as those that have been established for cancers and birth defects, can be helpful in selecting patients in an unbiased manner if reporting to them has been complete. Accurate ascertainment of the antecedent exposure is not easy. Interviewing about past exposures is subject to recall bias, and records of previous exposures—for instance, to drugs or to chemicals in the workplace—if they exist, are not always accessible or cannot be linked to the patient or control.[28] The data on exposure are analyzed to determine if the postulates are satisfied.

The alternative strategy—of beginning with a specific agent and determining whether disease occurs following exposure—is sometimes used. Longitudinal study of individuals in proximity to the accidental release of potentially toxic agents is one example. Postmarketing surveillance of drugs or other chemicals (e.g., pesticides) for toxic reactions is another. Randomized controlled trials in which a drug is administered to one group and a placebo is given to another are an experimental approach to the problem. However, unless the agent is widely used and manifests its toxicity rapidly and in a large proportion of those exposed, such studies can be very costly.

Genetic factors

The search for genetic factors can start with a case-control study as well. If a family history of the disease under investigation is found more frequently in cases than in controls, then a genetic factor may be contributory. Family factors can, however, also be due to a shared environment. Segregation analysis, which involves determining whether the distribution of disease within families is consistent with Mendelian patterns (axiom 10), can provide strong evidence for the presence of an allele at a single locus as a cause of the disease.[29] When more than one gene locus plays a role, or when environmental as well as genetic factors are needed, other approaches—twin, migrant, adoption, and multifamily studies—can indicate whether genetic components contribute significantly to the disease under consideration.[30] It is also useful to search for disease in inbred populations, in which a single mutation may be transmitted to multiple offspring whose descendants may show a higher frequency of the disease than is found in outbred populations.

In contrast to evidence that exposure to an environmental agent increases risk, findings suggestive of the operation of genetic factors tell nothing about which genes are implicated or how they operate to cause disease. But positive findings from such studies should encourage the search for discrete genetic factors by the techniques that will be described in chapters 3 and 4. The identification of a few families in which

Alzheimer disease appeared to segregate as a dominant disorder,[31] and of families in which bipolar affective disorder segregated as an X-linked disorder,[32] and a few others from an inbred population in which it segregated as an autosomal dominant disorder,[33] has permitted studies localizing disease-related genes to specific chromosomes.

In view of the possibility of variable expressivity, the absence of clinical disease may incorrectly classify an individual with a disease-causing genotype as unaffected. This is particularly a problem for late-onset disease; some people may be classified as not having the disease when, in fact, it simply has not become manifest. Occasionally, a routine laboratory test may have positive results in patients with the disease, or may define a subset of patients with the clinical entity. If the test is also positive prior to clinical manifestation, it may give a clue to the underlying genetic factor and may also be used to classify asymptomatic relatives as affected or unaffected. Følling's discovery that the urine of some patients with mental retardation gave a green color when mixed with ferric chloride solution eventually led to the discovery of the basic genetic defect in phenylketonuria (PKU). For a time the ferric chloride test was used to detect asymptomatic infants with the disorder. More recently, Goldstein et al. have found that the plasma cholesterols in first-degree relatives (but not the spouses) of hypercholesterolemic men who had myocardial infarctions were distributed bimodally—suggesting a single-gene origin. Further work by Goldstein and Brown established the discrete genetic defect for which they received the Nobel Prize.[34]

The alternative strategy—that of beginning with a genetically determined factor—can be used as it becomes increasingly possible to assay for enzymes and proteins and, as the human genome is mapped, different alleles at a gene locus. When variations are found within the population, it is possible that one or more of the variant forms play a role in specific diseases. Individuals with different forms can be followed prospectively to see if the presence of a specific variant or variants correlates with the occurrence of disease. Sometimes the way in which the gene is expressed will suggest the type of disease that might be expected. Enzymes that alter the chemicals found in cigarette smoke may play a role in carcinogenesis; individuals with one variant form may be more likely to develop lung cancer than individuals with another. Individuals with enzyme activities at each extreme of a unimodal distribution of activity may have different alleles.

By detecting individuals that do not show obvious clinical symptoms, laboratory tests may reveal Mendelian inheritance within a family in which some other members manifest disease. This is particularly helpful in the search for susceptibility-conferring alleles in families in which all of those at risk have not yet been exposed to the environmental agent.[35]

Shortcomings in the search

In the investigation of disease etiology, too little attention has been paid to two of the points I mentioned earlier: (1) the same disease may be caused by more than one agent, and (2) the same agent may cause more than one disease. I will give a few examples. After the thalidomide tragedy, many countries established birth defects monitoring systems so that they could rapidly detect the introduction of teratogens into the environment. However, these registries have *not* been responsible for sounding the first warning for any teratogen, although several have been introduced. Although methodological problems contribute to this failure, I believe a bigger reason has been the likelihood that the same birth defect can be caused by several different agents.[36] When a new agent is introduced, the number of new cases caused by it is relatively small compared to the number of cases contributed by other causes. Moreover, few teratogens are as potent as thalidomide; they will not cause birth defects in the offspring of most women exposed at the critical time.[37] Monitoring might be more successful if the test population was expanded and a more specific classification of malformations was employed so that only those likely to be caused by a single teratogen were included in any category.[38]

Investigators are not attuned to considering multiple factors. For instance, a recent report that young women who used phenacetin analgesics were 6.5 times more likely to develop bladder cancer than women who did not[39] failed to consider the possibility that women with the disease could have had a genetically determined variant enzyme that is known to metabolize the drug more slowly.[40] If this variant was found more frequently among women who developed bladder cancer than among women who did not, the relative risk for the women with that variant would be higher than 6.5.

Turning to the second point, physicians and others frequently fail to consider that two or more diseases can share a common etiologic factor. Recently, I was consulted about a baby born with an unusual malformation. Several of the mother's relatives (siblings and cousins) had also had babies with birth defects, but of types different from each other and from the malformation in this infant. The other physicians—including some geneticists—dismissed the relevance of this history; if the malformation was genetically induced, then the same malformation should have been apparent in each relative with the disease-causing allele. What these physicians neglected, and what physicians investigating possible causes frequently neglect, is that they may be dealing not with a disease-causing allele but with a susceptibility-conferring allele. The other factors needed before disease will occur may vary. The clinical entity that results from the presence of these factors in combination could well depend on the time of exposure and the nature of the other factors. If, in the example given, the susceptibility-conferring allele altered the activity of an enzyme that detoxified several drugs with teratogenic potential, the specific malformation could well depend on the time during pregnancy when those drugs were taken or on which of the drugs was taken. Different drugs that are detoxified by the same enzyme could attack different developing organ systems, resulting in different malformations. The time at which a drug is taken is known to influence the organ that will be malformed. Some detoxification enzymes with broad specificity are discussed in chapter 3.

Valuable leads to the role of a specific agent—either environmental or genetic—can be lost if investigators fail to recognize that an agent can cause more than one disease. Let us suppose that a variant form of an enzyme with relatively low activity has been found to segregate as a dominant trait. Let us also suppose that the enzyme, as in the previous example, catalyzes reactions involving several different substrates. The different substrates are capable of adversely affecting different organs; the particular effect is also dependent on the stage of life at which the exposure occurs. If only one of the possible adverse effects was looked for in family members in whom the activity of this enzyme was low, it is doubtful that a strong correlation with the possession of the variant enzyme would be found. But a complete survey of illnesses within families might turn up *several different* diseases that appeared more frequently in family members with the variant than in others. This has been documented for variants at the genes of the major histocompatibility complex (MHC). Within families, the presence of specific alleles at certain of the MHC loci predisposes members to more than one autoimmune disease.[41]

The same allele can predispose a person to quite different diseases (or different degrees of severity of the same disease), depending on the allele present on the homologous chromosome as well as on the alleles present at other loci. Unless advantage is taken of methods to distinguish the presence of different alleles, such possibilities could go completely unnoticed. Evidence for the modifying effects of other gene loci (epistasis) on the manifestations of single-gene disorders was recently reported for sickle cell anemia.[42]

Strategies for Reducing the Burden of Disease

Three strategies for reducing the burden of disease are possible: (1) preventing the disease or its manifestations from occurring in the first place; (2) effectively treating the disease after its manifestations appear; or

(3) avoiding the conception or birth of infants at risk for developing it. Strategies for avoiding the conception of infants at risk include adoption and the use of sperm or ovum donated by someone who is not at risk for having affected offspring. The principal strategy for avoiding the birth of an affected child is abortion. In chapter 5, I will examine each of these strategies as they pertain to genetic disorders. Here, I wish to point out that the strategies can be applied to both discrete and modulating factors on either a population or an individual level, and that their effects may not be as pronounced as one might expect.

Discrete factors

Because few common diseases today result from a single cause, it is unlikely that a strategy directed against one discrete factor would come close to eliminating the disease; there are few magic bullets, though one might be the marked reduction in the occurrence of lung cancer following a sharp curtailment of cigarette smoking. Mental retardation remains a significant problem (it is formally classified as a disease) despite the discovery of several discrete causes and the subsequent development of effective interventions for some of them, such as phenylketonuria. The removal of ubiquitous toxic chemicals, such as lead, from the environment can reduce morbidity, including mental retardation, and mortality, but other causes of the same clinical problems will persist.

Elucidating additional major genetic factors will reveal even further degrees of etiologic heterogeneity than has hitherto been suspected. As I will discuss in the next chapter, the presence of any one of several different disease-causing alleles, or of such alleles at a different locus (*genetic heterogeneity*), may result in the same clinical disease.

The ability to use strategies against discrete factors depends, of course, on knowing what those factors are. Following the discovery of the identity of a disease-causing allele, avoidance remains the only strategy available until additional research leads to effective means of preventing or treating the disorder. In the case of environmental agents, if it is possible to remove the agent from the environment, prevention may be possible. If removal is not possible, immunization can prevent diseases caused by infectious agents. When not everyone is immunized, the birth of exposed fetuses may sometimes be avoided. Abortion, for instance, is offered to women who have contracted German measles early in pregnancy, even though it cannot be predicted with certainty that the fetus is affected. Avoidance will also be offered to women at risk of transmitting the HIV virus for AIDS to their fetuses.

It is possible that the identification of the genes responsible for Alzheimer disease or bipolar affective disorder in a small proportion of all those affected with these disorders will eventually lead to the discovery of interventions that are effective in those with specific genetic defects, but it is much less likely that these interventions will be effective in other forms of the two disorders in which the same genes prove to play little or no role.

Modulating factors

For some diseases, alteration of modulating factors can have a beneficial effect. Changes in lifestyle may delay or reduce the occurrence of several diseases that are prevalent today. Pharmacologic agents (e.g., digitalis or cortisone, and perhaps aspirin) that do not alter the underlying cause—hence they are modulating factors—can improve the body's ability to withstand a wide variety of insults or compensate for the damage they have already wrought. As I have already mentioned, improvements of living standards played a role in reducing the prevalence of many infectious diseases. Laws that reduce speed limits, make the wearing of seat belts mandatory (or better yet introduce air bags), or make it more difficult to drive while intoxicated attempt to reduce the burden of injury by attacking modulating factors (some would call them distal causes), which will make accidents less likely to occur, or if they do occur, will reduce the chance of serious injury.

Even before the discrete gene has been discovered, one can, in the case of X-linked conditions, use avoidance on a modulating factor, sex. As there is a 50 percent chance that the male offspring of a female carrier of an X-linked condition will have the disorder, all male offspring (determined by prenatal diagnosis) can be aborted, even though only about half of them will be affected. This strategy was used by some women at risk for having children with hemophilia or Duchenne muscular dystrophy before the genes for these disorders were identified.

Making changes in populations or in individuals

Efforts to alter discrete or modulating factors can be directed at the entire population or at only high-risk individuals, such as those who already indulge in a potentially harmful habit or those who have a genetic susceptibility.[43] Strategies will be directed at populations when the prevalence of the factor they are designed to alter is high, when there is little resistance to the change, when the change is safe, and when no alternative approach is possible. (Economic factors influencing the choice of strategy will be considered in chapter 8.) The population may be limited to subgroups, such as workers exposed to a toxic substance, even though not all of them will develop disease. Changes involving lowering the amount of fat in the diet or encouraging people to exercise (both modulating factors) will be better tolerated by entire populations than an effort to get everyone to take a drug that may have undesirable side effects (although people are already taking megadoses of vitamins or aspirin to ward off illness, despite inadequate proof of their preventive efficacy).

Individual strategies will be undertaken when the conditions for population-wide strategies are not present, and when individuals at risk can be identified. Identification is made possible by determining the presence of potentially toxic substances or of genetic susceptibilities in apparently healthy people (who may go on to develop symptoms), or by the presence of particular high-risk behaviors (e.g., smoking, drinking). Recombinant DNA technology will increase the number of situations in which individual strategies will be used.

Individual strategies are not always independent of population strategies. To identify individuals at risk because they possess disease-causing or susceptibility-conferring alleles, one must examine whole populations.

Choices can be made between population and individual strategies, and people will differ in their preferences. Industrial employers may prefer to use the individual approach to identify workers at risk for harm from exposure to workplace chemicals rather than lower the exposure of all workers or use a less toxic but more costly substitute. Workers, on the other hand, may prefer a workplace that is safer for all of them. The owners of old tenement houses in which lead paint is still on the walls may prefer voluntary screening programs that identify individuals who are at risk, and the subsequent deleading of those individuals, over the removal of lead paint from the interiors of all houses. Families in those houses might prefer to get the lead out before any of their children are exposed. Tobacco growers and some smokers who find it difficult to kick the habit might prefer voluntary screening programs to identify those at high risk of lung cancer over further efforts to restrict smoking. In view of the dangers of cigarette smoking to nonsmokers, the latter may prefer population policies that prevent everyone from smoking in public places.

Policies directed at populations will certainly affect people who are not destined to develop the disease that may have inspired the policy. This is less likely for policies directed at individuals, but it is not out of the question. Because of variable expressivity, not all of the people who possess disease-related alleles will go on to develop the illness for which they are at risk. People will object to the infringement on their personal liberties by population-based strategies. Some individuals will object to avoidance strategies because they involve abortion or alternatives to the usual means of reproduction.

Summary and Conclusions

With few exceptions, the noninfectious diseases that are the leading causes of death and disability in the developed countries today each have complex etiologies. It is highly unlikely that every individual afflicted with any one of these diseases has developed it as a result of the same factors (etiologic heterogeneity). In most individuals with a disease, multiple factors will be responsible, but different combinations of factors will operate in different individuals. In addition to this heterogeneity, a specific factor or factors will have variable expressivity, depending on the presence of other factors that have yet to be identified. For many afflicted individuals, the specific factors responsible for their respective diseases have not been identified.

Factors incriminated in the etiology of a disease can be divided into discrete factors, for which causal relationships have been established, and modulating factors, for which associations have been observed but a causality has not been demonstrated. I divide discrete factors into two categories: genetic and environmental. A large number of genetic factors play a role in many diseases prevalent today. In some of those affected with a specific disease, the presence of disease-causing alleles at a single locus may be all that is needed to cause the disease. In others, the presence of susceptibility-conferring alleles at one or more loci will confer susceptibility to harm from exposure to external agents. In others, specific alleles at two or more loci will be sufficient to cause disease (multifactorial disorders).

Modulating factors include those for which causal relationships do not exist (they facilitate the disease-causing action of discrete factors) or have not yet been established. The search for causal factors begins either with studies of patients with a clinical entity or with studies of a discrete environmental or genetically determined factor. I have enumerated postulates that should be satisfied in establishing that a factor contributes to the causation of disease in which other factors also play a role.

Strategies to reduce the burden of disease can be directed at either discrete or modulating factors, or both. Because of the multiple factors involved in etiology, and differences in etiology between individuals with the "same" disease, no intervention directed at a single etiologic factor is likely to eliminate the disease. This is in contrast to the effect of "magic bullets" (immunizations and antibiotics) aimed at infectious diseases.

Strategies to reduce the burden of disease can be directed at entire populations or at individuals. As recombinant DNA technology leads to the identification of disease-causing or susceptibility-conferring alleles for a large number of diseases, strategies designed to detect healthy individuals who possess these alleles will become increasingly possible. Before examining these strategies in greater detail—and the problems some of them entail—I must first explain the role of genetic factors in common diseases and examine the techniques used to identify disease-related genes.

Chapter 3

The Role of Genes in Disease

Many people, including some scientists and physicians, will be incredulous to learn that genes, or more precisely alleles, contribute to the causation of common disorders as well as to rare ones. They might argue that, if this were true, these alleles would have been discovered already. Later in this chapter, I will show that reliance on indirect methods, which were the only ones available from the time of Mendel until the development of recombinant DNA technology, greatly slowed the rate of discovery and consequently slowed the development of tests for genetic disorders.

Methodologic limitations aside, two objections to an important role for genetic factors can be raised. One arises from the belief that little allelic diversity exists: except for those rare alleles that cause rare diseases, we all have the same alleles at most loci. It follows from this belief that genetic susceptibility cannot explain why some people succumb to a particular *common* disease while others do not; environmental differences must be the explanation. The other objection arises from the notion that deleterious alleles will not be passed from one generation to the next in sufficient frequency ever to account for common diseases. Although this is generally the case, there are a number of important exceptions, which I will consider after discussing genetic diversity and its role in disease.

Genetic Diversity

Considerable evidence for a marked amount of genetic variation now exists. An examination of specific proteins within human populations indicates that at 10–20 percent of the loci (axiom 1) for structural genes (axiom 5), two or more alleles are frequently observed.[1] Recombinant DNA techniques have revealed more alleles at some structural gene loci than were detectable by protein methods; it is likely that these techniques will uncover common variants at additional structural gene loci. (Recombinant DNA techniques have also uncovered extensive variation in segments of DNA that do not encode for proteins; these techniques will be described in chapter 4.)

Loci at which the most common allele has a frequency of .99 or less are, by definition, *polymorphic*. When an allele has a frequency of .01, about 2 percent of the population will be heterozygous for it.[2] When an allele has a frequency of .14, 2 percent of the population will be homozygous for it and about 24 percent will be heterozygous.[3]

The protein products of the different polymorphic alleles at a structural gene locus often differ in physical, chemical, and immunologic properties. The latter have been used to establish the presence of polymorphic alleles of several genes in the major histocompatibility complex (MHC), particularly at the HLA gene loci, and blood group loci. Allelically determined protein differences may be responsible for differences in the susceptibility to disease, as I will demonstrate shortly.

In addition to polymorphic alleles, "rare" alleles, with frequencies of less than .01, have been found at just over half of the structural gene loci examined indirectly by protein comparisons. Surveys of very large populations were needed to find them. (Fewer individuals were examined for variants at the loci for which no rare alleles were found.) Harris has estimated that about 1 in 1,000 individuals will be found to have a rare allele at a specific structural gene locus; if there are 30,000 gene loci for enzyme structure, each individual will have about 30 rare alleles.[4] Although most autosomal recessive disorders are rare, the alleles for them may occur frequently enough (in heterozygotes) to satisfy the definition of polymorphism.

Genetic diversity enhances protection

Having more genetically determined "options" to draw on could protect an individual from adverse agents in the environment. "Options" capable of being transmitted from one generation to the next arise as a result of mutations in germ cells (axiom 7). Gene duplication (axioms 7 and 8) followed by mutations in one of the duplicates could result in the formation of a gene with a different function. Additional mutations in either the original or the duplicated gene result in allelic diversity. If the particular allele resulting from a mutation (axiom 9) increases the likelihood that the individual will survive to reproduce (compared to others without the mutation), the mutation is likely to increase in frequency in succeeding generations.

The benefits of diversity are best exemplified by the immune system. The ability to synthesize specific antibodies against any one of a vast number of foreign substances (antigens) protects individuals from many infectious organisms and toxins. Both inherited and somatic cell mutation play a role in maintaining this extraordinary diversity.[5]

Allelic diversity at some of the MHC loci may also be advantageous. An immune attack by T-cells of the host's immune system is effectively launched only after a foreign substance (including bacteria or viruses) becomes associated with an MHC protein on the surface of other host cells. It is possible that having several different MHC proteins (due to polymorphisms) increases the chance that at least one of them will "recognize" the foreign substance. Because polymorphisms at several of the MHC loci are so extensive, the probability of heterozygosity at any locus is high, giving any individual a good chance of having the largest possible number of different MHC proteins.

Another consequence of the extensive polymorphisms at some of the MHC loci is that no two individuals, except for identical twins, are likely to have the same combination of alleles at the different loci. This difference plays an important role in distinguishing foreign organisms from self. One situation in which this distinction is important is the implantation and development of the embryo. It is interesting that couples who share alleles at the MHC loci have more spontaneous abortions and progeny with neural tube defects than those who have different alleles at those sites.[6] This may indicate another advantage of extensive polymorphisms.

The genetically determined array of structurally similar cytochrome P450 monooxygenase enzymes (they form carbon monoxide complexes that absorb light with a 450-nm wavelength) is another example of the benefits of genetic diversity. It is likely that the members of the modern family of these enzymes, which are capable of metabolizing a wide range of endogenous and exogenous compounds, arose by successive duplication and allelic diversification from one or more progenitor genes.[7]

Polymorphisms and disease

Diversity can backfire. Unless great care is taken to match donors and recipients, the MHC alleles in an organ or tissue transplanted from one individual are likely to differ from the recipient's and be recognized as foreign and rejected immunologically. This is also the case when a donor's blood group differs from the recipient's. These two examples represent adverse reactions initiated by humans in an effort to restore the normal function of the body. But polymorphisms can also have harmful effects without human intervention; Rh blood incompatibility can result in the death of an Rh-positive fetus in an Rh-negative mother.

Sometimes foreign organisms have, by mutation, developed mechanisms to "recognize" specific human polymorphic variants. Such mutations may enhance the survival of the infecting agent and consequently be propagated in subsequent generations of the agent. *Plasmodium vivax* malaria recognizes the Duffy blood group antigen, so individuals who possess it are much more susceptible to infection than those who do not.[8] Women with a polymorphic variant of blood group P to which *E. coli* bacteria may be more adherent are more likely to develop recurrent pyelonephritis in the absence of other predisposing factors than are women with other variants.[9]

Specific forms of polymorphic proteins coded by the MHC-D loci increase the likelihood of insulin-dependent diabetes mellitus but are not sufficient to result in the disease.[10] The mechanism of susceptibility is not yet known. Normally, the pancreatic cells that make insulin do not express the host's D alleles. One theory holds that a virus mimics certain forms of D polymorphic proteins. The entry of such viruses into the pancreatic cells of a host who possesses the alleles for those proteins could trigger an immune response against the cells. Another theory is that injury may trigger the cell to transcribe protein for the specific D allele. This protein may be juxtaposed on the cell surface to insulin produced by the cell, leading thereby to the production of antibodies against the individual's own insulin.[11] Antibodies against both insulin and pancreatic cells are seen early in the pathogenesis of IDDM.[12] Whether foreign agents play such a role in the associations between specific alleles at one or more of the histocompatibility loci and the occurrence of ankylosing spondylitis, psoriasis, and other diseases has not yet been elucidated.[13]

The product of a specific polymorphic allele at a different gene locus from those determining the blood groups or major histocompatibility antigens has been found to be associated with susceptibility to rheumatic fever; it may occupy a position on cell surfaces very close to, but distinct from, the binding site of group A streptococci.[14] A polymorphic variant of an enzyme that may play a role in immune responsiveness has been found to be associated with susceptibility to hemophilus influenza in Eskimos, in whom the prevalence of hemophilus infections is very high.[15]

Polymorphisms of genes whose products are involved in the metabolism of exogenous chemicals, including drugs, also have been implicated in diseases and drug reactions. At the "acetylator" locus, the product of one allele rapidly acetylates a number of exogenous compounds; the other acetylates at a slower rate. Homozygotes for the "slow acetylator" constitute about 50 percent of the white population and are at increased risk of developing peripheral neuropathy following prolonged isoniazid therapy, a lupus erythematosus–like reaction following treatment with certain drugs for cardiovascular disorders, and bladder cancer following exposure to arylamines (compounds used in the dye industry until recently).[16] The risk of diabetes is greater in rapid than in slow acetylators, and the risk of breast cancer also may be higher in rapid acetylators.[17] The mechanisms are unknown. Although the acetylator type increases the risk of various toxic reactions or diseases, the correlation is far from perfect; modulating factors play an important role. For instance, lupus erythematosus is much more likely to develop in slow acetylators receiving hydralazine (an antihypertensive drug) if they also have the DR4 allele at one of the MHC-D gene loci.[18]

Polymorphic forms of a receptor for aryl hydrocarbons—a large class of chemicals that includes coal tars found in cigarette smoke—differ in their ability to induce synthesis of aryl hydrocarbon hydroxylase (AHH), a P450 enzyme, in the presence of a hydrocarbon; the AHH converts the hydrocarbons to other compounds.[19] The risk of bronchogenic cancer is greater in smokers who are high inducers than in smokers who are low inducers. The compound formed by the action of the enzyme is more carcinogenic than the precursor. About 10 percent of the U.S. population are high inducers; they are either heterozygotes or homozygotes for the high-inducer receptor allele.

Smokers who possess the predominant form of a polymorphism for another P450 enzyme also are reported to be at increased risk for lung cancer.[20] With this form of the enzyme, they extensively metabolize several drugs (debrisoquine, phenacetin, nortriptyline, metoprolol). Those with the less common form of the polymorphism are poor metabolizers. About 40 percent of white Anglo-Saxons are homozygous extensive metabolizers, 53 percent are heterozygous extensive metabolizers, and 7 percent are homozygous poor metabolizers.[21] The pharmacologically effective dosages of drugs that induce this enzyme will differ between poor and extensive metabolizers.[22] Whether it is the extensive metabolizers or the poor ones who are more likely to develop toxicity from a drug depends on whether the drug itself or the product of the oxidation reaction is more toxic.[23]

Genetically determined differences in AHH activity may also play a role in teratogenicity. Only mouse embryo cultures derived from a high-AHH-inducer strain showed chromosomal abnormalities (sister chromatid exchanges) following incubation with benzo[a]pyrene, an AHH inducer.[24] When high-AHH-inducer male mice are mated with low-AHH-inducer female mice and the pregnant dam is then given benzo[a]pyrene, only the high-inducer fetuses show embryotoxicity. If the female is AHH responsive, all embryos show toxicity.[25] In humans, a high rate of activity of a placental AHH has been associated with a lower rate of congenital malformations in the infants of women who smoke. One explanation is that the organs of fetuses who have inherited an allele for high placental enzyme activity are protected from the teratogenic effects of cigarette smoke.[26]

A polymorphic form of the enzyme epoxide hydrolase, which detoxifies the epoxide of dilantin, an anticonvulsant drug, has been implicated in the occurrence of major congenital malformations. Fetuses who have inherited the form with reduced enzyme activity are at greater risk when their mother takes the drug early in pregnancy.[27] Because the rate of epoxide formation depends on AHH activity, it might be expected that fetuses who are slow AHH inducers as well as slow epoxide detoxifiers would be protected. This has not yet been tested.

An X-linked condition, glucose-6-phosphate dehydrogenase (G6PD) deficiency, which occurs in over 10 percent of American black males and commonly in males in Mediterranean countries and the Middle East,[28] results in hemolytic anemia following the ingestion of fava beans or certain drugs (including primaquine—an antimalarial—and several sulfur drugs).[29] Different alleles are responsible for the deficiency in different populations, but within each population the susceptibility-conferring allele is polymorphic.

Until recently, there was no evidence for a genetic susceptibility to the common type of Down syndrome, or trisomy 21, due to nondisjunction. (In nondisjunction, both members of the chromosome pair enter the same germ cell instead of only one [axiom 3].) Recently, however, the presence of a genetically determined chromosomal variation in the nucleolar organizing region of chromosome 21 of the parent in whose germ cell the nondisjunction occurred was reported to increase the risk of having a baby with Down syndrome approximately twentyfold. (The variant may occur in 2 percent of the population, qualifying as a polymorphism).[30] The other genetic or environmental factors that contribute to the actual occurrence of Down syndrome in the presence (or absence) of the variant have not been established. X-irradiation probably increases the risk of nondisjunction.[31]

The associations between common (polymorphic) alleles and disease that I have just described were all discovered without the use of recombinant DNA technology. That technology is already uncovering others. A susceptibility to having children with nondisjunction Down syndrome, independent of the one just described, has been reported using the new techniques.[32]

In considering the association between polymorphic alleles and disease, it is important to emphasize one other point: The frequency of the diseases associated with polymorphic alleles is almost always much lower than the frequency of the alleles; environmental and/or other genetic factors must be present before disease occurs. In other words, the pathogenic effects of the polymorphic alleles have low expressivity.

Many of the polymorphic susceptibility-conferring alleles discussed thus far determine the production of proteins whose primary function relates to the recognition or metabolism of exogenous compounds. Those that increase the likelihood of disease in one environment may help deter disease in another environment. They may be thought of as having multiple effects (pleiotropism), each of which depends on the environmental context. Even when they are present in double (homozygous) dose, they do not impair the integrity of essential functions. Males who are hemizygous for G6PD deficiency polymorphisms will not usually be adversely affected by the deficiency except in the presence of harmful oxidizing chemicals or drugs.

Alleles for rare diseases

Heterozygotes for alleles that cause rare recessive diseases occur much more frequently than affected homozygotes.[33] (The frequency of an allele for a recessive disease that occurs in 1 in 10,000 liveborn infants is .01, just qualifying as polymorphic.) Occasionally, the presence of a single (heterozygous) dose of an allele for a rare recessive disease of high expressivity will increase susceptibility to disease.[34] But the chance of disease is far from certain, and when it does appear it is usually of later onset and milder severity than the disease in homozygotes. Moreover, some of the manifestations of the disease in homozygotes may be totally lacking in heterozygotes who show any manifestations. In other words, the pathogenic effects of single doses of alleles for rare recessive disease have low expressivity.

When, for instance, alleles that produce defective low-density lipoprotein receptors are present in double dose, a very rare, severe form of familial hypercholesterolemia results, with the onset of coronary artery disease by adolescence. When only one of these alleles is present, the person has an 85 percent chance of developing coronary artery disease by age 60. About 0.2 percent of the population are heterozygotes for defective LDL receptor alleles. Five percent of coronary heart disease in men under 60 years of age occurs in them.[35]

Heterozygotes for homocystinuria, a rare recessive disorder, have been reported to be at increased risk for peripheral and cerebral occlusive vascular disease.[36] Homozygotes for ataxia-telangiectasia have a greatly increased chance of dying from cancer. Based on studies of blood relatives and their spouses, the risk of cancer in heterozygotes, although lower than in homozygotes, is estimated to be significantly greater than in the general population: 2.3 times higher for men and 3.1 times higher for women.[37] In another recessive disorder in which the risk of cancer is greatly increased and in which cells show increased chromosomal abnormalities (Bloom syndrome), cells of heterozygotes show changes that might also be associated with cancer.[38] Heterozygotes for an allele that results in alpha-1-antitrypsin deficiency may be at increased risk for chronic obstructive pulmonary disease, particularly if they smoke, but much less so than homozygotes.[39] Heterozygotes for a recessive form of osteogenesis imperfecta may be more liable to early osteoporosis.[40]

What Accounts for the High Frequency of Some Disease-Related Alleles?

The alleles for most recessive diseases are maintained in successive generations by matings between heterozygotes and homozygotes for normal alleles at the locus. Even when heterozygotes do manifest disease, their reproductive capability of transmitting the disease-causing allele may not be impaired, as I will discuss shortly. This capability maintains the frequency of such alleles, sometimes at polymorphic levels, but other mechanisms are at work as well.

The role of mutation

The relatively high frequency of Duchenne muscular dystrophy and hemophilia, both of which are X-linked disorders that impair the reproductive capability of males, depends on high mutation rates. These are accounted for by the exceptionally long length of the genes for these disorders and, consequently, the greater chance that mutations will occur within the gene sequence. Many of the mutations in hemophilia involve cytosine-guanine (CG) dinucleotide sequences, which are more prone to mutation than other dinucleotides. The ratio of CG to other dinucleotides is no greater in the gene for this disorder than in other genes, but the absolute number (due to gene length) is greater.[41]

New mutation plays an insignificant role in maintaining the frequency of polymorphic alleles or the alleles for autosomal recessive disorders. Examinations of siblings, parents, and grandparents of individuals in whom variant (nonlethal) alleles have been found almost never reveal new mutation.[42]

Balanced polymorphism

When heterozygotes for an allele that is harmful only in double dose are more likely than normal homozygotes to survive until adulthood and reproduce, the force driving gene frequency downward (lack of survival of the homozygote) will be balanced by the selective advantage of the heterozygote. In areas endemic for malaria, this is the case for the sickle cell allele, and perhaps also for alleles for G6PD deficiency and the thalassemias.[43] In areas where malaria has been eradicated, heterozygotes no longer have a reproductive advantage. Many generations will have to pass, however, before the allele is removed from the gene pool. Infectious agents have been extremely important in human evolution. Childs et al. reviewed a number of "tricks" that microorganisms use to gain a foothold in their human hosts.[44] Another form of balanced polymorphism, frequency-dependent selection, may have played a role here. When a human allele for a product that conferred resistance to an infectious agent became very high in frequency, mutations in the microorganism may have succeeded in breaching the defense. As a result of the "success" of the infectious agent, humans with the allele will now be less likely to survive than others, and the frequency of the particular allele will fall. The process will recur in subsequent generations, preventing any single allele from completely replacing the other. Epidemics that occur only once in several generations may result in an enrichment of "resistance-conferring genotypes," which in the absence of the infectious agent are neutral or deleterious.

"Balanced polymorphisms" may also result when individuals who lose some of their offspring because of a recessive disorder compensate by means of increased fertility, producing heterozygotes to normal homozygotes in a ratio of 2:1.

Another balancing mechanism involves preferential survival in the meiosis of gametes carrying one allele compared to another ("meiotic drive"), or preferential fertilization with gametes containing certain alleles that presumably are expressed in the gamete. These alleles, however, prove to be disadvantageous after birth. Such a mechanism is present at a mouse locus, but no evidence for it has yet been demonstrated in humans.[45]

The founder effect

In closed populations, the likelihood of matings between people with a common ancestor is greater than that in open populations. A mutation occurring in the ancestor, which is harmful only in double (homozygous) dose, may be transmitted in single dose through several generations and reach polymorphic frequency. As the frequency increases, however, the likelihood of matings between heterozygotes also increases. Disease will occur in one-quarter of such matings. If the reproductive capability of these affected homozygotes is impaired, as is the case for many recessive disorders, the allele will not be transmitted to subsequent generations; this tends to lower the frequency of the allele. Nevertheless, the allele continues to be transmitted to approximately half the offspring of matings between heterozygotes and normal homozygotes. The founder effect may account for the high frequency of the Tay-Sachs allele (about one in thirty) in Jews of eastern European origin.

Late onset

When a disease does not become manifest or disabling until middle adulthood or later, the alleles for it tend to pass to the next generation, thereby maintaining the frequency of the disease-causing or susceptibility-conferring allele. Alleles that cause disease in a single dose (dominance) cannot be maintained at a high frequency without fresh mutation if they impair reproductive capabilities. It is not surprising, therefore, that a higher proportion of dominant diseases whose frequency cannot be explained by new mutation have their onset in adulthood, and consequently impair reproduction less than recessive or X-linked disorders do.[46] The classic example of a late-onset dominant disorder is Huntington disease, which occurs in about 1 in 10,000 individuals. The allele is passed along before the parent knows that he or she is affected.

The appearance of the more common disorders in which alleles in single dose play a role often depends on the presence of other factors as well. Genetically susceptible individuals may not encounter these factors until fairly late in life. One such factor could be a drug used for an adult-onset disease. Environmental agents such as carcinogens, which may be encountered early, have a long latency period before their harmful effects become manifest in genetically susceptible individuals. Atheromatous plaques, which begin to form early in life, must reach a certain thickness and distribution before coronary heart disease results. Consequently, the susceptibility-conferring allele is likely to be passed to the next generation before the disease appears; reproductive fitness is not markedly impaired.

Environmental change

The environmental and social conditions during the vast period over which humans evolved as hunter-gatherers were strikingly different from conditions during the short period—far less than 1 percent of all human generations—since the discovery of agriculture. Thus, alleles that were advantageous or neutral for the hunter-gatherers but are disadvantageous for civilized humans may still be present in fairly high frequency because an insufficient number of generations have passed under the new social and environmental conditions to allow selective mechanisms to remove them. Neel postulated that this time lag accounts for the high frequency of non-insulin-dependent diabetes.[47] For hunter-gatherers, whose lives were marked by alternating periods of feast and famine, the ability to secrete maximum amounts of insulin might have been advantageous. When food is consistently abundant, as is true in affluent civilizations, this genetically determined ability may lead to diabetes. Similarly, the polymorphic forms that increase susceptibility to rheumatic fever or *Plasmodium vivax* malaria may have served a beneficial function before urbanization and the rise of infectious diseases, and enzymes that originally detoxified chemicals to which our ancestors were exposed (e.g., the combustion products of wood, or certain poisonous fruits) may, in fact, enhance the toxicity of chemicals in the modern environment.

The Illusion of High Allele Frequency: Allelic Diversity and Genetic Heterogeneity

A genetic disease of high prevalence may give the illusion of high allele frequency, when in fact the disease results from the presence of any one of several different alleles at the same locus or at a different locus. (In the case of recessive disorders, any pair of disease-causing alleles at a locus would have to be present.) The latter case is defined as "genetic heterogeneity," although sometimes allelic diversity is included as well. It seems unlikely that alleles at two different loci could each cause the same phenotypic disease, but the gene products of each locus (different polypeptide chains) may constitute a single protein. Moreover, because the different steps in a metabolic pathway are catalyzed by enzymes whose genes segregate independently, genetically determined defects in any of these steps could have the same pathophysiologic effect. The presence of genetic heterogeneity for recessive disorders is demonstrated in vitro when cells from one affected individual "correct" the defect (usually measured biochemically) in cells from another and in vivo when individuals with the same phenotypic recessive disease mate and have children who do not manifest the disease. However, there are relatively few human conditions in which either of these "tests" is possible. Close scrutiny of the historical, physical, and laboratory findings in patients with the same disease may reveal differences between affected families that suggest heterogeneity.

Heterogeneity has been demonstrated for albinism, several connective tissue disorders (mucopolysaccharidoses), xeroderma pigmentosum, ataxia telangiectasia, methemoglobinemia, phenylketonuria, congenital deafness, and blindness.[48] Several different mutations result in classical hemophilia,[49] thalassemia,[50] G6PD deficiency,[51] familial hypercholesterolemia,[52] and phenylketonuria.[53] Although selection operates to reduce the frequency of each disease-causing allele, their combined frequencies can be relatively high. The single mutations that account for all patients with sickle cell anemia and the common type of alpha-1-antitrypsin deficiency (PiZZ) may well be exceptions to the rule of heterogeneity.

The Burden of Genetic Diseases

I hope I have demonstrated to the reader's satisfaction that there is extensive genetic diversity in humans, that both rare and polymorphic alleles account for a small but not insubstantial fraction of common disorders, and that evolutionary and other mechanisms account for maintaining the frequency of these alleles in successive generations. Biochemical and recombinant DNA techniques have established the presence of disease-causing or susceptibility-conferring alleles for malaria, coronary artery disease, lung and colon cancer, chronic obstructive pulmonary disease, insulin-dependent diabetes mellitus, bipolar affective disorder, Alzheimer disease, and some congenital abnormalities. Single-gene abnormalities account for at least 7.5 percent of congenital abnormalities,[54] the leading cause of infant mortality in the United States. Due to its variable expressivity, an allele (or alleles) that results in Tourette syndrome may account for 10–30 percent of the cases of attention-deficit disorder and hyperactivity in young children.[55] As the contribution of infectious diseases to infant mortality and morbidity has dropped, that of genetic diseases has increased.[56] Moreover, a higher proportion of infections today than fifty years ago results from an underlying genetic susceptibility.[57]

A full count of the frequency of genetic disorders in a cohort of live births requires the reporting of all genetic abnormalities in the cohort as it grows older. This has been accomplished successfully by the Health Surveillance Registry of the Canadian province of British Columbia. The rate of genetic disorders appearing before the age of 25 years in more than one million consecutive live births was found to be greater than 5.3 percent. The vast majority were multifactorial disorders.[58]

Epidemiologic studies offer evidence that genetic factors operate in adult diabetes mellitus, hypertension, schizophrenia, breast cancer, Parkinsonism, some types of arthritis, gout, and duodenal ulcer.[59] For these conditions, and for those in which more specific evidence of a genetic role is available, methods in the pre–recombinant DNA era were insufficient to elucidate fully the genetic mechanisms involved. I turn now to a brief description of these methods and their limitations.

Finding the Genetic Basis of Disease

Until recombinant DNA techniques came along, geneticists relied on indirect methods and inference to sort out inherited factors involved in disease causation. The indirect methods fall into two broad categories. The first, which I call the *classical* approach, involves epidemiologic studies, segregation analysis, and other statistical approaches mentioned in chapter 2. The second, or *neoclassical* approach, uses laboratory analysis to detect biochemical and physiologic consequences of the presence of genetic differences. Usually, but not always, this method builds on observations made using the classical approach. In a small proportion of diseases in which genetic factors play a role, it can progress to the point of inferring that a gene for a particular protein is defective. Only through recombinant DNA techniques, to be discussed in chapter 4, can virtually any genetic defect be determined by direct analysis at the DNA level.

Refining the definition of disease

Laboratory tests may reveal biochemical or physiologic features in some but not all of those with a constellation of clinical characteristics, thereby delineating a subcategory of the disease that may be etiologically distinct. Two general approaches have been taken. The first is often called a "fishing expedition." Laboratory tests are performed on patients with a clinical disease entity (or, more often, on their fluids or tissues) without any clear idea of what abnormality might be present. The testing of urine or blood from patients with mental retardation for abnormal metabolites led to the discovery of phenylketonuria. When simple methods for determining amino acids in body fluids were developed, entire populations in institutions for the mentally retarded were tested in a search for subgroups with specific, but hitherto unknown, abnormalities. Because the method permitted the detection of abnormalities that might involve many different gene loci, it was more efficient than might be thought. One drawback in looking exclusively at populations with a particular handicap is that not every metabolic abnormality observed will be etiologically related to the handicap. Studies of healthy relatives or of healthy populations have revealed that some "abnormalities" are simply normal variants. In other instances, the abnormalities have been found to result from changes, such as diet, brought about by the institutionalization itself. In a few cases, however, the abnormalities have indicated a significant association with the handicap.

The second approach hypothesizes that the specific laboratory abnormalities found in some patients with a clinical entity may be genetically determined. For instance, Goldstein et al. separated survivors of heart attack into different subcategories on the basis of the specific lipid abnormality present. They found that in the blood relatives (but not spouses) of those with hypercholesterolemia, the plasma cholesterol concentrations had a bimodal distribution, which was consistent with a single-gene locus making a major contribution to plasma cholesterol concentration. This bimodal distribution of cholesterol was not present in the relatives of heart attack patients with other lipid abnormalities.[60] In subsequent studies using the neoclassical approach, Goldstein and Brown elucidated the defect in low-density lipoprotein receptors.[61]

Finding a laboratory abnormality in certain people with the disease under investigation provides a new phenotype to use in segregation analysis and other studies to determine the presence of genetic factors. If the laboratory abnormality is etiologically related to the disease, it may also be present before the disease becomes manifest, thereby providing a means for detection in the presymptomatic individual.

Methods and their limitations

Unfortunately, most enzymes and other proteins—the direct products of gene expression—cannot be detected in readily accessible tissues or fluids. If the search is restricted to such tissues and fluids, accumulations or deficiencies of substances that provide indirect evidence of an underlying genetic defect may sometimes be found, using, for instance, chromatography to detect abnormal concentrations of amino acids or other metabolites in blood and urine, and chemical studies to detect alterations in serum cholesterol and other lipids. The concentration of these and other substances that are not themselves primary gene products often depends on several genetically determined enzymatic and transport reactions, including absorption and excretion. Observed changes may be caused by some alteration unrelated to the disease under study, or may be the result rather than the cause of the disease process. Consequently, more direct methods of identifying alterations in gene product are desirable.

Enzyme assay provides a more direct approach.[62] However, the assay has to be performed on preparations of the organ or tissue in which the enzyme is active in normal individuals. Occasionally, radioactively or otherwise labeled compounds can be administered to patients and healthy controls and their respective fates followed in vivo. There is, however, a general reluctance to administer radioactive compounds. (Newer techniques, such as magnetic resonance imaging, may facilitate in vivo testing.) Although a biopsy of liver, kidney, lung, skin, muscle, and brain is possible, it is not without risk, and only a limited amount of material can be obtained by it. Despite these limitations, the basic defects in several single-gene disorders of amino acid and carbohydrate metabolism were discovered by enzyme assay.

Cell culture sometimes provides a way around the problem of access to tissue in which the enzyme system of interest is active. It also involves biopsy, but the cells become plentiful enough to serve as the source of innumerable experiments. Many metabolic pathways operate in cultured fibroblasts, obtained from skin biopsy, so they are a valuable tool for conducting enzyme assays. It is now possible to culture other tissues and organs as well as skin. Tumor cultures have played a major role in elucidating the origins of cancer, including the role of genes.

None of the methods described thus far involves a direct examination of the primary gene product, the protein or polypeptide chain. In 1949, Linus Pauling applied a new technique, electrophoresis, to the direct examination of the protein hemoglobin in patients with sickle cell anemia, normal subjects, and those whose blood sickled but who did not have anemia.[63] He showed that the hemoglobin band for patients with the anemia had a different electrophoretic mobility from that of the band for normal subjects, but that asymptomatic individuals whose blood sickled had both bands. Coupled with genetic analyses performed independently in the same year,[64] Pauling's findings resolved the longstanding puzzle of the inheritance of sickle cell anemia. Although the inheritance of sickling without anemia as a dominant trait was appreciated soon after the phenomenon was first reported in 1910, it had generally been believed that the occurrence of anemia in patients whose blood sickled was due to the presence of at least one additional factor, either environmental or genetic.[65] The finding that asymptomatic patients whose blood sickled had both sickle and normal hemoglobin suggested that they were in fact heterozygous, while those with sickle cell anemia were homozygous for the sickle cell allele.

Eight years after Pauling's discovery, Ingram reported that sickle hemoglobin had a valine substituted for a glutamic acid in one position of one of the polypeptide chains of the molecule. The charge difference between the two amino acids explained the differences in electrophoretic mobility.[66]

Electrophoresis made it possible for scientists to look for evidence of genetic disease at the level of the gene product. The technique was particularly useful for hemoglobin studies because its concentration in red blood cells was so high that no other protein obscured its electrophoretic mobility. When it came to examining other proteins, the technique proved less successful; several proteins had the same electrophoretic mobility, and the absence of one could not be detected because of the presence of others. In response to this problem, the techniques of enzyme assay and electrophoresis were combined.[67] Using this approach, investigators discovered several different alleles responsible for a deficiency of red cell G6PD.[68] The classical electrophoretic technique is limited to detecting soluble proteins found in blood, accessible tissues, or cultured cells. The recently developed technique of two-dimensional electrophoresis extends the search for interindividual differences to proteins of the cell matrix; solvents permit some insoluble proteins to be examined as well. Although this technique can detect protein polymorphisms, it cannot discern the function of the proteins.[69] Use of the technique has not yet resulted in the detection of variant proteins associated with the presence of disease.

Immunologic techniques that detect very small differences in proteins (due to alterations in amino acid sequence or to sugars attached to specific amino acids) have proved valuable in allowing scientists to confirm the role of suspected proteins in genetic disorders. Common to these techniques is the preparation of antibodies against a highly purified protein (antigen) that is suspected of being defective in the genetic disease of interest. The failure of tissues that normally contain the protein to react with the antibody or to give a normal reaction suggests that the patient from whom they were obtained has a defect in that protein. Monoclonal antibodies afford still greater specificity than conventional antibodies. The success of the immunologic methods depends on one's ability to purify the protein suspected of being defective in a genetic disorder, and having accessible tissues from normal and diseased individuals in whom the protein is present. There are many diseases for which these conditions cannot be met. The importance of the immunologic techniques is exemplified by their identification of tissue antigen polymorphisms at the HLA loci in the major histocompatibility complex (MHC) discussed earlier in this chapter.

The Use of Neoclassical Methods for Genetic Testing

The methodologic limitations in identifying genetic factors in disease have imposed even greater limitations on genetic tests. Obviously, tests can be used only for those conditions for which a measurable genetic factor has been discovered. But even then the experimental methods used to elucidate the genetic factor may not be adaptable to routine clinical testing, for at least three reasons.

First, the test will not provide meaningful information when it is performed on readily accessible tissues such as blood, urine, or, in the fetus, amniotic fluid cells or chorionic villi. This will be the case if the defective enzyme is not active in accessible tissues or if the concentrations of related compounds are not altered in such tissues. More invasive tests involve some risk—for example, in vivo radioactive studies or organ biopsy. They might be used in patients who are already symptomatic, particularly when they confirm or exclude a specific diagnosis that has a bearing on management or future reproductive plans. They are less likely to be used in healthy individuals to predict future illness, except when the risk is very high, as in relatives of people with severe, single-gene disorders. Invasive tests will not be used for screening of the general population.

Second, even when the test provides meaningful information on accessible tissues, it may not do so in time to benefit the patient. Compounds that accumulate in blood or urine as an indirect consequence of a genetic defect may not be detectable until after irreversible damage has occurred. Such tests may be helpful in confirming or excluding a diagnosis after symptoms appear and, consequently, in alerting others in the family to their risks, but they will not influence the management of the patient.

Third, an abnormality in the substance being measured may result from a number of factors, only one of which is an alteration in the gene of interest. Cholesterol elevations are an example. Even measurements of enzyme activity will be influenced by a variety of factors. Other protein variants measured by neoclassical techniques may not always be associated with disease. The association between a particular polymorphism and disease will usually be less than perfect. Despite the fact that possession of a specific allele (B27) at the HLA-B locus of the major histocompatibility complex increases the chance of ankylosing spondylitis over 100 times, only about one in seven persons with the antigen will ever get the disease.[70] The remainder will be false positives.

As I will show, the first two problems are eliminated by tests at the DNA level. Fewer false positives will result from DNA-based tests than from neoclassical tests, but because of variable expressivity, disease will not always occur when the results are positive. Moreover, recombinant DNA technology will lead to the identification of a greater proportion of alleles capable of producing disease than will be ascertainable by neoclassical tests. This will result in fewer false negatives. When, however, extensive genetic heterogeneity exists, DNA-based tests will still fail to detect some people who will develop disease.

Summary and Conclusions

By examining proteins obtained from different individuals within healthy populations, investigators have found genetically determined variant forms occurring frequently at several gene loci. The occurrence of two or more variant forms, the least common of which occurs in at least 2 percent of the population, has been designated a polymorphism. Most variants are "neutral"; they neither protect from nor predispose to disease. As I will show in chapter 4, this extensive genetic variability, which is even more pronounced when DNA is examined, is critical in localizing and identifying genes whose presence up to this time could only be inferred.

The presence of one or more polymorphic forms of some proteins has been associated with an increased chance of developing a variety of common diseases, but other genetic or environmental factors are often needed as well. Some alleles that cause severe disease in homozygotes may cause milder or later-onset disease when only a single dose is present. Although recessive diseases are rare, the frequency of heterozygotes for some of them approaches 2 percent. The combined frequency of disorders due to rare alleles and polymorphisms is substantial.

Since disease-causing or susceptibility-conferring alleles are subject to natural selection, the high frequency of some them seems a contradiction. However, alleles that cause disease only in double (homozygous) dose will not impair the reproductive capabilities of those who possess them in single dose. Sometimes, as with the sickle cell allele, a single dose may be advantageous. This balance permitted the sickle cell allele to attain polymorphic frequency. Today's environment is quite different from that under which the human genome evolved; alleles that were beneficial in the earlier environment may be harmful today, but not enough generations have lived in the new environment to cause a reduction in the frequency of such alleles.

For some diseases, more than one allele is capable of causing the disease; thus, the frequency of each disease-causing allele is not as high as it would be if only one allele accounted for all of those with the disease. For relatively common X-linked disorders, such as hemophilia and Duchenne muscular dystrophy, which impair reproduction, new mutation partially accounts for the high frequency of disease-causing alleles.

With the indirect techniques described in this chapter, great strides have been made in discovering the inherited basis of metabolic disease. The most recent edition of the compendium on the subject, published in 1983, lists approximately 140 different disorders in which an enzyme or other protein defect has been demonstrated.[71] Most of them are due to defects at different gene loci; if the different alleles at a single locus that are responsible for different clinical manifestations are included (e.g., the different hemoglobinopathies), the number is considerably higher. A recent report indicates that there are over 140 disorders of connective tissue alone.[72]

The continued application of these techniques will undoubtedly uncover additional disorders. These tests are limited, however, by the availability of tissue in which the gene is active. Moreover, in order to prove that an abnormality plays an etiologic role, one must detect the presence of that abnormality prior to the onset of overt disease, thereby eliminating the possibility that it is a consequence rather than a cause. If cells in which the abnormality can be detected cannot be obtained easily and safely, it is doubtful that asymptomatic individuals will be investigated.

Even when indirect methods uncover etiologic genetic factors, they will not always provide useful genetic tests to diagnose or predict disease. For such methods to be effective genetic tests, the gene in question must normally be expressed in accessible tissues at stages in the life cycle that will yield maximum benefit to the person being tested. Because tests based on neoclassical methods fail to measure the genetic defect (or defects when there is heterogeneity) directly, most of them will result in false positives and false negatives.

Only a small fraction of the genes that play a role in human diseases have been elucidated. What is needed is a method to look for allelic differences at the gene level, for then cells in which a suspect enzyme or other protein is expressed would no longer be needed. Genetic lesions will be discovered even when there are few clues as to what the basic defect might be. Hitherto undiscovered single-gene disorders will be amenable to examination at the DNA level, as will multifactorial disorders in which, as is probable in many common diseases, a few loci exert major effects.[73] Moreover, direct DNA examination will facilitate the unraveling of genetic-environmental interactions. Once the gene locus or loci involved in a specific disease have been established, genetic tests for those at risk will be possible using the most accessible nucleated cell.

Chapter 4

Finding Gene Loci and Alleles Implicated in Disease

By facilitating the discovery of the gene loci responsible for disease causation or susceptibility, recombinant DNA technology will lead to a marked expansion of genetic testing. In this chapter, I first describe how the technology is used to determine whether a gene that has already been characterized is responsible for genetic disease. The characterization will usually result from an analysis of the gene product, but may also result from DNA analysis. Then I describe the linkage approach for locating and identifying genes that are responsible for single-gene disorders, but whose function is still unknown. Both methods exploit properties of the genome that previous methods could not: the presence of a full complement of genetic material in nucleated cells from any tissue or organ, and the frequent presence of DNA polymorphisms along the genome.[1] Next I examine the use of recombinant DNA techniques to locate the genes responsible for multifactorial disorders. I conclude with a discussion of some of the pitfalls in finding genes.

The Candidate-Gene Approach

The clinical and biochemical findings relative to a specific disease may well suggest a particular "candidate" protein that is defective. However, examination of that protein may be extremely difficult or impossible in a living person with the disease because of the inaccessibility of the organs or cells in which the protein is present. For instance, defects in the visual pigment rhodopsin might account for some forms of inherited blindness. Since rhodopsin is present only in the eye, it is difficult to obtain from living people. Even if the protein could be examined, the quantity available would be insufficient to distinguish differences between normal and abnormal subjects. With recombinant DNA technology, sufficient DNA can be obtained from small amounts of accessible tissues, such as white blood cells, to determine whether the gene for the candidate protein is different in those with disease compared to unaffected individuals. Examination of this "candidate" gene requires that total genomic DNA—obtained from readily accessible cells—be chopped with *restriction endonucleases* into fragments of variable length so that they can be separated by electrophoresis. The nucleotide sequences of the candidate gene will be contained on one fragment, or on more than one if the endonuclease chops within the gene. A *probe* containing sequences that are complementary to that of the gene is then added to the electrophoretically separated fragments. Because the gene's sequence is likely to be unique, the probe will probably bind (hybridize) to only those fragments that contain the DNA of the candidate gene. Such duplexes can be visualized. If the candidate is, in fact, the disease-causing gene, the length of the fragments obtained from patients with the disease may differ from the length of the fragments obtained from unaffected individuals. If no difference in fragment lengths is found, other methods can be used to determine if the nucleotide sequences differ. These steps will now be considered in greater detail.

Restriction endonucleases

Approximately two hundred different restriction endonucleases (REs) have been discovered. Each of these enzymes recognizes a specific sequence of nucleotide pairs. Usually these sequences are four or six nucleotide pairs long. Each such sequence will occur approximately once in one to twenty kilobases (kb) along the chromosomes (1,000 nucleotide pairs = 1 kilobase). An RE cleaves the bonds between two of the nucleotides in the sequence. Some REs cleave both strands of DNA between the same nucleotides. For others, the cleavage points are offset by a few nucleotides, leaving "sticky ends," as shown at the bottom of figure 4.1.[2] Each RE will cut the DNA at points recognized only by that RE. (A few REs require specific sequences of eight nucleotides for cleavage; these occur much less frequently, approximately once in 20,000–100,000 nucleotide pairs.)

REs cut genomic DNA into fragments of different lengths. The length of each of these *restriction fragments* depends on the number of nucleotide pairs that reside between the restriction sites. Fragments of different lengths can be separated electrophoretically, the longer fragments migrating less distance in an electric field than the shorter fragments.

Constructing the probe

Probes for candidate genes can be constructed from mRNA for the protein of interest. Single-stranded DNA in which the nucleotide sequence

FIGURE 4.1

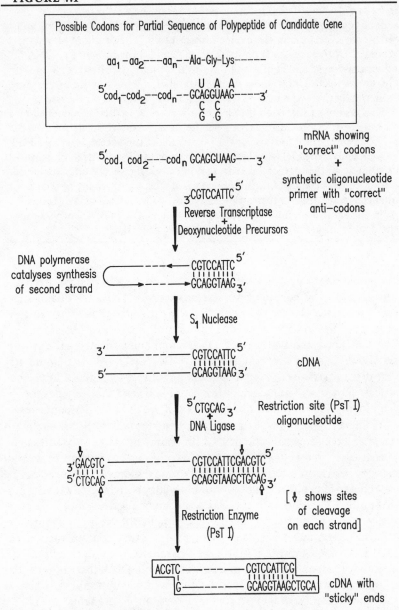

Preparation of complementary DNA (cDNA) for recombination. The amino acid sequence of at least part of the protein of interest is known. Because more than one triplet can code for the same amino acid, several different oligonucleotides are possible (shown in the box at the top). Each will have to be synthesized. The oligonucleotide containing the correct anticodons will be recognized by mRNA containing the complementary codons and will serve as primer for its reverse transcription. The resultant single strand of DNA loops back on itself at one end. In the presence of DNA polymerase, a strand complementary to the first is synthesized. S_1 nuclease cleaves the loop, and a double strand of cDNA containing the same exon nucleotide sequences as the gene for the protein is synthesized.

To accomplish insertion into a vector whose DNA has been opened by a specific restriction enzyme, Pst I (see figure 4.2), nucleotide sequences that are complementary to those at the open ends of the vector must be added to each end of the cDNA. This can be done by synthesizing an oligonucleotide with the correct sequences. With DNA ligase, the oligonucleotides are added to the ends of the cDNA. As is the case here, many of the sequences recognized by restriction enzymes are palindromes; when read from the same direction (e.g., the 5' end), the nucleotides of both strands of the double-stranded molecule have the same sequence.

---

is complementary to that of the mRNA can be synthesized from the mRNA with the enzyme *reverse transcriptase*. A short "oligonucleotide" sequence of deoxynucleotides, which is complementary to a sequence on the mRNA, is needed to "prime" the reverse transcription.[3] The addition of another enzyme, DNA polymerase, results in the synthesis of double-stranded "complementary DNA (cDNA)" (see figure 4.1). One of these strands is complementary not only to the mRNA but also to at least part of the sequence of the candidate gene that encodes for the protein. cDNA, therefore, can be used as a *probe* for those sequences.

As I have already indicated, the cells that synthesize the protein of interest and consequently the mRNA for it may not be readily accessible. In that case, a probe for the candidate gene in an animal can be used to identify restriction fragments of the human candidate gene that can be expected to have sufficient sequence homology to hybridize with the animal probe.[4] The human fragments can then be used as probes. Alternatively, if at least part of the amino acid sequence of the human protein is known, oligonucleotides can be constructed that contain the correct anticodons for a short part of it. The oligonucleotide will then bind to a fragment from an RE digest of human genomic DNA that contains the complementary sequence. Hybridization will occur even if only part of the sequence of the fragment is complementary to the probe.

The restriction fragment that binds to an oligonucleotide probe will almost certainly not contain the sequence of the entire candidate gene. But it can be used as a probe to search for fragments, obtained with other

REs, that contain the same sequence but extend farther on one or both sides of it than the original fragment. These in turn can be used to search for additional fragments extending farther from the original oligonucleotide sequence. This process is known as *chromosome walking*.

The genomic fragments with overlapping sequences serve as probes not only of the exon gene sequences, which encode for protein, but also of promoter and intron sequences. Mutations in promoters can impair the start of synthesis, and mutations in introns can affect the correct splicing of exons (axiom 5b). That such mutations account for disease is evident from studies of the mutations in thalassemia.[5]

Intron sequences are not contained in mRNA or the cDNA prepared from it. But once cDNA is prepared, it can be used in the same way as oligonucleotides to search for complementary fragments from libraries of cloned DNA fragments, which ultimately become the probes for the candidate gene.

Cloning probes

Cloning is a means of increasing the supply of a segment of DNA so that it can be used as a tool in a variety of experiments or in "manufacturing" large amounts of the protein for which it encodes. The first step in cloning involves insertion of the segment, such as a human cDNA or a restriction fragment, into *vectors*—plasmids (molecules of circular DNA from bacteria) or viral DNA (figure 4.2). This is accomplished by treating the vector with an RE so that an opening is formed. The segment to be inserted must also be treated with the same RE so that it will bind to the exposed sites in the vector in the presence of a ligating enzyme. In some molecules of the vector, the human DNA takes the place of the excised vector fragment (right side of figure 4.2). In others, the ends of the vector ligate without insertion of the foreign DNA (left side of figure 4.2). Next, the vector is incubated with bacteria. The process can be arranged so that an average of only one vector molecule infects each bacteria. The vector then multiplies within the bacteria, and the bacteria themselves multiply. The result is the production of a large number of molecules of the segment of human DNA. Clones of bacteria that contain the human DNA insert can be distinguished from those that do not. One method, entailing the interruption of an antibiotic resistance gene by a cDNA insert, is shown in figure 4.2. The probe is prepared from the colonies of bacteria (clones) that contain the human DNA insert.[6]

Fragments from an RE digest of DNA from the entire human genome can be treated so that each fragment is incorporated into a separate vector. The bacteria into which the different vectors enter are then separated

FIGURE 4.2

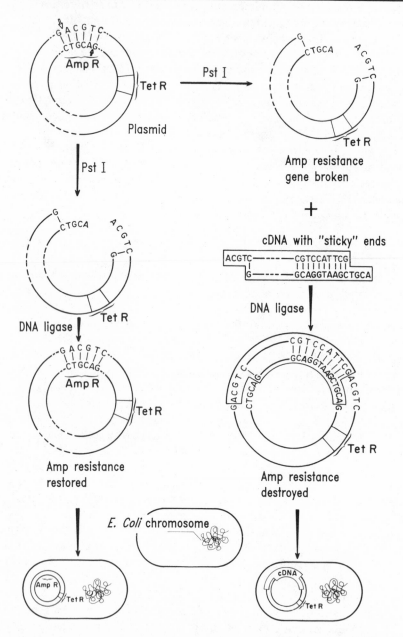

Recombining two species of DNA. The circular DNA of the plasmid shown here contains two antibiotic-resistant genes, one conferring resistance to ampicillin (**Amp R**), the other conferring resistance to tetracycline (**Tet R**). The Amp R gene contains a site for cleavage by the restriction enzyme Pst I. Incubation with Pst I opens up the plasmid at the restriction site, thereby disrupting the Amp R gene. If the cDNA described in figure 4.1 is now incubated with the open plasmids in the presence of DNA ligase, the cDNA will be inserted into some of the plasmids (*right side of figure*), destroying resistance to ampicillin. The ends of those plasmids into which cDNA is not inserted will join, restoring the Amp R gene (*left side of figure*). The plasmids are then inserted into bacteria that lack both ampicillin and tetracycline resistance. The conditions of the experiment are adjusted so that on average only one plasmid enters each bacterium. The clones resulting from the multiplication of each bacterium are examined for ampicillin and tetracycline resistance. Those containing the recombined cDNA are resistant to tetracycline but not to ampicillin. cDNA probes are obtained from these clones.

---

so that a clone for each restriction fragment is produced. This can also be accomplished for a mixture of cDNAs. The DNA derived from a clone can be probed for the presence of a human sequence complementary to that of the candidate gene. The DNA from clones containing complementary sequences can then serve as a probe for the candidate gene.

Identifying restriction fragments containing the gene sequence

To determine which RE fragment from a digestion of human genomic DNA contains the nucleotide sequences complementary to the probe for the candidate gene, one must separate the fragments. The procedure used most often is called Southern blotting, after its inventor, E. M. Southern (see figure 4.3). In the first step, the fragments obtained from an RE digest of DNA from a single individual are separated according to their size by electrophoresis on agarose gel. In the second step, the gel is "blotted" onto a filter membrane that binds DNA fragments (in the same positions relative to each other as on the agarose). Next, a solution containing the probe is poured over the membrane. Both the probe and the fragments are denatured—that is, separated into single strands that are capable of hybridizing with each other. The probe binds only to fragments containing a complementary sequence. Prior to blotting, the probe is modified by the addition of radioactive phosphorous or of biotin. These labels permit visualization of the probe-fragment hybrid.[7] With either technique, nothing is seen in the regions of the other (nonhybridized) fragments, even though they are still present on the membrane.

FIGURE 4.3

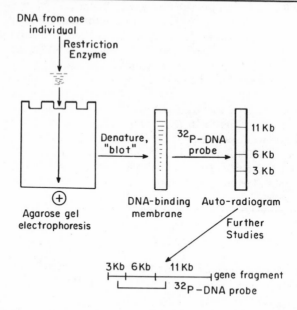

The Southern blot method. A restriction enzyme digest of DNA of the entire genome from one individual is placed on the top of one slot of an agarose gel. Upon electrophoresis, fragments of smaller size (fewer nucleotides) move faster toward the anode than larger ones. If visualized at this stage, fragments of a given length would appear as a band across the gel. Following electrophoresis, the DNA on the gel is denatured (so that hybridization with a complementary probe is possible) and blotted onto a nitrocellulose or nylon membrane; the bands on the blot occupy the same positions relative to each other as those on the gel. Single-stranded, radioactive probe is poured over the membrane. It binds only to the bands containing complementary sequences; the rest washes through. X-ray film is then laid on top of the nitrocellulose. The radioactive bands will appear as dark lines after the film is developed. (As described in the text, biotin can substitute for the radioactive label.)

One possible chromosomal arrangement of the three fragments that constitute the 20-kb sequence is shown at the bottom of the figure. (The actual arrangement requires studies with additional restriction enzymes and perhaps other probes.) Hybridization with the 3-kb and 11-kb gene fragments occurs even though the probe does not contain the full length of complementary sequences. cDNA probes will not contain all of the sequences present in the structural gene fragments obtained from a genomic digest; intron sequences were eliminated before mRNA, from which the cDNA was made, was released into the cytoplasm.

Finding disease-causing alleles

The big question is whether the mutation that causes the disease of interest resides in the candidate gene. Southern blots will provide an answer for some mutations, but when they do not, other methods will be needed before the gene can be struck from the list of candidates.

Mutations involving restriction endonuclease sites, insertions, and deletions. Southern blots of DNA obtained from an individual with the disease of interest are compared to those from unaffected individuals, who are frequently members of the family of the affected person. If the mutation is at a restriction site, and prevents cleavage by the RE, one longer fragment will be found in patients with the disease instead of the two shorter ones found in normals (figure 4.4). In sickle cell anemia, for instance, the single-nucleotide substitution that constitutes the disease-causing mutation destroys an RE site.[8] Alternatively, the mutation could add a new restriction site, resulting in two shorter fragments instead of one longer one. Mutations that involve insertions or deletions of several nucleotides within a restriction fragment will, by changing the length of the fragment, also be detectable. A deletion of 5 kb in the low-density lipoprotein receptor gene accounts for one type of familial hypercholesterolemia.[9]

It would be amazing good fortune if the first RE used did detect a single-nucleotide substitution responsible for the disease under investigation. Digesting with other REs could reveal a difference on Southern blots between the DNA from diseased individuals and that from normal individuals if the RE sites had been affected by the mutation. However, many disease-causing alleles result from single-nucleotide substitutions that do not involve restriction sites.

Tightly linked polymorphisms. Southern blots sometimes show that people with the disease of interest have the same form of a commonly occurring normal variant at a restriction site detected by the candidate-gene probe more often than controls, and that obligate heterozygotes have the variant form on one of the chromosomes carrying the disease-related gene. (These *restriction fragment length polymorphisms* [RFLPs] will be discussed at greater length in the section on the linkage approach.) The variant site shown in figure 4.4 could be due to a tightly linked RFLP rather than a disease-causing mutation. If so, some healthy people would have the same variant. Until the RE that digests the sickle cell mutation directly was found, tightly linked polymorphisms were used to detect the presence of the sickle cell allele.[10] They have also confirmed the presence of mutations in the gene for phenylalanine hydroxylase in patients with PKU.[11]

FIGURE 4.4

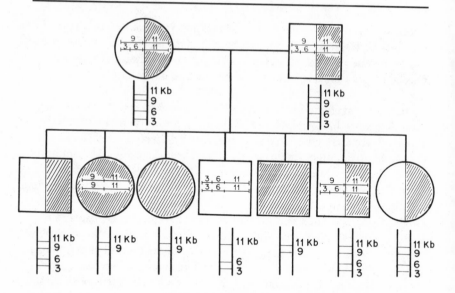

Southern blots using a candidate-gene probe. In these two generations of a family with an autosomal recessive disorder, fully shaded circles and squares indicate affected females and affected males, respectively. The parents are obligate heterozygotes, shown as half-shaded circles and squares. Each family member's Southern blot is shown below his or her symbol; the arrangement of the allelic sequences on homologous chromosomes is shown inside the symbol for selected family members. The contiguous genomic fragments are the same length as those shown in figure 4.3, except that one allele in each parent, and both alleles in the affected siblings, lack one restriction enzyme site. This results in the appearance of a 9-kb fragment in their respective blot patterns. The blots in the three affected children are identical, and different from those observed in their unaffected siblings and parents. Each of the affected offspring is homozygous for the mutation that eliminated the restriction site. This is consistent with the possibility that the mutation is responsible for the disease, or that the disease-causing mutation is very close to that site and tightly linked to it. Confirmation requires study of additional families. The heterozygote status of unaffected siblings also is established by Southern blots.

Oligonucleotide probes. Probes of up to twenty nucleotides that are *perfectly* complementary to a sequence of the candidate gene from healthy individuals will hybridize to the normal allele, but not to an allele that differs from it by as little as one nucleotide. The technique has been used to identify the mutation in alpha-1-antitrypsin deficiency[12] and some thalassemias. A disease-causing mutation outside the region complementary to the oligonucleotide probe will not be detected with this technique. It is possible to construct several oligonucleotide probes for different sequences along the gene's length, but the method requires knowledge of the gene's nucleotide sequence. The binding can be visualized by Southern blots; only the band that hybridizes with a labeled oligonucleotide probe will be visible.

Polymerase chain reaction. Recently, an elegant method for amplifying a specific segment of a gene has been reported.[13] The method involves constructing complementary oligonucleotide polymers for short regions of the gene that flank the sequence of interest; one oligonucleotide binds to one DNA strand, the other to the complementary (noncoding) strand. The distance between the flanking regions can be 0.1–3.0 kb.[14] The polymers are allowed to hybridize to denatured (single-stranded) genomic DNA, and then DNA polymerase and deoxynucleotides are added. The polymers serve as primers for the enzyme, which catalyzes the synthesis of two new strands, one from each direction. Both contain the region of interest. The mixture is again denatured, allowing for the hybridization of additional oligonucleotides to all four of the strands now present, and when DNA polymerase is again added, a doubling of the strands containing the region of interest occurs. When the process is repeated, each cycle doubles the number of strands present; hence the name polymerase chain reaction (PCR). The procedure has been modified so that only the region of interest is amplified.[15]

The DNA containing the amplified region can be treated with REs that are capable of detecting mutant from normal alleles if the two differ in RE sites. The bands can be separated by gel electrophoresis. Since the amplified bands are present in such high concentration, a stain for DNA will make them, but not the background (nonamplified) DNA, visible; Southern blotting is not necessary. Alternatively, labeled oligonucleotide probes for sequences between the flanking regions can be constructed. These can be applied to the entire DNA containing the amplified segment. Only if there is a perfect match between the probe and the sequence in the DNA, however, will the probe hybridize so that it can subsequently be made visible. These methods have been applied to detecting patients with thalassemia,[16] hemophilia,[17] and phenylketonuria.[18]

Ribonuclease treatment of RNA-DNA heteroduplexes. The use of oligonucleotide probes or primers requires knowledge of at least part of the sequence of the candidate gene. However, that knowledge is not necessary for the method described here, or for the following method, denaturing gradient gels. In ribonuclease treatment, a labeled RNA probe is synthesized (by transcription) from the DNA of the candidate gene obtained from a healthy individual. The probe is then hybridized to denatured DNA from patients and controls. This is followed by digestion with ribonuclease (RNAase). RNAase will digest all the RNA except those sequences that are hybridized to the DNA. Any ribonucleotide in the hybridized RNA that is not complementary to the nucleotide on the DNA will be cleaved by RNAase. The digest is then electrophoresed under conditions that separate (denature) the RNA-DNA duplex, and the bands are made visible. If the controls have perfect RNA-DNA duplex hybrids, only one RNA band will be seen. If, however, there is a single mismatch between the RNA and DNA, two RNA bands, whose total length will equal that of the single band in the controls, will be observed. By analysis of the RNA, one can then locate the mutation and identify the nature of the nucleotide change.[19] This method has been used to detect mutants in thalassemia.[20] It has been modified to detect mismatches between labeled RNA complementary to normal mRNA and mRNA from patients with diseases in which the mRNA is known to be present in the cells of accessible tissues.[21]

Denaturing gradient gels. If a double-stranded DNA fragment obtained from a person with the disease of interest differs by as little as one nucleotide pair from normal, it will denature at slightly different concentrations of denaturing chemicals than the fragment from the normal control. This will also be true of perfect duplex hybrids between a probe and a DNA fragment compared to duplexes in which there is one mismatch due to mutation. Such differences can be detected by electrophoresing the fragments in gels containing a gradient in the concentration of denaturing agents. As soon as a fragment reaches a concentration at which it denatures, its mobility is greatly slowed. Thus, fragments that differ in the conditions under which they denature will migrate different distances in the gel. Mutations in thalassemia have been distinguished by this method.[22] Neither the denaturing gradient method nor the RNAase heteroduplex method will detect all mutations. However, each will discover some missed by the other. Because each is limited to segments of less than 1.5 kb, several different experiments must be performed to cover an entire gene.

Direct sequencing. The most direct approach to finding a mutation is to compare the sequence of the gene in normal and affected individuals. This approach was impractical until the discovery of the polymerase chain reaction. The PCR made it possible to amplify a segment of the DNA that could easily be obtained from a single individual to a quantity sufficient to permit direct sequencing. Sequencing requires a labeled oligonucleotide primer that is complementary to one end of the DNA segment whose sequence is of interest. Polymerization is carried out in four separate reaction tubes. Each contains the primer, the denatured segment of DNA that is being sequenced, the four deoxynucleotides, and a DNA polymerase. One tube contains a sequence-terminating adenine nucleotide analog, the second contains a cytosine analog, the third a guanine analog, and the fourth a thymine analog. When polymerization is complete, each tube will contain a mixture of new fragments of different length; each of these fragments will terminate with the analog in that tube. The products of the four tubes are electrophoresed side by side (four channels) in a medium in which the distance migrated by each fragment depends on its length. When the bands are made visible, the sequence is determined directly by observing in which channel the shortest fragment is present, in which the next-shortest is found, and so on. If the shortest visible fragment (the one that migrates fastest during electrophoresis) is in the "adenine" channel, an adenine nucleotide begins the sequence after the primer. If the next-shortest visible band is in the thymine channel, then thymine comes next. This method has been used to find two previously undescribed mutations for thalassemia.[23]

The Linkage Approach

So little is known about the biochemical derangements underlying many single-gene disorders that no candidate genes suggest themselves. This is the case for cystic fibrosis, retinitis pigmentosa, Huntington disease, adult polycystic kidney disease, and many other single-gene disorders. We also have very few clues as to which genes play a role in common diseases such as Alzheimer or bipolar affective disorder.[24] Another means of finding the genetic lesion is needed. The presence of DNA polymorphisms scattered throughout the human genome permits the localization of disease-related genes to specific regions of specific chromosomes. In theory, the locus of at least one of these polymorphisms will be close enough to the locus of the gene responsible for the disease of interest that crossing over between the two is less likely to occur than if the two were unlinked (axiom 3). Consequently, within families in which different forms of the polymorphism exist, individuals with the disease will be more likely than unaffected individuals to inherit one particular form of the polymorphism. Linkage to polymorphisms has already localized the genes at which alleles reside for all of the diseases mentioned earlier in this paragraph and several others. I will now examine this approach in more detail.

Restriction fragment length polymorphisms

At positions 100–500 nucleotides apart on the human genome the nucleotide pair will frequently vary—for instance, an adenine-thymine pair will be present instead of a guanine-cytosine.[25] A plausible explanation for the high frequency of these variants is their neutrality; one variant is neither more helpful nor more harmful for survival and reproduction than the other. Support for this explanation comes from the observation that these variants are more likely to occur in regions of the genome that do not encode for structural genes—that is, they are more likely to be found in introns, pseudogenes, and sequences between genes of no known function (axiom 5c) than in sequences that are known to encode for proteins.[26] They are also called "silent" mutations. Some RFLPs have been found in or very close to structural genes—for instance, the insulin gene and some oncogenes.

Approximately one in twenty of these variants (or one every 2–10 kb along the genome) will involve RE sites and will therefore show up on Southern blots of DNA treated with the appropriate restriction enzyme. When the site is present on a chromosome, two bands will be present. The length of these bands (in kilobases) will equal the length of the one long band that is present on chromosomes from which the site is absent. Because of the high frequency of both forms of the polymorphism, many individuals will be heterozygotes; they will possess both forms of the single-nucleotide polymorphism. Consequently, in Southern blots of their DNA, three bands (two short and one long) will be present. (Compare, for example, the left-most heterozygote in figure 4.5 and the left-most homozygote, diagramed above it.) These fragments of different length are called *restriction fragment length polymorphisms* (RFLPs).

Sometimes more than one RFLP is detectable with the same probe. This is illustrated in figure 4.5, where two polymorphic loci appear 5 kb apart. Four different combinations of the polymorphic forms are possible. These combinations are called *haplotypes*. Individuals inherit one haplotype from each parent. Ten different pairs of haplotypes are possible, four homozygous and six heterozygous. The extensive individual differences detectable by haplotypes are very important in the linkage approach.

The number of nucleotides between two adjacent RE sites can vary due to the presence of different numbers of a repeating oligonucleotide sequence. The number of these *tandem repeats* is genetically determined and transmitted in Mendelian fashion, as is the case with other RFLPs. As a class, they have been called *variable number of tandem repeats* (VNTRs). Probes have been prepared for several different genomic fragments that contain tandem repeats. Each such probe identifies a single

FIGURE 4.5

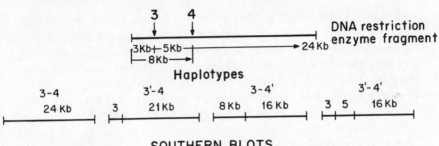

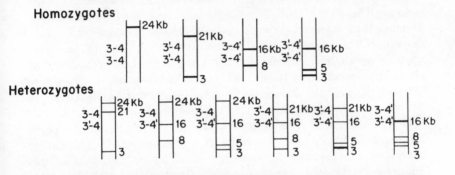

Use of restriction fragment length polymorphisms to establish haplotypes.
In the 24-kb segment of a chromosome at the top of the figure, the arrows
designate single nucleotide loci 3 and 4, at which common polymorphisms
occur. One form of each polymorphism is recognized by a restriction enzyme. Allele 3 is not recognized by the enzyme, but allele 3' is. Similarly,
allele 4 is not recognized, but 4' is. Four different combinations of locus 3
and 4 are possible, as shown in the second row. Each of these combinations
is a haplotype. Since the restriction enzyme digest of each haplotype has a
unique band pattern on a Southern blot, each of the ten different combinations of homologous chromosomes also gives a unique pattern. Thus
the alleles present at positions 3 and 4 on each chromosome can be determined in every case: the homozygous patterns are shown in the top row of
blots, the heterozygous patterns in the bottom row. The use of these RFLPs
in establishing linkage is illustrated in figure 4.6.

locus at which the number of tandem repeats varies. At some loci there
may be just two different numbers of tandem repeats; at others there may
be as many as twenty. The chance of heterozygosity and of different genotypes is very high. At least seventy-seven probes for VNTRs at different
positions along the genome have been discovered thus far.[27]

Mapping the human genome

The chance of localizing a disease-related gene by the linkage method depends on one's having polymorphic markers close to the gene. Considerable effort is being made by academic centers and commercial enterprises to identify RFLP polymorphisms and determine their position on specific chromosomes.[28] With funds from the NIH, a probe repository has been established to facilitate the exchange of probes between investigators.[29] The sequencing of large segments of DNA will also facilitate establishing relationships between markers.[30] The number of RFLPs mapped is rapidly approaching 1,000.

The mapping of markers requires probes for different sequences of the genome. These are obtained by cloning different restriction fragments obtained from digests of the entire human genome or from isolated chromosomes. The second method immediately establishes the chromosome on which the fragment is located. The problem has been that not all chromosomes can be isolated.[31] It is also possible to map a sequence of DNA to a specific subchromosomal region by hybridizing labeled probes to spreads of chromosomes *in situ*.[32]

DNA from several different individuals must be examined by a probe for a specific fragment to determine if it contains RFLPs. Once polymorphic fragments have been identified, their linkage to other RFLPs can be readily established by studies in healthy families in which DNA from members over three generations is available.[33] The approach is the same as that described next for linkage between polymorphisms and disease-related genes.

Relation of polymorphisms to loci at which disease-causing alleles exist

In a family in which several members are affected with the same dominant disorder, we can be confident that the mutation is the same in every affected member. Barring crossing over, which I will discuss shortly, the disease-causing allele and one form of a linked polymorphism (or one haplotype) will be transmitted together in meiosis. In Mendelian terms, they will cosegregate. However, the same form of the polymorphism will probably not be found in those with the disease in other families.[34] In families with recessive disorders, two different mutations at the same locus can cause the disease because of allelic diversity, and each can be linked to a different form of the same polymorphism. Even when identical mutations on the maternally and paternally inherited chromosomes account for the recessive disease, the form of the RFLP (or haplotype) to which it is linked may differ on the maternal and paternal chromosomes (see note 34). This is different from the process shown in figure 4.4.

Dominant disorders. Cosegregation of a polymorphic "marker" and an allele for a dominant disease is shown in figure 4.6. The individuals who possess the disease-causing allele are known because they have overt disease. Table 4.1 tabulates the number of times each of the alleles shown in figure 4.6 was present in the family members studied. None of the alleles at positions 3 or 4 was responsible for the occurrence of disease; each was present in healthy family members as well as those with disease. Table 4.2 tabulates the number of times each possible haplotype of alleles at adjacent loci was present in the family members studied. One haplotype, 3'-4, was present exclusively in the individuals with disease. This is consistent with linkage of the mutation causing the disease to the 3'-4 haplotype. The number of observations in this study was small, however, and the association could have resulted from chance. The finding of linkage to haplotypes of positions 3 and 4 (but not necessarily the 3'-4 haplotype) in studies of other families would confirm the association, as would a demonstration of linkage to other markers known to be linked to positions 3 and 4. At the same time, linkage to other polymorphisms unlinked to positions 3 and 4 should be excluded.

Heterozygosity in the polymorphic marker is critical to establishing linkage. If the individuals in the pedigree shown in figure 4.6 were all homozygous at loci 3 and 4, it would be impossible to establish linkage. In many of the RFLPs discovered thus far, the least common variant occurs in at least 10 percent of healthy individuals, and often there are more than two variants; the lower the frequency of the most common allele, and the greater the number of alleles, the greater the likelihood of heterozygosity. Compared to known gene product (protein) polymorphisms (discussed in chapter 3), which also can be used for linkage studies, there are many more DNA polymorphisms (RFLPs, including VNTRs), and there is more extensive diversity in most of them.

One of the first diseases localized by linkage with RFLPs was Huntington disease. Reviewing this accomplishment by Gusella et al. may make the linkage approach clearer. Their first requirement was obtaining DNA from several affected and unaffected members spanning three generations of two different families. The DNA from each member of each family was digested with REs that had previously been found to reveal polymorphic markers on the normal human gene map. One of these markers, G8, proved to be associated with the presence of HD in both families. Completion of the family studies revealed that, despite the finding that one affected person did not have the same form of the polymorphic marker (i.e., recombination had occurred), the odds that the HD locus would be linked to the marker were greater than one trillion to one![35]

Despite the many similarities of the HD in one family to the HD in the

FIGURE 4.6

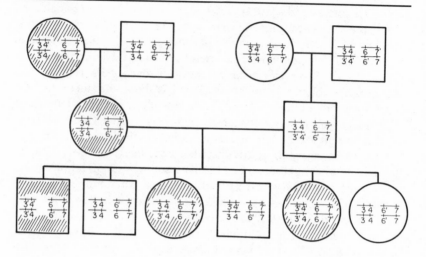

Pedigree of a family with an autosomal dominant disease. Shading indicates affected members. The frequency of alleles is shown in table 4.1, the frequency of haplotypes in table 4.2.

Table 4.1 Number of Times Each Allele Shown in Figure 4.6 Was Present in Family Members Studied

	Allele							
	3	3'	4	4'	6	6'	7	7'
Family members with disease	3	7	7	3	6	4	5	5
Family members without disease	9	5	9	5	6	8	7	7

Table 4.2 Number of Times Each Haplotype of Closely Linked Alleles (Figure 4.6) Was Present in Family Members Studied

	Haplotype							
	3-4	3-4'	3'-4	3'-4'	6-7	6-7'	6'-7	6'-7'
Family members with disease	2	1	5	2	1	5	4	0
Family members without disease	9	0	0	5	0	6	7	1

other, differences occurred as well. The question remained, therefore, whether linkage to the G8 marker would be found in additional families. At least ten additional families have now been studied. In all of them there was linkage to the marker, although as was expected, the linked G8 haplotype differed from family to family.[36] *In situ* hybridization and other techniques localized the markers linked to HD to the terminal end of the short arm of chromosome 4.[37]

Recessive disorders. Allelic diversity complicates the use of linkage to locate the genes for recessive disorders, but it does not prevent its use. One way around this problem is to find large kindreds in which all disease-causing alleles have been derived from one person in an ancestral generation (founder effect; see chapter 3). Within each such family the individuals who have the disease will be homozygous for the same allele, and all heterozygotes will have the same form of the polymorphism at a marker locus linked to the disease-causing allele, barring crossing over. The search for linkage, then, is similar to that described for a dominant disease.

Another way to get around allelic diversity is to use families in which at least two siblings with overt disease are available for study. All affected sibs within any one family will have the same pair of disease-causing alleles and, barring crossing over, will share haplotypes at a polymorphic locus linked to the disease. (The linked haplotype on one chromosome in the offspring with disease need not be identical to the haplotype on the homologous chromosome.) The parents and healthy siblings will not have the same pair of markers at the linked locus as the siblings with disease. (The parents and heterozygote siblings will have one of the haplotype markers linked to the disease-causing allele). This approach has been successful in locating the cystic fibrosis "gene" to the long arm of chromosome 7.[38]

Crossing over (recombination)

In the family pedigree shown in figure 4.6, no crossing over between the haplotype and the disease-causing allele occurred. (See axiom 3 and figures 1.2 and 1.3 for a review of meiosis and crossing over.) With existing markers, studies of additional families are likely to show crossing over (assuming linkage to the markers in those families). This will also be the case for recessive disorders. The proportion of meioses in which recombination between a polymorphic marker and a disease-related gene will occur depends on the nucleotide distance between the marker and the gene. When recombination is observed in 5 percent of meioses, the two loci are said to be 5 *centiMorgans* (cM) apart.[39] At 5 percent recombination, 95 percent of individuals with the disease would show linkage to positions 3 and 4, and 5 percent of healthy family members would show linkage as well. Recombination in 50 percent of observed members is indistinguishable from the association that would be expected if positions 3 and 4 and the disease-related gene were unlinked—that is, if they were either far apart on the same chromosome or on different chromosomes. Whether the odds for linkage are higher than those for nonlinkage is determined mathematically from the observed associations in all families known to have the disease.[40]

The frequency of crossing over between a marker and a disease-related gene can be used to locate a gene more precisely. To return to the family shown in figure 4.6, let us assume that two new polymorphic markers, 2 and 5, have been found linked to the disease-related gene (figure 4.7). To which of these markers is the disease-causing allele closest? If it is closer to locus 2, then in families in which the disease exists, the probability of crossing over between locus 2 and the locus for the disease-causing allele will be less than that between the disease locus and locus 5. The reverse would hold if the disease-causing allele were closer to locus 5. This more precise localization is one way of narrowing the distance between a known fragment on a chromosome and the actual location of the disease-related gene and it facilitates identification of the gene.

Figure 4.7 makes another point. Under the hypothesis that the disease-related locus is situated between the two markers, the chance for double crossovers (right-most case) is much less than that for single crossovers between the disease-related locus and either marker (middle two cases). Consequently, if two flanking polymorphic loci were available, it would take a smaller number of families to establish (or exclude) linkage than it would if only one marker was available.[41] For both dominant and recessive disorders, families with multiple affected members may be difficult to find, so this is an important practical consideration.

Identifying Genes Once They Have Been Localized

The localization of a disease-related gene to within 5 cM (about five million nucleotide pairs) of a polymorphic marker locus is still a long way from identifying the gene itself. With a higher map density of RFLPs, a still closer marker might be found, but as the markers get closer to each other, recombination between them will be observed so rarely that it will be impossible to determine confidently the sequence of marker loci on the chromosome or to position the locus between any two of them. Even if the distance between the nearest marker and the locus were 2 cM, this space would still be great enough to contain 40 genes of an average size of 50 kb. Chromosome walking techniques, mentioned in the section on

FIGURE 4.7

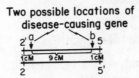

Two possible locations of
disease-causing gene

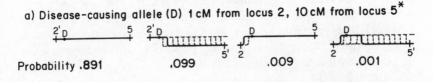

a) Disease-causing allele (D) 1 cM from locus 2, 10 cM from locus 5[*]

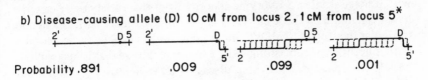

b) Disease-causing allele (D) 10 cM from locus 2, 1 cM from locus 5[*]

[*]Location of crossover shown by shift in line level. Some other sites of crossover are shown with dashed lines.

Use of crossing over (recombination) in gene mapping. The disease-related gene is flanked by two polymorphic loci, 2 and 5, which are 11 cM apart. Two polymorphic alleles, 2 and 2', and 5 and 5', occur respectively at these loci. Haplotype 2'-5 is observed in first-generation members with disease, before any crossing over occurs. If the disease-causing allele is at position (a), close to locus 2, then affected offspring of the affected parent will have fewer crossovers between locus 2 and position (a) (which would result in the association of disease with alleles 2 and 5) than between position (a) and locus 5 (which would result in the association of disease with alleles 2' and 5'). Consequently, the 2'-5' combination will be observed in those with disease about eleven times more frequently than the 2-5 combination. If, however, the disease-causing allele is at position (b), close to locus 5, then affected offspring will have fewer crossovers between position (b) and locus 5 than between locus 2 and position (b). Consequently, alleles 2 and 5 will occur in people with disease about eleven times more frequently than alleles 2' and 5'. Regardless of where the disease-causing mutation is, the presence of alleles 2 and 5' in those with disease will be very rare; it requires a double crossover. This demonstrates the benefit of three-point mapping.

the candidate-gene approach, are not practical to cover this distance. Other approaches are needed.

The use of chromosomal abnormalities

Sometimes individuals with single-gene disorders are found to have a chromosomal abnormality. A deletion or a break in the DNA sequence of the gene that leads to the translocation of genetic material from elsewhere in the genome could disrupt normal transcription of the gene. Large deletions (spanning several genes) and translocations are detectable by karyotyping. When they are found in patients with a single-gene disorder, they may indicate the site of the disease-related gene, particularly if the same site is deleted in unrelated individuals and if they are consistent with linkage studies. Karyotypic abnormalities that satisfy these criteria have been found on the X-chromosome in some patients with Duchenne muscular dystrophy (DMD),[42] and on chromosome 13 in some patients with inherited retinoblastoma (RB), a tumor of the eye that leads to blindness.[43] One patient with three diseases—DMD; retinitis pigmentosa (RP), which causes blindness by the third decade of life; and chronic granulomatous disease (CGD), a disorder of phagocytic cells that impairs host defenses against infection—was found to have a deletion on the X-chromosome in the same region as that in which other DMD deletions had been reported.[44] The gene loci for the three diseases are linked.

Karyotypically observed deletions can stretch over several million nucleotide pairs. Probes for the deleted region that are prepared from normal DNA, however, can detect smaller deletions in other patients with the disease. Investigators at Harvard's Children's Hospital hybridized the DNA of the patient with CGD, RP, and DMD with DNA from complete X-chromosomes (without deletions).[45] They prepared probes from the unhybridized region of the intact X to detect deletions in other DMD patients. Some of these deletions were considerably shorter, and thus narrowed the region of the DMD locus still further.

Having probes for the region of the deletion provides a starting point for the search for the gene of interest in DNA from normal individuals. Chromosome walking techniques have been used to identify restriction fragments in and adjacent to deletion sites in CGD, DMD, and RB. Some of the probes for these fragments will hybridize with segments of the disease-related gene. The question is, which ones?

If we assume that in normal individuals the disease-related gene is transcribed in at least some organs (i.e., is a structural gene), we can perform a sequence of experiments to identify it. First, since it is likely that the nucleotide sequences of exon portions of the gene will be conserved from species to species, the human probes for the region of the deletion can be tested to see if any of them hybridize to DNA from other species. This approach has been used with positive results in studies on RB[46] and DMD.[47] In the case of DMD, the nucleotide sequences of two conserved fragments were determined. They were found to contain *open reading frames*: properly oriented sequences for splicing exons and transcribing a large number of consecutive codons. They became excellent candidates to probe for the structural gene.

Second, efforts can be made to hybridize the probes with RNA or cDNA prepared from mRNAs (see the earlier section on candidate genes) in cells in which the gene is normally transcribed. Hybrids were found with "RB" probes in cultured normal retinal cells,[48] with "DMD" gene probes in fetal skeletal and heart muscle,[49] and with "CGD" probes in normal phagocytic cells.[50] The DMD and CGD probes did not bind the mRNA or cDNA obtained from normal cells from organs or tissues in which the gene was not expected to be transcribed. Although RB probes hybridize with RNA in a variety of tissues and other tumors, they fail to bind RNA or DNA in some retinoblastoma cells, while in some others they yield hybrids of altered size compared to normal.[51] This is consistent with the hypothesis that absence of the normal gene [or failure to transcribe a normal message] is important in retinal tumorigenesis. Probes for transcribed sequences did not hybridize to genomic DNA or to mRNA in phagocytic cells from some patients with CGD, while in some others the hybridized fragment was structurally altered.[52] A cDNA probe for the DMD locus failed to hybridize to genomic DNA from some boys with DMD.[53]

Third, once an mRNA or cDNA from normal cells is found that hybridizes with probes for fragments in the deleted region, the amino acid sequence for which they encode can be determined. From this sequence, information about the shape of the protein can be deduced and homologies to other sequenced proteins sought. The protein of the DMD gene resembles that of another skeletal muscle protein, actinin, but has other domains as well.[54] Knowledge of the sequence permits construction of synthetic polypeptides, which can be used to make antibodies that may cross-react with the protein in normal cells. It is also possible that mRNA can be translated in an experimental cell system; the resultant protein would then be used to produce antibodies. Such studies in DMD have been used to localize the protein to sites within muscle cells.[55] This information may help explain the protein's function. Through the use of antibodies, the protein product of the RB gene has been found to be a phosphoprotein with DNA-binding capacity which resides in the nucleus of normal retinal cells. The phosphoprotein is missing in retinoblastoma cell lines.[56] Antibodies against the CGD protein were recently found to bind to one of the polypeptide chains of neutrophil cytochrome b.[57] The defect in X-linked CGD consequently appears to be due to a defect in this polypeptide. The gene and its function have been identified!

Probes for a disease-related gene will detect small deletions (by the different size of their restriction fragments) that are not visible karyotypically. They will not, however, detect point mutations that do not alter restriction sites. Some of these point mutations might be discovered due to their altering the gene product sufficiently to interfere with its binding of antibody against the normal gene product. The techniques described under the candidate-gene approach (e.g., oligonucleotide probes and the RNAase heteroduplex method) can be used to find additional mutations.

Moving long distances along the genome

Gross chromosome abnormalities will probably prove to be the exception rather than the rule for most genetic disorders, but methods are needed that will permit investigators to span the distance between the nearest linked marker, which will probably be at least 2 cM away, and disease-related genes of interest. The largest DNA fragment that can be incorporated into currently available vectors is about 50 kb long.[58]

A relatively new technique, *pulsed field gel electrophoresis* (PFGE),[59] permits investigators to examine much longer fragments—up to two million nucleotide pairs (2,000 kb) in length. If a known marker linked to a disease-causing gene is at one end of such a long fragment, and another is found toward the other end which is more tightly linked to the disease-related gene than the known marker, as measured by a lower frequency of crossing over, then the disease-related gene must be closer to the new marker. This technique recently permitted investigators at St. Mary's Hospital Medical School in London to narrow the region of the genome that contains the gene locus for cystic fibrosis (CF) to approximately 1 cM from the "met" locus,[60] whose linkage to CF had been established by the techniques described in the previous section. Using PFGE, they found an 820-kb fragment of DNA that contained the "met" locus about 150 kb from one end and two new RFLPs close to the other end.[61] Initially, no crossing over was observed between these two RFLPs and the CF locus, indicating that they were more tightly linked to the CF locus than was the "met" locus.

The St. Mary's group thought they had identified the CF locus near the two new RLFPs; they found conserved sequences and a high frequency of guanine–unmethylated cytosine dimers, which have been observed to cluster around the ends of some structural genes.[62] Further study, however, failed to reveal differences between the sequences from normal individuals and those with cystic fibrosis. Moreover, crossing over between the new markers and the CF gene were reported.[63] Nevertheless, the group did establish that the CF gene is closer to the two new markers than to the "met" marker. It should be possible to use the techniques described in the previous section to find mRNA transcripts for this region, or the techniques described for the candidate-gene approach to determine if there are particular mutations associated with cystic fibrosis.[64]

The work of the St. Mary's group suggests that there may be one predominant CF mutation. The evidence for this comes from the finding that one form (allele) of each of the two new linked RFLPs was associated with the cystic fibrosis allele (as was the haplotype of the two forms) much more often than would have been expected from the frequency of these alleles in the population. This *linkage disequilibrium* suggests that the cystic fibrosis alleles in the many unrelated families in the study had descended from a single mutation arising on the chromosome with the particular haplotype.[65]

Multifactorial Disorders

A disease may become manifest because of the presence (in appropriate dosage) of a disease-causing allele at a single locus, in which case it is Mendelian or single-gene in origin. The same manifestations may result from a susceptibility-conferring allele at one locus and an environmental exposure, or from the simultaneous presence of susceptibility-conferring alleles at several loci (no one of which alone would cause the disease). In these cases the disease is multifactorial. Finally, the manifestations may result entirely from environmental exposures. For common disorders, particularly those of adult onset, multifactorial patterns will predominate.[66]

Identification of the single-gene locus operating to cause disease in rare families manifesting Mendelian inheritance of a common disease could result in the discovery of a hitherto unknown or unsuspected protein or enzyme that also plays a role in the pathogenesis of multifactorial forms, either because it is altered—due to the presence of a susceptibility-conferring allele—or because it is part of a metabolic pathway in which other components are altered (on either a genetic or an environmental basis). Linkage studies of the type already described have succeeded in locating the gene locus at which disease-causing alleles reside in families with Mendelian forms of bipolar affective disorder,[67] Alzheimer disease,[68] and colon cancer (familial polyposis).[69] The gene and gene product have been identified for familial hypercholesterolemic heart disease.[70] Whether these discoveries will contribute to elucidating the etiology and pathogenesis of multifactorial forms remains to be seen.

In the case of many common disorders, no families in which a disease follows the Mendelian pattern of inheritance will present themselves. Nevertheless, there will be families in which a disease or a related group of diseases cluster. Although shared environmental factors may account for or contribute to the clustering, linkage studies may reveal a marker allele or haplotype that occurs with greater frequency in those with these diseases than would be expected in the general population. According to Lander and Botstein, loci at which alleles increase the risk of disease at least tenfold should be detectable by linkage analysis.[71] When the simultaneous presence of alleles at a few loci is needed to detect disease, linkage studies may also be fruitful provided that the frequency of any of the disease-causing alleles is not too high.[72] A number of common disorders probably involve alleles at only a few loci exerting a major effect.[73]

The candidate-gene approach can also be applied to the discovery of at least one of the gene loci involved in multifactorial disorders. This was attempted a few years ago for non-insulin-dependent diabetes mellitus (NIDDM). Because insulin secretion is inappropriate in NIDDM, it is plausible to hypothesize that one genetic lesion resides in the insulin gene or in a nucleotide sequence adjacent to it that regulates the transcription of the gene and consequently insulin synthesis. Although early work using probes for the insulin region suggested that a polymorphism in a sequence flanking the gene was associated with NIDDM,[74] subsequent work has not borne this out.[75]

In view of the alteration of lipoprotein concentrations in some patients with heart disease, genes for the apolipoproteins become reasonable candidates. One form of an RFLP linked to the apolipoprotein A-I gene locus has been reported to be associated with low levels of apo A-I and coronary artery disease.[76] Almost one-third of patients with coronary artery disease possess this form compared to only 4 percent of disease-free controls. An association between one form of an RFLP for the apolipoprotein B gene and coronary artery disease also has been reported.[77] Other, genetic abnormalities of apolipoprotein have been associated with coronary heart disease as well.[78] Tests at the DNA level may ultimately prove to be better predictors of coronary artery disease than lipid or apolipoprotein measurements, but they will not be perfect either; 20–30 percent of men who are heterozygotes for LDL-receptor deficiency escape premature coronary artery disease.[79]

Recombinant DNA techniques may provide better discrimination than neoclassical methods in elucidating susceptibility-conferring alleles at loci already incriminated in multifactorial diseases. For many years investigators have known that certain forms of polymorphic cell surface proteins specified by alleles at loci of the major histocompatibility gene complex (MHC) increase the risk of insulin-dependent diabetes mellitus (IDDM). The use of DNA probes reveals considerably more allelic diversity than the serological methods that were used to detect protein variants. In other words, one type detected serologically may actually consist of several different types that can be distinguished by comparison of their respective DNAs. What is most important is that specific alleles determined by direct DNA analysis show better correlations with disease than do the serologically determined markers.[80] As will be discussed in chapter 5, this improves the ability to predict risk of IDDM.

Facilitated by the polymerase chain reaction, DNA sequencing has now revealed that the codon for the fifty-seventh amino acid in the beta chain protein specified at the DQ locus of the MHC correlates most strongly with susceptibility or resistance to IDDM.[81] Individuals who are homozygous for DQ alleles encoding for amino acids other than aspartic acid at position fifty-seven have marked susceptibility to IDDM.[82] However, they do not all develop diabetes. Those who are heterozygous for such alleles are at moderate risk. The risk is lower in those who have alleles for aspartic acid at position fifty-seven. The region of the protein in which this amino acid alteration is found plays a role in triggering antibody production. This is consistent with theories that the susceptibility to IDDM conferred by alleles at the D loci involves immune response mechanisms (see chapter 3).

The presence of serologically determined polymorphic variants at some loci of the MHC increases the risk for several other diseases, including different types of arthritis, celiac disease, myasthenia gravis, systemic lupus, and narcolepsy. It is possible that DNA analysis will uncover alleles whose presence increases the risk of developing these diseases more than the presence of serologically determined cell surface protein markers does.

Pitfalls in Finding Disease-Related Genes

Some of the obstacles to localizing and identifying loci at which disease-causing or susceptibility-conferring alleles reside reflect methodologic problems that are rapidly being overcome. The advances made in technology and in the probes developed since the Huntington "gene" was mapped have been phenomenal. Other problems are inherent in the genetic diseases themselves, most notably genetic heterogeneity and variable expressivity. These, too, can be at least partially overcome.

An insufficient number of informative probes

The candidate-gene approach is limited to the number of proteins for which gene probes can be constructed. As more proteins are identified—

either by biochemical techniques or as a result of identifying more structural genes by linkage—the number of probes for genes of known function will grow.

The low density of highly polymorphic markers on the human gene map limits the effectiveness of the linkage approach. The more widely spaced polymorphisms are along the genome, the greater the chance of crossing over occurring between them and the disease-related genes to which they are linked. This lowers the odds of linkage and requires a larger number of families before investigators can establish linkage with statistical confidence. The requisite number of families may not be available.

It is not that RFLPs and variant proteins do not exist in abundance, but simply that discovering them is a painstaking task; many RE fragments from many different individuals from large multigenerational families, not necessarily with genetic diseases, must be tested with many different probes before informative loci are discovered. The assignment of markers to specific regions of chromosomes accelerates the process of mapping additional markers. The number of RFLPs discovered and mapped over the last few years has increased enormously.

The difficulty of finding informative families

Even with an increased map density, an insufficient number of informative families in which the disease of interest has occurred, and in which both healthy and sick individuals can be studied, may limit the effectiveness of linkage studies. On the other hand, statistically significant linkage can be established in one family alone if the pedigree is very large and many family members with disease are available for study. This has been possible for Huntington disease[83] and bipolar affective disorder.[84] The problem remains of confirming the association in other families, which might be done by linkage or by direct tests for disease-causing alleles after the gene has been identified.

The number of consanguineous (inbred) families needed to map a gene for a recessive disease is much lower than the number of outbred families needed for the same map density.[85] The reason for this is that the offspring of consanguineous matings are much more likely to be homozygous not only for the disease-causing allele but also for polymorphic markers adjacent to it. Although increased homozygosity might also be observed at unlinked regions (on the same or other chromosomes), it is highly unlikely that the same regions would be involved in unrelated offspring of different consanguineous matings. Therefore, finding one region that is homozygous in several such offspring greatly increases the odds that it contains the disease-related gene.

Another problem is false paternity. If the presumed father of a child with a recessive disorder is not the biological father, it will be impossible to confirm linkage even when two siblings are affected. RFLP typing of the father can be done to establish paternity, but this would be very costly on a routine basis when attempting to establish linkage.

Variable expressivity

Although the range of expressivity of a genetic disorder is less within families than between them, it can still be striking for some diseases. Age of onset (particularly for adult-onset conditions) and clinical manifestations may vary. For instance, in the family in which a "gene" for bipolar affective disorder was localized to chromosome 11, members counted as having the disorder had one of at least three different types of psychiatric disorders (all of them with affective components).[86] There is considerable interfamily variation in neurofibromatosis. The localization of the gene in several unrelated families to a region of chromosome 17 suggests that this is more likely due to variable expressivity than to genetic heterogeneity.[87] This is confirmed by extensive intrafamily variation.[88]

Variable expressivity affects the candidate-gene and linkage approaches. If some people who have not yet manifested the disease have a detectable disease-causing mutation in the candidate gene, that mutation may be overlooked as a cause of the disease. In linkage studies, very strict criteria for who has the disease may exclude families that in fact are informative. On the other hand, loose criteria may result in the misclassification or inclusion of families that actually have another defect (genetic heterogeneity; see below). Adjustments for the likelihood of expressivity (usually called "penetrance" by geneticists) at different ages can be used when including asymptomatic family members in linkage studies.

Allelic diversity

As has already been discussed, different mutations at the same gene locus may be responsible for a specific disease. This should not interfere with linkage studies, but it may affect analyses of candidate genes. It is not certain that probes for a candidate gene will detect all disease-causing mutations. The finding that a large proportion of people with the disease do not have the detectable mutation(s) might suggest that the candidate gene is not implicated when, in fact, other, disease-causing mutations occur at the same locus but go undetected. This can be overcome through the use of techniques that detect multiple mutations. The analysis of sequence data can often indicate whether the mutation(s) will affect the transcription of a structural gene or its amino acid sequence. If they do, this further supports their causal nature. (The observed mutation may,

however, be a variant that is tightly linked to the disease-causing mutation and will not affect gene function.) Final proof that the candidate gene
is involved will come from finding an abnormal gene product in patients
with the disease.

Genetic heterogeneity

Diseases with very similar manifestations may be caused by one or
more alleles at one locus in some families but by alleles at a different
locus in others. A number of examples were cited in chapter 3. Unless
linkage can be established in one or a few large families, heterogeneity
may interfere with finding disease-related genes. The determination of
linkage will depend on adding together the logarithm of the odds for linkage (LOD score) in the individual families studied (see note 40). When
heterogeneity is present, some families will have negative LOD scores for
linkage to one specific locus while others (in which the disease is linked
to that locus) will have positive scores. Consequently, the sum of the
scores may be less than 3, the usual cutoff to determine significant linkage. The simultaneous search for linkage to one *or* another of several
markers scattered throughout the genome in families included in a study
is one way around this problem.[89] This will be made possible by having a
high-density map of RFLPs throughout the genome. For some instances
of disease, through careful history, physical, and laboratory findings it
may be possible to separate diseases due to mutations at different loci.
Linkage studies can then be performed on each separately.

Because of genetic heterogeneity, the finding of a disease-related locus
in one or a few families by either the candidate gene or the linkage approach does not automatically mean that the same locus is implicated in
other families.

Summary and Conclusions

Recombinant DNA technology permits the search for the genetic basis
of disease to proceed directly at the gene level. In the candidate-gene approach, a mutation in an identified gene, usually of known function (i.e.,
one that is responsible for the synthesis of a well-characterized protein),
is suspected of being responsible for the disease of interest. DNA probes
are constructed that will hybridize to the candidate gene. Suspicion that
the gene harbors the disease-causing mutation increases if the DNA that
hybridizes with the probe from affected individuals has a different nucleotide sequence from that of the DNA from unaffected individuals.

In the linkage approach, no specific gene need be suspected. Probes are constructed for genomic sequences (RFLPs) that differ between normal individuals. Such differences are detected because they change the length of fragments that hybridize with the probe following digestion with restriction endonucleases. Within a family in which a genetic disease occurs, one form of a polymorphic sequence that is linked to the disease-causing gene locus will be found in affected family members and another form will be found in unaffected members. The availability of RFLPs mapped to different positions on the human genome makes it likely that genes that play a major role in any one of a large number of diseases can be localized to a specific region of a specific chromosome. Eventually, the gene will be identified and its function determined.

There is no doubt that recombinant DNA methods offer a much greater opportunity to identify disease-causing alleles than earlier methods did. At the present time, the application of these methods is limited by the number of probes available. This limitation is rapidly being overcome, but finding suitable families in which to conduct linkage studies presents a more persistent problem. Finally, the possibility of variable expressivity, allelic diversity, and genetic heterogeneity for genetic diseases may make it difficult for investigators to localize or identify disease-related genes. And even when genes are localized, these phenomena will interfere with the ability to predict correctly that a person has a disease-causing genotype or one that places his or her offspring at risk.

Chapter 5

Genetic Testing in Health Care

Genetic tests can be used in people who are already sick to determine if a specific genetic disease is present and in apparently healthy people to predict the risks of future disease in them or their offspring. In the first part of the chapter I describe the types of genetic tests that will be used in health care, how their ability to yield correct answers (test validity and reliability) is measured, and how genetic heterogeneity and variable expressivity influence validity. Diagnostic uses pose fewer problems of validity and raise fewer ethical and legal questions than predictive uses, but despite their importance to clinical medicine, they are not dealt with at length here.

The information gained from genetic tests must be of some use in order to justify testing. For some diseases, tests will facilitate the prevention or amelioration of clinical disease. For others, neither will be immediately possible, although the discoveries that led to the tests may eventually lead to effective interventions. Until such interventions are developed, some parents will use genetic test results to avoid the conception or birth of an affected infant, while others will use them to prepare for the birth of such an infant.

In the second part of the chapter I examine the uses to which genetic tests are put to benefit the individual being tested. I briefly mention uses that may benefit third parties, but I postpone discussion of some of those uses until chapter 8.

Predicting Genetic Risks in Families and Populations

Genetic tests can be performed in families at risk once disease-related genes have been localized to specific regions of specific chromosomes. Testing on a population basis (genetic screening) without regard to family history—for example, the testing of pregnant women, newborns, specific ethnic groups, or workers in certain industries—becomes possible only after the disease-causing or susceptibility-conferring alleles have been identified.

Family-centered testing

Linkage methods used when the disease-related gene locus is unknown. Probes for the markers to which a genetic disease has been linked can be used to determine who is likely to harbor the disease-causing allele in families in which the disease has already occurred.[1] Southern blots will indicate whether apparently healthy members (or fetuses) contain the same allele or haplotype at the marker locus as is carried on the chromosome with the disease-causing allele. If so, the inference is that these family members carry the disease-causing allele. The particular marker allele or haplotype linked to the disease-causing allele will differ from one family to another. Consequently, prediction is not possible without the participation of several members of the family under study. Sometimes the chromosome containing the disease-causing allele can be determined from studies in obligate carriers.[2] Often, however, DNA from affected offspring is needed, particularly for autosomal recessive disorders.

A number of problems are associated with the ability to conduct and interpret linkage tests. First, obtaining DNA from informative family members may be difficult. The family member requesting genetic tests may not want to involve members of the extended family, or those members may not be willing to cooperate. Persons with the disease may already have died. For this last reason, geneticists are suggesting that families arrange for the indefinite banking of DNA from patients with genetic diseases, even diseases for which the genes have not yet been localized.

Second, misinformation regarding the family pedigree creates problems. DNA from the father of an affected person is often needed. If the presumed father is not the biological father, erroneous results in the linkage studies are possible. (Occasionally, linkage studies will suggest that the putative father is not the real father.)

When these problems do not arise, yet a third problem is possible: the genotypes of important family members may not be informative. Unless certain family members are heterozygous at linked marker loci, it will not be possible for geneticists to distinguish the chromosome on which the disease-causing allele resides from the homologous one. As more RFLPs are mapped, there will be more linked polymorphic markers to choose from; the probability that a key family member will be heterozygous for at least one of them will be high.

Unavoidable errors in interpretation also are possible. The most important is due to the risk of crossing over (recombination) between the marker and disease-related gene loci in one of the germ cell precursors of the person in whom risk is being predicted. The occurrence of crossing over will be undetectable until the prediction can be confirmed clinically and will mean that some at-risk individuals will be classified as not at risk while others who are not at risk will be classified as at risk. The frequency with which such mislabeling occurs depends on the distance between the marker and the locus at which the disease-causing allele resides. The availability of markers on both sides of the locus will reduce the frequency of errors.

When the markers used for linkage studies are common polymorphisms and when only one previous case of an X-linked disorder has occurred in a family, failure to recognize that the case may have arisen by new mutation may lead to erroneous prediction.[3] An error would be particularly likely if, by chance, the affected child with the new mutation inherited an RFLP allele that was different from that inherited by his unaffected siblings. A fetus or infant carrying the same RFLP as the affected child would not be affected.

The possibility exists that the disease in a family under study is the result of a disease-causing allele at another locus (genetic heterogeneity). Careful history taking and physical examination may distinguish one form of the disorder from others, but subtypes suggesting heterogeneity are not always found, and when they are, they may not be due to genetic heterogeneity. In small families particularly, linkage studies could indicate that the subject whose risk is being assessed has the same markers as the affected person, but because the disease is due to a mutation at another locus, the subject may not, in fact, be affected. This is less likely to occur when more than one marker is used and when several affected members are available. Genetic heterogeneity is suggested when two affected siblings do not share the same haplotype for linked loci or when an affected and an unaffected sibling do share the same haplotype.

Despite these shortcomings, linkage studies are already being offered to families with single-gene disorders in which the gene has been localized but not identified. These disorders include Huntington disease, cystic fibrosis, adult polycystic kidney disease, X-linked retinitis pigmentosa, fragile X mental retardation, and neurofibromatosis.[4]

The use of linkage methods for disorders in which at least two gene loci are implicated compounds some of the problems encountered in identifying single-gene disorders. The possibility of crossing over arises independently for each of the loci. To build any statistical confidence that the markers were truly linked to susceptibility-conferring alleles, one would have to study more than one affected member in a family, and many unaffected members as well. Linkage studies for alleles at multiple loci will predict risk with much less certainty than those involving only one locus.

Direct tests. The availability of direct tests for disease-causing alleles will eliminate the problem of recombination when tests are carried out in families in which the disease of interest has already occurred. Due to the possibilities of allelic diversity and genetic heterogeneity, one must always make sure, however, that the detectable disease-causing allele(s) is present in the person manifesting clinical symptoms. If its presence is demonstrated, the detection of the same allele in an asymptomatic family member or fetus (in disease-causing dosage) is much more likely to predict correctly the subsequent appearance of clinical disease, while its absence is almost certain to rule it out, than detection of the allele when the same test is used in populations (see below). It would be extraordinary if different mutations caused the same disease in one family.[5]

Linkage methods used when the disease-related gene locus is known. Sometimes the disease-related gene, but none or not all of the disease-causing alleles, will have been identified. In these cases, polymorphisms in or very close to the gene can be used to predict disease.[6] Until recently, none of the mutations that cause PKU were known, but the gene had been identified. Within most families with a child with PKU, RFLPs very tightly linked to the mutation sites could be used to determine which maternal and paternal chromosomes carried the disease-causing allele. If a fetus carried both of these chromosomes, the probability was over 99 percent that it was affected; if it had only one, it would be a carrier; and if it had neither, it would be a normal homozygote for the PKU "gene." When none of the known disease-causing alleles can be found in a person with disease, a search for cosegregation of the polymorphic markers known to be tightly linked to the disease-related gene may permit prediction in other family members.

Until probes for the DMD "gene" were made, diagnosis depended on studies of linkage to RFLPs within the locus and to some close to it. Crossovers were still observed, however.[7] This is not surprising, since the DMD gene spans two million nucleotides on the X-chromosome.

When an RFLP is very close to the disease-related gene, linkage disequilibrium may be observed between one form of the RFLP and the disease-causing allele. This has been demonstrated to be the case for sickle cell anemia (for which the gene is known),[8] and has been reported for cystic fibrosis (for which the gene has not yet been identified).[9] It suggests that all disease-causing alleles arise from a single mutation. Although detection of the form of the polymorphism that is in linkage disequilibrium with the disease-causing allele would not provide reliable prediction of disease or carrier status, since many more people will have the polymorphic form than have the disease, its absence would reduce the chance of carrier status relative to the general population. This might be important information for someone contemplating marrying a carrier with a recessive disease like cystic fibrosis.[10] Once the disease-causing allele has been identified, much better tests for carriers will be developed.

Testing in populations: Genetic screening

DNA-based tests. Over seventy genes that are known to be responsible for hereditary disorders have been cloned.[11] Southern blots can be used to test for disease-causing deletions or rearrangements (which occur, for example, in thalassemia, hemophilia, familial hypercholesterolemia, Duchenne muscular dystrophy, congenital adrenal hyperplasia, growth hormone deficiency, and osteogenesis imperfecta) or point mutations at RE sites (in, for example, thalassemia, sickle cell anemia, and hemophilia). For other known point mutations (including alpha-1-antitrypsin deficiency, thalassemia, PKU, and osteogenesis imperfecta), oligonucleotide probes can be used. (That one disease is mentioned in more than one of these three categories indicates both allelic diversity and genetic heterogeneity.)

Use of the polymerase chain reaction speeds up and simplifies tests for disease-causing alleles involving both Southern blotting and oligonucleotide probe analysis.[12] Additional advances will soon make it feasible to use these tests in populations. Wherever allelic diversity and genetic heterogeneity are detected, tests will be needed to discover the various forms unless false negatives can be tolerated.

Direct tests for multifactorial disorders also are possible. When two or more genes contribute to disease expression, but only one locus is examined, the future occurrence of disease will depend on whether susceptibility-conferring alleles are present at other loci. Nevertheless, the risk of developing disease will be greater for that individual than for individuals who lack a susceptibility-conferring allele at the first locus. The person can be told his/her relative risk, just as persons are advised of the likelihood of disease following an environmental exposure.[13]

Gene-product and other tests. If a disease-related gene is transcribed normally, then tests can be constructed to search for the gene product. These tests have one major advantage over DNA-based tests: with significant allelic diversity or frequent new mutation, one test for an altered gene product may indicate the presence of all of them. For then the different mutations capable of causing the disease must each alter the structure and the function of the gene product. Many alterations in structure can be detected by a single electrophoretic or immunologic test. Alterations in function can be detected by a single enzyme assay or test for an excess of the substance whose metabolism depends on the defective enzyme or for a deficiency of the product of that enzymatic reaction. Evidence of defective gene product, however, may not be present in accessible tissues (e.g., blood, urine, or fetal cells from amniotic fluid or the chorionic villi) at a stage in the life cycle when prediction would be useful. Moreover, compared to DNA-based tests, the chance is greater with tests for gene product that an alteration *other than* the specific genetic defect that is being sought will give an abnormal result, or that the defect will not be detected.[14]

Direct tests for mutations or gene-product tests can be used for genetic screening. A committee of the National Academy of Sciences has defined genetic screening as a search in a population of apparently healthy individuals for those with genotypes that place them or their offspring at high risk for disease.[15] For most disorders, genetic screening will result in a greater reduction in the incidence of specific diseases in the population than can be achieved by family-centered testing, which requires that a disease already have struck. With genetic screening, carriers who have never had a child can be identified, as can newborns or adults who have not had an affected relative. At a time when many couples are limiting the number of their offspring, first occurrences will constitute a significant proportion of all cases of that disease in the population.

The Validity and Reliability of Tests

Before undertaking screening, the health care provider should be aware of the validity and reliability of the test. The validity of a test, or its ability to distinguish those with abnormalities from those without them, can be quantified. Reliability is harder to quantify, and generally depends on the laboratory performing the test.

The parameters of sensitivity, specificity, and predictive value (figure 5.1) are used to validate a clinical test by answering the following questions:

What proportion of people with the disease will the test detect? (Sensitivity)

What proportion of people without the disease will have normal (negative) results? (Specificity)

What proportion of people with positive results will develop the disease? (Predictive value of a positive result)

Sensitivity and specificity are independent of each other and of disease prevalence. The predictive value of a positive result increases with increasing disease prevalence. A highly specific test will yield more false positives when prevalence is low than when prevalence is high. This explains why a test used for screening inherently has lower predictive value than the same test when used for diagnosis. The greater chance of false

FIGURE 5.1

Parameters of the validity of genetic tests.

		Disease: Present	Disease: Absent
Test Result	Positive	A	B
	Negative	C	D

A = True positives: those with positive test results who *will* manifest the disease.
B = False positives: those with positive test results who *may* or *may not* have the genetic defect but who *will never* manifest the disease.
C = False negatives: those with negative test results who *will* manifest the disease.
D = True negatives: those with negative test results who will never manifest the disease.

Sensitivity = the probability that the test will be positive in someone who will manifest the condition (**A/A** + **C**).
Specificity = the probability that the test will be negative in someone who will not manifest the condition (**D/B** + **D**).

Predictive value positive = the probability that a person with a positive result will manifest the disease (**A/A** + **B**).
Predictive value negative = the probability that a person with a negative result will not manifest the disease (**D/C** + **D**).

positives with screening is due to the lower prevalence of the disorder in the general population than in people with symptoms and signs suggestive of a specific disorder.

The usual method of determining validity

The sensitivity of a new test is frequently determined in people who already manifest the disease of interest. For genetic tests, families in which the disease follows Mendelian inheritance (and therefore has high expressivity) are often used. Measured in this way, sensitivity and specificity may not be the same as when the test is used for predictive purposes in apparently healthy people.

Gene-product tests. An abnormality that shows up in people in whom the disease is manifest may not yet be present in asymptomatic people with a disease-causing genotype. This is true for PKU. When screened on the first few days of life, infants with PKU do not always show elevated levels of phenylalanine. Consequently the sensitivity of the test is lower at this point than when it is performed at a later age.[16] The problem is less likely to occur when the structural gene product (enzyme or protein) is measured directly, but the concentrations of these can change with age, too. Although tests can detect the small amounts of hemoglobin S present in newborns with sickle cell disease, the proportion among newborns is much less than that in older infants. For tests that measure continuous variables, such as enzyme activity or metabolite concentration, sensitivity can be increased by changing the concentration defined as "abnormal." This almost always diminishes the specificity of the test.[17]

Tests at the genetic (DNA) level. When disease-causing alleles are determined by linkage or directly, the clinical stage of the disease has no relevance to the sensitivity, but then other factors—genetic heterogeneity and variable expressivity—gain considerably more importance. The tests may prove positive in all or a large proportion of the reference families with Mendelian inheritance, but when applied for predictive purposes to more families (linkage studies) or to populations (direct tests), the same test may prove negative in people destined to develop the same clinical (phenotypic) disease. The reasons will be genetic heterogeneity (for both linkage and direct tests) and allelic diversity (for direct tests that do not detect all mutations).

By selecting reference families with high expressivity, investigators can be confident that virtually all of those with the disease will have positive test results. (That is one reason for selecting families with high expressivity.) But when tests are applied in families in which inheritance patterns suggest multifactorial origin, or in the general population, there is much less assurance that every time the disease-causing genotype is encountered it will ultimately result in clinical disease; expressivity may be variable.

The problem lies in knowing how often genetic heterogeneity (and allelic diversity) will lower sensitivity, and how often variable expressivity will lower specificity and the predictive value of a positive test result, before launching widespread testing. For most diseases for which new DNA-based tests are developed, so little will be known initially about the pathogenesis of the disorder that it will be impossible for investigators to confirm the prediction that clinical disease *will* develop with another independent test. Only the subsequent appearance of disease—which in the case of adult-onset disorders may be many years after screening—will provide confirmation.

The appropriate determination of validity

When widespread use of DNA-based tests is contemplated, the validity of the tests should be determined in a large number of unrelated people with clinical manifestations of the disease and in others who are past the age at which the disease usually appears and who have no signs of the disease. For rare diseases this requires surveying very large numbers of people to be confident of the results. Moreover, some adjustment will be needed for people with the disease who would have been in the groups surveyed but who have already died.[18]

Another method of validation entails following all of the people tested to see how many with negative results remain free of disease and how many with positive results develop the disease. If the disease is rare and of late onset and the test is used for screening entire populations, this will be a long and costly undertaking. Most of the people who are followed will never develop the disease. Although somewhat more feasible for common, late-onset disorders, this prospective approach will still take many years.

Some information on test parameters may be gained by comparing the rate of positive test results in asymptomatic people to the rate of occurrence (incidence) of the disease in a population with the same age distribution. If the positive rate of the genetic test is much higher than the observed incidence, the expressivity of the disease-causing genotype is low; not everyone with it goes on to manifest the disease. If the positive rate of the genetic test is much lower than the observed incidence, then heterogeneity is at work; some people develop the disease as a result of factors that are not detected by the genetic test.

Unfortunately, accurate estimates of the incidence of diseases, particularly rare ones, are seldom available. (One of the few is the Health Surveillance Registry of British Columbia—see chapter 3.) They require extensive epidemiologic surveys. In addition, the absence of definitive diagnostic or predictive tests (before the discovery of direct tests for disease-causing genotypes) will lead to disagreements about classifying individuals as having the disease.

Another way of validating tests may become possible if blood samples from which DNA can be obtained are collected on sample populations representing all ages. The DNA from each sample would then be isolated and stored indefinitely. As a new test was developed, the DNA from each specimen could be analyzed. This would immediately indicate the frequency of the disease-causing genotype, which could be compared to the incidence of the disorder, if it was known. If the frequency of the disease-causing genotype is not known, the individuals with positive results, and a representative sample of those with negative results, could be contacted and examined by predetermined criteria to see if they had manifestations of the disease. For those who died, the cause of death could be determined.

Intervention before validation

Intervention before a test is validated may interfere with validation. At the same time, if the effectiveness of the intervention is not established, failure to validate may interfere with assessing its effectiveness. Consider a dietary modification that is hypothesized to prevent the manifestations of coronary artery disease in those with a disease-causing genotype for which a direct test has been developed. The diet is given to everyone with a positive test result. Let us assume that after a long follow-up fewer people with "positive" test results had heart attacks than would have been expected. Although this could be due to the effectiveness of the diet, it could also be due to low expressivity of the genotype. These two effects could be disentangled if a randomized trial was undertaken in which only some of those with positive test results were given the diet.

A randomized trial of this type is currently under way to validate newborn screening for cystic fibrosis (CF) and at the same time to determine whether the early intervention made possible by screening improves the outcome.[19] All newborns are screened, but the test results are calculated and reported for only a randomly determined group. If the diagnosis in this group is confirmed, these newborns receive comprehensive management for CF. Infants with CF in the other group (and false negatives in the first group) are diagnosed clinically. When infants in the second group reach the age of 4 years, their test results will be determined, those with positive results will be tracked, and the nutritional and respiratory status of patients with CF in the two groups will be compared. By 4 years of age, all patients with cystic fibrosis should be symptomatic.

A difficult problem of validation arises in the use of new tests for prenatal diagnosis when the expressivity of the disorder is unknown. Some fetuses not destined to develop clinical disease may be aborted. Expressivity can, however, be determined in an older population first. If it is incomplete, parents would have to decide whether they wanted to take the chance of aborting a fetus that was not definitely going to develop disease.

Reliability

The reliability of a test is gauged by its ability to measure accurately that for which it was designed, and to give consistent results when repeated on the same specimen by one or more technicians. Tests that prove reliable in late developmental or pilot stages often prove less so when they are used routinely. Many laboratories offering medical tests are multipurpose and their personnel will not have as much in-depth familiarity with or time to devote to one particular test as those who developed the test. In addition, the volume of specimens received and the need for rapid turnaround increase the chance of error. Specimens may be mixed up. Rather than repeat the tests, laboratories may report equivocal results as either positive or negative. The tests themselves are subject to error. Incomplete digestion of DNA may fail to yield the expected restriction fragments on Southern blots, as will faulty hybridization. An astute technician can detect such problems, but in busy, multipurpose laboratories such errors do slip through. It is unclear how common these laboratory errors will be as genetic testing employing recombinant DNA technology proliferates. Correctly interpreting the Southern blot also poses problems to the inexperienced.

The quality of clinical laboratory performance is measured in several ways. The ways most often used are personnel requirements, performance standards, on-site inspections, and proficiency testing. Proficiency testing usually involves the periodic distribution of specimens to laboratories, which then conduct the test, sometimes with the knowledge that they are being evaluated (open testing) and sometimes without such knowledge (blind testing). In general, laboratories perform better in open than in blind programs.

Preventing or Ameliorating the Manifestations of Genetic Diseases

There is little point in performing genetic tests for predictive purposes unless some benefit will accrue. This by itself, however, is not a sufficient justification for testing, for if the same benefit could be gained from treatment following clinical diagnosis—waiting for symptoms to appear, using the tests as a diagnostic (rather than a predictive) tool, and on confirmation of diagnosis, instituting therapy—there would be little point in screening. The costs of predictive testing and of treating some people (false positives) unnecessarily—both of which could be eliminated by relying on clinical diagnosis—could exceed the benefits.

The response to postsymptomatic treatment of many single-gene disorders is rather dismal, reflecting the fact that irreversible damage has often occurred by the time symptoms appear. Using seven different outcome measures—life span, reproductive capacity, somatic growth, intellectual development, and social adaptation (learning ability, capacity to work, and cosmetic effect)—Hayes et al. reviewed the evidence for the effectiveness of treatment for 351 disorders selected at random from McKusick's catalog of human single-gene phenotypes.[20] Treatment resulted in improvements in life span in 15 percent, in elevated reproductive capacity in 11 percent, and in better social adaptation in 6 percent of the disorders studied. Of the 351 disorders reviewed, 65 were inborn errors of metabolism, for which the basic defect was known in most cases. Within this group, intervention gave complete relief in 12 percent of the cases, a partial response in 40 percent, and no improvement in the remaining 48 percent. Several of the inborn errors for which postsymptomatic treatment had the best effect were those involving susceptibility-conferring alleles in which the first encounter with the harmful agent did not cause irreversible damage.

Whether presymptomatic therapy, which might be possible following the identification of asymptomatic, affected individuals by genetic testing, will be more effective remains to be determined. It is important, therefore, to examine the benefits of prevention and the use of avoidance.

Primary prevention

Preventing disease itself constitutes primary prevention. Diseases in which environmental as well as genetic factors play a role could be prevented by removing the environmental factor. This could be done by removing the agent from everyone's environment, in which case there is no point in identifying those who are genetically susceptible. Identifying those with susceptibility-conferring genotypes and selectively lowering their exposures is another approach.

Substituting a normal allele for the disease-causing allele in germ cells is one form of primary prevention. It would have to be preceded by identifying parents who carry the disease-causing allele, either by their having previously affected children or by genetic screening that identifies them as carriers. If the substitution succeeded, the normal allele would replicate with the rest of the genome, being passed to all daughter cells, including the germ cells for the next generation. The procedure would be done in vitro—that is, the ovum or sperm would be manipulated outside the body. Excising a gene from a single germ cell and inserting a new gene in its place have not been accomplished. However, the addition of a normal allele, without removing the disease-causing one, is possible. Unless inserted in its customary position on the genome, the donated allele almost certainly would not be induced to transcribe, or would be repressed from transcribing, in a manner necessary for normal development of the embryo. (An exception would be genes for enzymes that are synthesized at a steady rate throughout development.) Inserted into an "incorrect" position, the donated allele could disrupt other genes, thereby preventing their expression. Or it could activate genes prematurely or unnecessarily. Cancers may well originate from such inappropriate activation. If the donated allele is transcribed, the number of copies made could differ from the number required for optimal translation and, consequently, expression. Finally, successful manipulations might interfere with the fertilization of the cell or, if they were carried out in a zygote (already fertilized), with successful implantation into the uterus.

Aside from these technical problems, there are ethical constraints. In virtually no situations today are *all* the zygotes resulting from any mating inevitably affected. The only situation in which that can be envisioned is the very unlikely mating between two homozygotes for the same autosomal recessive disease.[21] In all other matings of high-risk couples, at least 50 percent of either partner's germ cells will carry the normal allele. This means that the manipulations described in the preceding paragraph will often be carried out on normal cells, unless affected germ cells were first distinguished from unaffected ones. But if such a distinction could be made, it would be far easier to arrange the fertilization of the unaffected germ cells than to correct the affected ones! Although this may not be possible in the foreseeable future, it may be possible following in vitro fertilization to determine at a very early stage in development (eight or sixteen cells) whether the zygote is affected.[22] Then, only unaffected zygotes could be implanted. I classify this as "avoidance" (see below) rather than primary prevention.

Secondary prevention

Preventing the manifestations of disease (secondary prevention) in those who possess a disease-causing genotype is possible. For defective enzymes or proteins involved in the transport of small molecules, reducing exposure to an exogenous substrate when its accumulation causes the disease, or providing the product of the impaired reaction when a deficiency of product is harmful, may be effective. For some disorders the function of an impaired enzyme can be boosted by the administration of cofactors such as vitamins,[23] or excessive enzyme activity can be inhibited. In some diseases, the defective protein can be replaced or the defective gene can be supplemented by a normal one. Secondary prevention has also been attempted for a few genetic disorders for which no specific means of overcoming the genetic defect have yet been discovered but for which some general measures may ameliorate the disease.

The success of these interventions depends on a number of factors. First, there can be no irreversible damage at the time of the intervention. In some genetic diseases, irreversible changes will begin in utero, and intrauterine therapy will be needed. In others, in which the mother compensates for the defect in the fetus through the placenta, changes will not begin until the neonatal period. Therapy started in the neonatal period can be effective. Second, the therapeutic agent must reach the tissue or organ where it can prevent damage. For instance, the administration of a substance that is needed to overcome a deficiency in the central nervous system but that does not cross the blood-brain barrier will not be effective. Third, the intervention must be safe and acceptable. The complications from some regimens may be such that letting the disease appear—particularly if it does not occur until a few years after detection—is preferable to intervention in an apparently healthy infant or child. Special diets may be so restrictive, or the side effects of drugs so uncomfortable, that therapy cannot be maintained in effective doses. Because of the risk they entail, despite the possibility that they might succeed in improving the outcome in symptomatic individuals, organ transplants are unlikely to be attempted in apparently healthy individuals with disease-causing genotypes detected by genetic testing.

The ability of gene therapy (the insertion of genes into somatic cells) to improve outcome may depend on its use in asymptomatic individuals. Much progress has been made in this modality,[24] but its application is likely to be restricted to a few conditions. Many of the problems raised in the discussion of inserting normal genes into germ cells—appropriate regulation and expression without disrupting the function of other genes —must be solved here, too. Other problems arise as well. The cells with the normal allele must provide sufficient amounts of normal gene product, and that product must be able to reach those parts of the body where its action is necessary to prevent disease. It is not likely to work in dominant disorders in which one normal gene is already present. The protein produced by the foreign, but normal, allele may also induce an immune reaction. The diseases for which gene therapy will first be attempted are all extremely rare and severe. I doubt that this type of intervention will ever become practical for common diseases.

Let us now examine a few examples in which secondary prevention or amelioration might follow predictive genetic testing.

Newborn screening. The success of newborn screening in preventing or greatly reducing mental retardation due to phenylketonuria (PKU)[25] indicates that early treatment can be effective in single-gene disorders. Treatment after symptoms appear accomplishes little.[26] Newborns throughout the United States are screened for PKU (and for congenital hypothyroidism), and in some states they are screened for sickle cell anemia and cystic fibrosis, as well as for a few rare single-gene disorders (galactosemia, maple syrup urine disease, homocystinuria, biotinidase deficiency, and congenital adrenal hyperplasia).[27] A recent National Institutes of Health consensus development conference concluded that newborn sickle cell screening can lead to a reduction of lethal infections in infants and children with sickle cell anemia by facilitating the early administration of prophylactic penicillin.[28] Evidence is accumulating that identification of newborns with cystic fibrosis by screening may improve their nutritional status.[29] Whether it will also reduce the frequency and severity of respiratory infections, which usually cause early death in this disease, remains to be determined.

The newborn screening tests for these few diseases detect changes in the quantity or quality of small molecules or proteins in a dried blood spot obtained from asymptomatic infants with the disorders. There are other severe disorders for which early intervention improves the outcome, but for which presymptomatic detection is not possible using the neoclassical methods described in chapter 3. One group of such disorders are those in which the removal of ammonia, a toxic end product of protein metabolism, is impaired.[30] Tests based on recombinant DNA technology could detect the disease-causing alleles that are present in the DNA of all nucleated cells, including white blood cells. The technological hurdles to permit its wide-scale use in newborn screening are being overcome rapidly. With the polymerase chain reaction described earlier, sufficient DNA can be obtained from the white cells in the dried blood spot to perform tests at the DNA level.[31] Thus it will be possible to expand the number of disorders on which newborn screening can be performed. DNA-based tests will also be able to detect disease-causing alleles that current tests sometimes miss. Tests that depend on the accumulation or deficiency of some molecule in the infant soon after birth may be falsely negative if performed too early. This is a problem when newborn infants are tested very early.[32] Even when screened a week after birth, some infants with homocystinuria are missed.[33]

Insulin-dependent diabetes mellitus. Insulin-dependent diabetes mellitus (IDDM) is frequently diagnosed only after a child develops life-threatening manifestations. If it were possible to detect individuals at risk for IDDM before symptoms appeared, the chance of early death could be reduced and, possibly, the long-term prognosis improved. As discussed in chapters 3 and 4, susceptibility-conferring alleles at loci of the major histocompatibility complex (MHC) increase the risk of IDDM. Neoclassical tests to detect the polymorphic proteins that increased risk lacked the specificity needed to make them useful for prediction; there were too many false positives. By detecting the susceptibility-conferring alleles directly, DNA-based tests provide much greater specificity and predictive value; the chances that someone with one of the susceptibility-conferring alleles will develop disease are much higher, perhaps in the order of 10–20 percent.[34] The technique can be used to screen infants or young children for the susceptibility-conferring allele. Those in whom it is present can then be monitored closely by urine glucose measurements or for the appearance of insulin or pancreatic cell antibodies. It may also be possible to suppress the production of insulin antibodies, although the risk of toxicity of the most effective drug, cyclosporine, makes it too dangerous to use in children who may never develop IDDM.[35] If certain viruses are found to trigger the autoimmune response leading to diabetes,[36] then children at risk could be vaccinated to protect them from infection.

Coronary artery disease. Cholesterol screening of children and adults is fairly widespread, but as pointed out in chapter 2, relatively few men with elevated cholesterol concentrations (and other risk factors as well) develop coronary artery disease prematurely. It is quite possible that tests for different susceptibility-conferring alleles (see chapter 4) will be of greater specificity and predictive value. Efforts to lower the dietary intake of fats could be focused, perhaps with greater effectiveness, on those in whom such tests are positive. Low-fat diets may be harmful for persons with low cholesterol levels[37] and for children.[38]

The effects of diet alone in lowering plasma cholesterol and the risk of heart disease are not very impressive.[39] The addition of a resin that blocks cholesterol absorption from the intestine does result in some reduction of mortality from coronary artery disease. There are, however, slight increases in mortality from other causes by the same ages, so total mortality in diet-treated groups compared to controls has not differed.[40] Discovery of the low-density lipoprotein receptor defect in familial hypercholesterolemia led to the development of drugs that inhibit cholesterol biosynthesis. These drugs are much more effective in reducing lipid abnormalities than diet alone.[41] They have not been in use long enough to indicate an effect on mortality, nor has the safety of their long-term use been established. Until these data are available, and until it can be shown that most individuals identified by screening to be at risk for coronary artery disease actually suffer the disease, the routine use of drugs following the identification of at-risk persons by screening will be hard to justify.

A stronger case can be made for diet and drug intervention in asymptomatic siblings and offspring of patients with coronary disease in whom genetic factors have been identified by testing.

Cancer. In some families, malignant melanoma, cancer of the colon, retinoblastoma, and Wilms tumor are inherited as dominant disorders. A strong genetic component accounts for breast cancer. Unfortunately, by the time people with these disorders are found to have cancer, the malignancy is advanced and therapy is drastic and not always effective. By identifying people at risk for these disorders early on, genetic tests might lead to a better outcome. People at risk could be monitored for signs of cancer. Infants with an inherited retinoblastoma allele could have frequent ophthalmological examinations. Early detection of tumor might spare them the loss of an eye. Young women at increased risk for breast cancer could receive mammograms more frequently than is currently recommended for the general population. People with familial adenomatous polyposis, who are at higher risk for colon cancer, could undergo periodic colonoscopic examination to detect early malignant changes. If certain drugs prove to have the ability to reduce the risk of cancer, as was recently reported for isotretinoin in people with the recessive disorder xeroderma pigmentosum,[42] people at risk might benefit from taking them. Whether these or other early interventions will improve the outcome in those with genetic predispositions remains to be established.

In chapter 3, I described polymorphic variants that increase the risk of lung cancer. Testing for these polymorphisms could be used to indicate to

Table 5.1 Projected Sequence of Discoveries in Detection and Management of Genetic Disorders

Stage	Research discovery	Practical application
I.	Disease-related gene localized to region of a chromosome	Diagnosis and prediction in families; avoidance of conception or birth of affected offspring
II.	Disease-related gene identified; tightly-linked polymorphisms or disease-causing alleles determined	Diagnosis and prediction in families *and* populations; avoidance of conception or birth of affected offspring
III.	Function of gene discovered	Diagnosis at the gene product level ? Conventional therapy
IV.	Recombinant DNA technology used to manufacture gene product	? Therapy with gene product
V.	Experimental gene therapy	? Gene therapy

people what their risks of developing lung cancer would be if they smoked. Those who proved to be at increased risk might be persuaded to give up smoking, while those who were found not to have the genetic predisposition might continue the habit, believing they were immune to harmful effects. Yet cigarette smoking has multiple harmful effects; those who are not genetically predisposed to one may be at risk for others.

Drug reactions. Genetic differences in the way people metabolize certain drugs may explain the adverse effects of drugs on some recipients,[43] or in the case of pregnant women, on some fetuses.[44] By testing individuals for susceptibilities before prescribing drugs with known genetic interactions, physicians could prevent some harmful reactions in their patients.

When Prevention or Treatment Is Not Yet Possible

For many disorders, neither drugs nor diets nor lifestyle changes have yet been found that markedly improve the outcome of those born with the condition. In this category are early-onset disorders such as cystic fibrosis or Duchenne muscular dystrophy, and late-onset ones such as Huntington and Alzheimer disease. The trajectory of discovery for these and other diseases is already clear (table 5.1). With recombinant DNA techniques, the disease-related gene will first be localized and then be identified. In the next stage, more will be learned about pathogenesis; the knowledge may suggest effective conventional therapies. Once disease-related genes have been isolated and cloned, recombinant DNA technology can be used to produce human enzymes, polypeptides, or proteins that can be administered to replace the defective ones. It may even be possible to enhance the activity of a protein (or some other property) by modifying the nucleotide sequences in the recombinant gene for the protein.[45] If none of these interventions is successful in preventing, ameliorating, or treating the disorder, gene therapy might sometimes prove successful.

As hopeful as this scenario sounds, each act may take years, and there may be no grand finale. Some diseases may prove intractable despite considerable gains in knowledge. Even in the early stages, however, predictive genetic testing will be possible. Some people will want to undergo testing to prepare for untreatable illness either in themselves or in their offspring. Others will use the tests as their rationale for avoiding the conception or birth of affected offspring. Predicting diseases for which management remains costly because effective interventions have not yet been developed will also be important to third parties such as insurers and employers. Health and life insurance companies may insist on genetic tests for costly, untreatable diseases and deny insurance or charge higher premiums to those in whom disease-causing or susceptibility-conferring alleles are found. They may do the same for couples at risk of having affected offspring. Employers who pay for their employees' health insurance may deny employment to those who are likely to raise the group premium the employer must pay. I mention the interests of third parties here as a consequence of the time lag between the availability of predictive tests and effective interventions. I will discuss them at length in chapter 8.

Avoiding the conception of affected offspring

Individuals who have been identified as carriers for autosomal recessive conditions can select sex partners who are not carriers or, if they are already married to carriers, refrain from having children. Women who are carriers for X-linked disorders or individuals who have dominant conditions also can refrain from procreating. Such individuals can choose to adopt children.

Sperm or ovum donation gives couples at risk for having children with genetic disorders the opportunity to have unaffected children whose genetic endowment comes from one of them (in contrast to adoption, when neither of them contributes). When both members of a couple are carriers for autosomal recessive disorders, or when the man has a dominant disorder, the couple can use artificial insemination with sperm from a donor. Couples can use ovum donation when they both are carriers for a recessive disorder, when the woman has a dominant disorder, or when the woman is a carrier for an X-linked disorder. Ovum donation can be accomplished in several ways. A noncarrier woman can be inseminated with sperm from a carrier's partner and then carry the pregnancy to term ("surrogate mother"). Or, following artificial insemination of a woman willing to donate a fertilized ovum, the embryo can be transferred to the carrier's uterus. A donor's ovum can also be fertilized in vitro by sperm from a carrier's partner and then implanted in the carrier's uterus.

Fewer than 1 percent of all artificial inseminations performed are for genetic indications,[46] but as more genetic conditions become predictable, the number will undoubtedly increase. There does not seem to be a scarcity of men willing to provide sperm, or of women willing to serve as embryo donors or surrogate mothers. A few in vitro fertilization programs have donor egg programs.[47]

When donated ova or sperm are used to avoid the conception of a fetus with a single-gene disorder, and when tests are available, the donor should be tested as well, to make sure that he or she is not a carrier of the condition whose avoidance is being sought. With the potential expansion of genetic tests, this should be increasingly possible. Potential donors and recipients should also be tested to determine if they are heterozygotes for recessive disorders that occur frequently in their ethnic or racial group. It may soon be possible to perform genetic tests on early embryos (following successful in vitro fertilization or prior to embryo transfer) before implanting them in a woman's uterus. Surveys of practitioners offering artificial insemination and of sperm banks in the late 1970s and early 1980s indicated that scant genetic screening of sperm donors was done and that decisions regarding the acceptance or rejection of donors for genetic reasons indicated faulty knowledge on the part of the practitioners or inconsistent policies.[48] Parents who wish to adopt and adopting agencies may use genetic tests on potential adoptees (see chapter 8).

Prenatal diagnosis and abortion

Prenatal diagnosis followed by the abortion of an affected fetus permits *both* members of an at-risk couple to contribute to the genetic endowment of their offspring but still not bring an affected infant into the world. Couples who elect to abort affected fetuses following prenatal diagnosis can conceive again, confident that eventually they will have an infant without the disorder. Some women at risk of having infants with serious disorders would not undertake pregnancy if prenatal diagnosis were not available or would terminate every time they became pregnant.[49]

In dominant disorders 50 percent of fetuses are affected on average. The risks are 25 percent for autosomal recessive and X-linked disorders. Prenatal diagnosis is also possible for chromosomal abnormalities and some conditions of complex etiology, such as spina bifida. Multifactorial disorders in which a small number of loci are implicated will be diagnosable prenatally once tests are developed to detect the responsible alleles at each of the loci. The risks for multifactorial disorders are lower than those for single-gene disorders. For instance, if single doses of specific alleles at three unlinked loci are needed for a disease to appear and testing demonstrates that between them the parents have one dose of each of the alleles, the chance that all three will be passed to any one child is 12.5 percent. The risks for Down syndrome (at any maternal age) are considerably lower than 12.5 percent.[50]

The most widely used method of prenatal diagnosis in the United States is amniocentesis. A needle is inserted through the mother's abdominal wall into the amniotic fluid that bathes the fetus and a small amount of fluid is extracted. For most tests, the number of cells in the amniotic fluid is insufficient for direct analysis, but enough cells can be obtained by growing them in tissue culture for approximately three weeks. The procedure is usually performed between the fifteenth and eighteenth week of pregnancy, although amniocentesis at twelve to fourteen weeks is currently being investigated. The later in pregnancy an abortion is induced, the greater the risk to the mother. The chance of miscarriage from amniocentesis performed after the fifteenth week is less than 1 percent.

Chorionic villi sampling (CVS) is a relatively new method of obtaining fetal cells. It is most safely performed between the ninth and eleventh weeks of pregnancy. In the most widely used procedure, a catheter is inserted through the vagina and cervix and guided by ultrasound until the tip rests against the chorionic villi on the edge of the placenta. With gentle suction, a few villi are extracted. An alternative, transabdominal CVS is currently being evaluated. Either procedure yields a sufficient number of chorionic villi cells to permit genetic tests and chromosomal analysis; it is not usually necessary to set up tissue cultures. Thus, a diagnosis can be established within a few days, in contrast to the three-week delay following amniocentesis. The earlier stage of pregnancy at which CVS can be performed makes it preferable to amniocentesis for many women. Moreover, when abortion is indicated, the procedure is safer because it can be performed earlier in the pregnancy. The safety of CVS itself—particularly the rate of miscarriage associated with it—is being evaluated in several countries, including the United States. It appears to carry slightly more risk to the fetus than amniocentesis.

A noninvasive method of obtaining fetal cells would present no risk to the fetus, in contrast to both amniocentesis and CVS. It is known that fetal trophoblast cells are released into the maternal circulation in the early stages of pregnancy. The problems of using them for prenatal diagnosis (which are now being investigated) include separating fetal from maternal cells and being able to assay the fetal cells directly or, if they are of insufficient quantity, being able to culture them.[51]

Today, prenatal diagnosis is used most frequently not for single-gene disorders but for Down syndrome and neural tube defects. It is now accepted obstetric practice to offer prenatal diagnosis to pregnant women 35 years of age or older because of the increased risk of Down syndrome. Examination of the chromosomes of fetal cells (karyotyping) reveals an extra chromosome 21 when the fetus has Down syndrome. Most fetuses with open defects of the neural tube can be detected because their mothers have elevated levels of alpha-fetoprotein (AFP) in their blood between the sixteenth and eighteenth weeks of pregnancy. Because of a high probability of false positives, the blood test must be followed by studies of the amniotic fluid.

Prenatal diagnosis of single-gene disorders is most frequently performed following the identification of couples at risk (by genetic testing) for thalassemia, Tay-Sachs, and sickle cell anemia. As a result of the availability of DNA testing, prenatal diagnosis in families in which cystic fibrosis, Duchenne muscular dystrophy, and hemophilia have occurred is increasing rapidly; these are among the most common single-gene disorders. Prenatal diagnosis is also being used for Huntington disease, a late-onset disorder, but to my knowledge the procedure has not been used in families in which either bipolar affective disorder or Alzheimer disease appears to be inherited as a single-gene trait.

Genetic markers that indicate increased risk of multifactorial diseases —such as MHC-D alleles for insulin-dependent diabetes or particular forms of RFLPs linked to apolipoprotein genes for coronary artery disease —could also be used for prenatal diagnosis. The chance that a fetus would eventually manifest a multifactorial disease would be less than the virtual certainty that could be predicted for fetuses affected with single-gene disorders of high expressivity.

Target Groups and Ages at Which Genetic Testing Is Performed

The strategy or strategies that will be used to reduce the burden of a genetic disease determine the stage of life at which testing is performed. For secondary prevention, presymptomatic tests have to be performed at an age that permits the institution of therapy with maximum effectiveness. The prevention of hemolytic anemia in the Rh-positive offspring of Rh-negative women (who have Rh-positive mates) requires the administration of Rh immunoglobulin during or after the woman's first pregnancy. Consequently, it is important to determine a woman's Rh status early in her first pregnancy. The best outcome for infants with phenylketonuria depends on identifying them in the newborn period and starting treatment promptly. For genetic susceptibilities to harmful reactions from drugs, chemicals, cigarettes, alcohol, and high-fat diets, testing should be conducted before the person is exposed to the potentially harmful agent. This could be before hospitalization or surgery or the administration of certain pharmacologic agents in ambulatory patients; before employment; or before dietary, smoking, or drinking habits are established.

For the avoidance of single-gene disorders, the testing of prospective parents for carrier status prior to pregnancy gives both of them the option of avoiding the conception and birth of an affected child. Whether such testing should be performed before one selects a mate—that is, before marriage (in conventional terms)—depends on personal and cultural factors. For individuals for whom neither "artificial" means of avoiding conception nor abortion is acceptable, mate selection may be heavily dependent on genetic testing. Among some Hassidic Jews, Tay-Sachs carrier status is taken into consideration in arranging marriages.[52] On the other hand, premarital identification of sickle cell status had little effect in reducing the number of matings between heterozygotes in an area of Greece in which the frequency of sickle cell anemia was quite high.[53] Sickle cell carrier status also can be determined in both partners early in pregnancy, thereby permitting prenatal diagnosis in high-risk couples. As mentioned earlier, the avoidance of chromosomal disorders (e.g., Down syndrome) and multifactorial disorders (neural tube defects) depends on testing in pregnancy.

Sometimes it is possible to limit testing to a subgroup within a population. Older pregnant women are at greater risk of carrying a fetus with Down syndrome, so they are given the highest priority in prenatal testing. Some genetic diseases are much more frequent in fairly well defined ethnic populations: thalassemia in people whose origin was around the Mediterranean and in parts of Asia, sickle cell anemia in blacks, Tay-Sachs in Ashkenazi Jews. Although testing for the specific condition will have a higher yield when limited to these groups, unquestionably some individuals at risk will be missed.

Other Uses of Human DNA Probes

I have chosen to focus this book on the use of human DNA probes to predict genetic diseases that can be transmitted from one generation to the next because of alterations in the genetic material in germ cells. Human DNA probes are already being used for other purposes, and additional ones might be anticipated. I briefly mention them here. I will not deal at all with DNA probes of microorganisms that are being used to detect infectious diseases in humans.

The diagnosis and prognosis of cancer

A number of lines of evidence are converging to suggest that the alteration of any one of a number of normal human genes in somatic cells can result in unregulated cell growth and ultimately in cancer.[54] The normal genes are called *protooncogenes,* several of which play a role in cell growth. Point mutations within these genes, or disruption of the normal gene sequence by translocations or deletions, transform them into *oncogenes,* thereby rendering them no longer subject to normal inhibitory mechanisms.

Much of this understanding has resulted from the application of recombinant DNA technology, which is now also being employed for diagnostic and prognostic purposes. Specific DNA changes (detected by Southern blots or other techniques) in tumor cells have been used to classify tumors more precisely than was possible with earlier techniques. This refined diagnosis permits physicians to choose the treatment regimen that has been most effective in tumors with the same alteration. Recombinant DNA techniques can also be used to follow the course of cancer in patients. An amplification of protooncogenes in some tumors has been found to be associated with invasive or metastatic stages of malignancy.

Another class of genes, termed *antioncogenes*, also plays a role in cancer. Although their precise mode of action is unknown, they serve to restrain unregulated cell growth. The germline mutation in retinoblastoma, discussed in chapter 4, represents the loss of one functional antioncogene allele. The tumor develops when, as a result of somatic cell mutation, the antioncogene allele on the homologous chromosome is rendered functionless. This same mechanism has now been demonstrated to occur in a large proportion of colorectal cancers.[55] In familial adenomatous polyposis, the first mutation occurs in a germline cell (and is therefore present in all of the individual's somatic cells), but the second occurs in a specific somatic cell, resulting in malignant transformation. Monitoring for such changes may assist in the early detection of cancer in predisposed individuals. Interestingly, the same region of chromosome 5 that bears these mutations is altered in several patients with nonfamilial colorectal cancer, suggesting that the inactivation of both alleles at a locus on chromosome 5 by two separate somatic mutational events results in cancer. Evidence for antioncogenes has been reported for certain lung and breast cancers as well.[56]

The finding of such changes in individuals with tumors opens up the possibility that analyzing cells from organs that are prone to cancer (and are fairly accessible) may indicate the loss—on a somatic cell basis—of one functional antioncogene. Individuals in whom this occurs will be at higher risk for cancer. Although many technological barriers remain to be overcome, such tests might be useful in people who have been exposed to known or suspected mutagens. It may also turn out that inherited predispositions, such as germline mutations in antioncogenes, occur sufficiently often to justify screening for them.

Identity testing

An individual's unique genetic make-up can be demonstrated by Southern blots, using probes for highly variable regions such as those containing variable numbers of tandem repeats. Testing for an individual's RFLP profile can be put to a number of uses.

Forensic. Sufficient DNA can be obtained from semen in rape victims or from blood, skin, or hair found at the scene of a crime for a forensic pathology laboratory to perform restriction endonuclease digests and Southern blots. These blots can then be compared with the blots of DNA of suspects. A match of these patterns indicates with over 99.99 percent certainty that the two specimens came from the same person. This rate is far higher than that obtained using blood groups or histocompatibility antigens. Much smaller amounts of tissue are needed to obtain the necessary DNA. Moreover, the DNA in dried samples is stable for many years. Courts are beginning to accept these tests as admissible evidence in criminal cases.[57]

Familial relationships. The RFLP profile can also be used to establish familial relationships. This arises most frequently in paternity suits. Comparison of the Southern blots of a child with those of the mother and putative father will establish paternity when all of the child's bands can be accounted for by bands in the mother and the putative father. If the child has inherited an RFLP that is not found in either the mother or the father, the most likely explanation (barring technical error) is nonpaternity. Paternity testing may be useful in linkage analysis when the identity of a child's father is in doubt.

The profile has been used to determine whether a child who is alleged to have been stolen from his or her biological parents is actually related to them. It can also be used to establish relationships with putative grandparents. DNA from the remains of otherwise unidentifiable bodies can be compared with that from people who might be related in an attempt to establish identity.

Transplantation. DNA analysis is used to establish compatibility between potential donors and recipients of organs such as kidney, heart, or liver. Once good matches have been established, it may be important to make sure that the donor does not have the same disease as the recipient. This can be determined by genetic testing. Many patients with adult-onset polycystic kidney disease will need kidney transplants in their forties or fifties. Because their siblings are more likely than unrelated individuals to be tissue compatible, they are logical candidates for donating kidneys. But these siblings also have a 50 percent chance of having the disorder if they are too young to show evidence of the disease. Because their kidneys will eventually manifest damage in themselves or a recipient, they are not suitable donors.

Maladaptive behavior

The discovery of a gene for bipolar affective disorder provides evidence of a genetic role in this complex behavioral disease. Although genetic testing may ultimately help people overcome the adverse effects of disease-causing genotypes, it may, in the meantime, be used against them. Police departments, schools, and employers may search for genotypes not in order to determine their disease-causing properties but because they are deemed socially maladaptive. Could the finding that someone who commits a violent crime possesses the genotype for bipolar affective disorder be used to build a stronger case against the person or, if he or she is convicted, to argue for longer sentencing because, allegedly, the biological basis makes recidivism more likely? Or could such a finding be used to say that the person was not acting volitionally (insanity plea)? Could people who are found to have a genotype for dyslexia be denied educational opportunities or jobs?

A significant association between a specific genotype and a maladaptive behavior may not be causal in nature. An increase in the proportion of men with an extra Y chromosome (XYY) in some mental-penal institutions suggested to some that this karyotype predisposed to criminal behavior.[58] This finding could also be due to an enhanced likelihood of being caught during misbehavior, or to a greater likelihood of being sentenced once apprehended.

Even if there is a causal relationship, variable expressivity is likely. Most males born with the XYY karyotype develop normally, without evidence of aberrant behavior.[59] Approximately 96 percent of XYY males will never come to the attention of penal authorities.[60] Unless the expressivity of a specific genotype (as measured by maladaptive behavior) proves to be high, many innocent people will be punished.

If *predictive* testing for such genotypes becomes widespread before the expressivity is established, the results may be used to discriminate unfairly in education or jobs. For instance, even the mere label of having a reading disability may interfere with the lives of children, by altering the way their parents raise them and their teachers educate them.

Summary and Conclusions

DNA-based genetic testing has already been introduced into health care. Linkage studies are being used in families in which disease has already occurred to predict the likelihood of disease in those at risk who are still asymptomatic and, by prenatal diagnosis, in fetuses at risk. Heterozygotes in these families also can be detected by linkage. Direct tests for disease-causing alleles are being used primarily in families in which a disease has already occurred, but also in prenatal diagnosis following the detection of couples at risk by heterozygote screening programs (sickle cell anemia, thalassemia). With further simplification of the technology, DNA-based tests can be used to test apparently healthy people without regard to their family history of the disease in question. This search in a population is known as genetic screening. Human DNA probes have been used for purposes other than predicting future disease (which is the focus of this book). These include classifying cancers and providing prognostic information, establishing identity in criminal cases or familial relationships in paternity suits and other situations, and looking for a biologic basis of maladaptive behavior. Additional uses not primarily for the benefit of the individual being tested are discussed further in chapter 8.

The validation of genetic tests is essential before their widespread, routine use is undertaken. Genetic heterogeneity can reduce the sensitivity of genetic tests; people with negative test results can still develop the disease. Physicians caring for people with early symptoms for which a genetic test result was negative may be slow to make the diagnosis because they assume the genetic test excluded it. Variable expressivity can reduce the specificity and predictive value of such tests; people with positive test results may never manifest the disease. The proportion of people treated unnecessarily will remain unquantifiable until the specificity and predictive value of the tests are determined. It is doubtful that any single test will be perfectly sensitive and specific. But unless we know how imperfect genetic tests are, it will be impossible to weigh their benefits and risks and decide rationally whether they should be used in health care and under what circumstances. Another important consideration in this regard is the reliability of the tests under conditions of routine use. Poor-quality laboratories performing the tests is another reason for erroneous test results.

Genetic testing of apparently healthy individuals as a part of general health care will not be undertaken unless some benefit accrues to those being tested. In the case of a few disorders, interventions prior to the onset of symptoms can prevent their occurrence or reduce the severity of the ensuing illness. For many genetic disorders, however, no effective intervention has yet been discovered. In these instances, predictive testing can warn people of what is in store and possibly prepare them for it. The tests can also be used to detect individuals or couples at risk of having offspring with disease. This knowledge can be used by them to avoid the conception or birth of affected offspring. By choosing to adopt, or by substituting an ovum or sperm (in an alternative reproductive technique such as in vitro fertilization or artificial insemination) from someone who does not carry the disease-causing allele for the germ cell of the heterozygous mate, couples at risk can still raise children. Prenatal diagnosis and the abortion of affected fetuses are the means by which avoidance of birth is accomplished.

Recombinant DNA technology will lead to the development of tests for many disorders long before it will provide sufficient knowledge on how to prevent or ameliorate the manifestations of disease. For many of these disorders, avoidance will be the major reason for testing. The extent to which genetic tests will be used for avoidance and the issues posed by such use are discussed at length later in this book.

Technology Transfer: From Research to the Commercial Development of Genetic Tests

The application of recombinant DNA methods to routine (as opposed to research) genetic testing depends on the *transfer* of these methods to organizations that will develop practical applications and then *transmit* them widely. (Transferal and transmittance might be viewed as analogous to the processes of transcription and translation.) In the United States, transfer is a two-phase process. In the first, knowledge from basic research, much of which has been government-supported, is acquired by privately financed biotechnology companies that will use the knowledge in the development of practical applications. (There are exceptions to this pattern; some not-for-profit organizations develop practical applications, and biotechnology companies obtain some support from the government to undertake basic research.) This phase has been facilitated by recent changes in one U.S. patent law and by arrangements between private industry and universities.

In the second phase, knowledge gained from basic research is channeled by biotechnology companies into genetic testing instead of or in addition to other applications of recombinant DNA technology. The extent to which this channeling occurs depends on the profitability of genetic tests. This in turn depends on the costs of test development and on the ease of transmittance of the tests to health care providers and ultimately to consumers. I will deal with the problems of transmittance, or "diffusion" as it has been called, in chapter 7. In this chapter, I examine transferal—the availability of recombinant DNA technology to biotechnology companies and the interest of such companies in genetic tests—and whether the process satisfies societal interests.

Basic Research and Technology Transfer

Without basic research, DNA-based tests would never have been developed. Additional basic discoveries will not only improve testing capabilities but also provide an understanding of the pathogenesis of disease, on which advances in prevention and treatment depend. Much of basic science involves "filling in the details" after new paradigms are postulated.[1] Techniques for high-resolution gene mapping and the identification of disease-causing mutations exemplify such basic research, which is more likely to derive support from public funds than from private investment. As I will show, support for basic research is tenuous. Paradoxically, this may facilitate technology transfer in the short run. If current trends continue, however, the fountains of basic knowledge from which transferable technologies spring may slow to a trickle.

Support for basic research

Since World War II, a very large proportion of basic research in genetics in the United States has been conducted with funds from the federal government, primarily from NIH. When restriction enzymes were discovered and used to recombine segments of DNA in the 1970s, NIH support increased still further. The number of extramural projects (those awarded to investigators not employed by NIH) for which a key descriptor was "genetic manipulation" rose from 546 in 1978 to 1,588 in 1982, with a commensurate tripling of their support to $185 million.[2]

As a result of the sale of the Hughes Aircraft Company to the General Motors Corporation for $5 billion in 1985, the Howard Hughes Medical Institute (HHMI) positioned itself to be a major contributor to certain areas of basic biomedical research. Its anticipated awards in excess of $300 million a year by 1990[3] are equivalent to approximately 10 percent of NIH's entire current budget for extramural research. In contrast to NIH, however, which judges research on its individual merit, HHMI has picked out four program areas in which it will concentrate its support. Genetics is one of these areas. (Immunology, neuroscience, and metabolism are the other three.)

Although dwarfed by HHMI, tax-exempt foundations have also contributed to the support of research in genetics. The March of Dimes Birth Defects Foundation and single-disease organizations such as the Cystic Fibrosis Foundation have contributed to research related to genetic diseases. Although single-disease organizations are more interested in research related to a specific disease, their major concern is finding the basic defect and seeing the pathogenic mechanisms elucidated so that effective treatment or prevention, if not a cure, can be found. Heavily influenced by parents and relatives of patients with specific diseases, they are often uneasy about supporting the development of tests whose major results are prenatal diagnosis and abortion. It is difficult for many parents who have lovingly raised children afflicted with genetic disorders to accept the proposition that those who are similarly afflicted should not be born at all.

The role of universities

The majority of the NIH research budget and almost all of the grants provided by HHMI and private foundations go to investigators at universities. The Reagan administration tried repeatedly to reduce federal expenditures for non-defense-related research. Congress withstood many of these attempts, but the nation's budget deficit may lead future administrations to try similarly to lower research expenditures. Pressure from the commercial sector also has eroded federal support for university-based research, although to a smaller extent. The Small Business Innovation Development Act, passed by Congress in 1982, requires that federal agencies with extramural budgets of over $100 million expend a small percentage of their budget on grants to small businesses, which it defines as those with 500 or fewer employees. The percentage increases to 1.25 by 1988.[4] Many of the grants and contracts awarded by NIH under this program have gone to new, small biotechnology companies.

The biotechnology industry has also called on NIH to expand its support of generic research—which focuses on developing the processes needed for large-scale production—which in turn would help it develop commercial applications more rapidly.[5] As Dr. Ruth Kirchstein, director of the National Institute of General Medical Sciences (NIGMS), has pointed out: "If greater emphasis were to be given to generic applied research, de-emphasis must be placed elsewhere. Should it be on the more free-ranging creative undertakings? If so, what does this portend for the long-range future competitive position of the United States?"[6]

The precarious nature of federal support has led universities to obtain other support for their research activities. According to an OTA report, "[the] universities are seeking money from their relationships with industry, motivated in part by a reduction, or fear of reduction, in Federal funding."[7] Some of these pathways may undermine the basic nature of university-based research, although at the same time they will facilitate technology transfer.

Patents. Prior to 1980, the federal government held most of the patents on work supported with public funds, including that at universities, and freely offered licenses on them.[8] In 1980, amendments to the Patents and Trademarks Act, for which many academic institutions lobbied, permitted universities (and other federal grantees) to retain the title to inventions arising from research funded by the federal government. This gave them the right to obtain patents and grant licenses from which they would be entitled to derive royalties.

The emerging biotechnology industry—the recipients of technology transfer—benefited from the amendments. Under the pre-1980 policy, a company had less incentive to use discoveries made in the universities with federal support because competing companies also had access to them. After the law was amended, a university could grant an exclusive license to a patent resulting from federally supported research. The licensee would have sole rights to the invention for seventeen years. (Licensing arrangements do not have to be exclusive, however. Some discoveries are of such fundamental importance that should patents be awarded, it would be to the advantage of the holder [e.g., a university] to grant nonexclusive licenses. Then all of the companies that would profit from using the discovery would have access to it for the price of a license from the patent holder.)

The current eagerness of universities to sell the rights to patents represents a substantial change in policy. Until recently, according to one Patent Office official, many universities viewed patents as "sort of immoral and not in keeping with their role in society."[9] The policy enunciated by Harvard in 1934 exemplifies the earlier attitude: "No patents primarily concerned with therapeutics or public health may be taken out by any member of the university, except with the consent of the president and fellows; nor will such patents be taken out by the university itself except for dedication to the public."[10]

In December 1980, Stanford University obtained a patent on the process of cloning DNA in bacterial plasmids. In the next four years it received close to $3 million in licensing fees and royalties.[11] Stanford has not granted exclusive licenses on this patent. In the area of genetic testing, the Massachusetts General Hospital (affiliated with Harvard), in whose laboratories the probes for markers of Huntington disease were developed, licensed the probes to Integrated Genetics, Inc. Stanford also applied for a patent to cover the use of RFLPs to detect gene loci implicated in human diseases. If the patent is granted, Stanford has agreed to give exclusive rights to it to Collaborative Research, Inc.[12]

While reiterating that recipients of NIH support "have first right to all inventions developed at their institutions with funds from the Federal Government," NIH recently cautioned investigators that "all unique biological materials developed with NIH funding [should] be readily available to the scientific community after publication of the associated research findings or announcement at conferences. Restricted availability of these materials can impede the advancement of basic research and the delivery of medical care to the nation's sick."[13]

Commercial support. The recognition that recombinant DNA technology has vast practical implications has led some large, established companies, such as Monsanto and Hoescht, to provide long-term, multi-million-dollar support for research at major universities or affiliated hospitals in return for the option to obtain exclusive licenses to patents resulting from company-supported research.[14] The agreements give the companies the opportunity to review manuscripts before publication and to play a role in selecting investigators. On a less grand scale, many of the new, small biotechnology companies have provided support to university-based investigators. In 1984, an estimated 46 percent of all firms in the biotechnology industry provided between 16 and 24 percent of all funds for biotechnology research and development at universities.[15] Commensurate with this, an estimated 23 percent of faculty engaged in biotechnology research received industrial support. (For faculty engaged in chemistry and engineering, the figure was 43 percent.)[16] Increasingly, universities themselves are going after private capital and developing profit-making corporations. Michigan State University has created Neogen to seek venture capital for limited partnerships for developing and marketing discoveries made at the university; the university will receive money from the company's successful commercialization of products.[17]

State and local governmental support. There are approximately 500 programs in 45 states in which state and local governments have provided incentives for industry to move into geographic areas in proximity to universities, thereby stimulating university-industrial relationships. Some of these programs are in the area of biotechnology.[18] For instance, in 1984 the mayor of Dallas appointed a Biotechnology Task Force from which the Dallas Biotechnology Development Corporation emerged. This for-profit corporation will raise capital to invest in research at the University of Texas Health Science Center at Dallas that has commercial potential. It will market the resulting products and technologies to companies in the area. The income will be shared equally between the corporation and the university.[19]

By mid-1987, at least twenty-five states had state biotechnology centers, and funds from the state government were the primary source of support in most.[20] Other sources were the federal government, private industry, and private foundations. The combined budget of these state centers is about $80 million, with most of the funds going to support research (frequently at universities in the state), and smaller amounts being used to promote economic development, training, and education.

Internal transfer. Many university-based investigators are closely affiliated with clinical genetics units. Often their research can be applied to the development of genetic tests, which are then offered to patients or their relatives as a clinical service. Initially, the investigators' research grants absorb the costs of such development and services, but as the demand grows and the relevance of the tests to the research diminishes, investigators must charge for these services. The revenue generated from such testing is sometimes large enough to support clinical and laboratory personnel and even the research itself. This has proved to be the case for genetics laboratories that perform chromosome analysis (karyotyping), and it is beginning to happen at a few university-based laboratories that offer DNA-based tests for genetic disorders. These laboratories are already competing with biotechnology companies that sell diagnostic services.

As the demand for genetic services increases and opportunities at universities level off or diminish, physicians who have received advanced training in genetics (usually through fellowships) and who have obtained full-time university appointments will establish their own genetics specialty practices, either independently or in conjunction with other physicians. This has already started.[21] Such practices may include testing laboratories.

Commercial research and development

Many of the biotechnology companies that have been created since 1976 are "specializing in research-oriented phases of development."[22] A survey of biotechnology companies in 1983 indicated that the industry was employing about 5,000 individuals in research and development activity, about 2,000 of whom had Ph.D.'s.[23] By 1985, these numbers had swelled to 12,000 and 4,000–5,000 respectively.[24] The vast majority of biotechnology companies spend much more money on in-house research and development than on university-based research.[25]

University-affiliated molecular biologists played a role in the founding of some of the young biotechnology companies and hold equity in them. It is not always easy to separate the research being conducted with the advice of these faculty members at the biotechnology companies from what might be performed in their university laboratories.[26]

Potential problems of university-industrial relationships

The salaries offered by biotechnology companies are usually higher than academic or government (NIH) salaries. Tenure-track faculty positions, moreover, are not increasing as rapidly as job opportunities with biotechnology companies. Consequently, scientists are being lured into industry. The loss of scientists to industry was documented in a recent report in the *New York Times*, which reported that Gary Takata, a venture capitalist, "persuaded an entire laboratory of National Cancer Institute scientists . . . to form their own company." While at NIH, they had to chronicle their work in professional journals. If they continued to do so, their work "would soon be taken over by private companies." Rather than let others capitalize on their discoveries, they were willing to postpone publication until they could capture the commercial rights. The report cites other examples as well.[27]

An academic brain drain could reduce the number of scientists willing to remain in nonprofit institutions to work on less commercially rewarding topics. Commercial support for university-based research, as well as efforts by university administrators and faculty to generate patents attractive to industry, could also diminish interest in research activities whose practical applications are not apparent. Thirty percent of faculty members receiving support from biotechnology companies have reported that commercial application influenced their choice of research topic; 70 percent of these thought industrial support placed too much emphasis on applied research, and 44 percent thought it posed "the risk of undermining intellectual exchange and cooperation within departments."[28] One-third of the companies providing support to graduate students or postdoctoral fellows stipulate that "they must work on problems or projects defined by the company, work for the firm during the summer, or work for the company after completing their training." The typically short duration of industrial support may also shift the focus of university research toward applied work.[29] In addition to concern that NIH is being pressured to shift its support to applied research, the director of NIGMS has pointed out that the current lure of researchers to industry could deplete the supply of competent teachers, who are needed to train a new generation of scientists capable of producing further advances in the basic sciences.[30]

The potential for commercial gain could also lead to increased secrecy, thereby retarding the rate of scientific progress. About one-quarter of the faculty members receiving support from biotechnology companies have reported that the results of their research supported by the companies are "the property of the sponsor and cannot be published without their [sic] consent."[31] Several companies do not permit their scientists to publish findings until patents are filed. Information on methods or materials that might be used legally by competitors to develop separate products can be held as trade secrets and never published. Scientists at five of the biotechnology companies I visited (see below) were almost all unwilling to have their respective companies contribute human gene probes to the NIH-sponsored repository (see chapter 4), even though probes from the repository cannot be used commercially.

An investigator at the Los Alamos National Laboratory told me that while his group submitted chromosome-specific probe libraries to the repository, it did not identify DNA segments that had commercial value for chromosome testing. Under an arrangement with the Department of Energy, which supports the research at Los Alamos, applications for patents on such probes can be filed by the University of California. This raises the question of whether societal benefits are being realized optimally by means of commercial development. Much of the research on which commercial development is based has been supported by the public through federal research grants. The temporary sequestration of discoveries based on that research in order to facilitate private financial gain delays the public's benefit from its investment. A more troublesome question is the extent to which the public pays twice for new applied technologies, first by supporting the basic research that was transferred to the corporate sector, and second by paying the companies' own development costs. The amounts that companies must pay for the licensing of patents that resulted from publicly supported research bears little relation to the public investment in that research.

The Use of Transferred Technology for Genetic Tests

The discussion so far has concentrated on the transfer of basic research findings that have many practical applications. Recombinant DNA techniques are being used in the production of proteins and hormones (e.g., interferon and insulin), vaccines for human and animal diseases, chemicals and enzymes for improving industrial processes and agricultural production, and the genetic engineering of microorganisms that could improve agricultural productivity. A number of companies are working on recombinant DNA techniques for diagnosing infectious diseases and cancer. Are biotechnology companies using, or planning to use, recombinant DNA technology for the development and distribution of genetic tests?

The interest of biotechnology companies in genetic testing

To determine interest in and attitudes toward genetic testing, in 1985 and early 1986 I conducted extensive interviews at six companies known to be developing probes of human DNA and examined annual reports and other statements provided by the companies.[32] I spoke with scientists who either worked for the companies or served as consultants or board members, as well as with business or marketing representatives. The interviews provided the framework for two sets of questionnaires. The first was designed to identify companies that were constructing human DNA probes—and for what purposes—and those that had completely rejected or abandoned human DNA probe construction—and for what reasons. The second or follow-up set consisted of two versions. One was sent to companies that had indicated an interest in tests for genetic and chromosomal disorders. It attempted to elicit the companies' plans for developing and marketing tests. The other was sent to companies that had rejected or abandoned test development. Through these follow-up questionnaires, I attempted to learn more about the factors that influenced the companies' decisions and what might lead them to reconsider. Both versions contained questions attempting to elicit attitudes toward the regulation of tests, and the potential uses and consequences of genetic testing.[33]

The first questionnaire was sent to 118 American-based companies that were working with recombinant DNA and developing or producing diagnostics, according to the directories published in *Genetic Engineering News*. By the end of 1986, 85 companies (72 percent) had replied (table 6.1). Forty-two of these said they were constructing human DNA probes, and 8 said they planned to within five years. The purposes of human probe construction are listed in table 6.2. Twenty-two of these 50 companies said the purpose of the probes was to test for genetic or chromosomal disorders. (Two of the 22 were not developing probes. One was using protein data bases to identify probes; the other was using probes in a clinical reference laboratory.)

The first version of the second questionnaire was sent to these 22 companies (table 6.3). Of the 19 that replied, 1 company refused to answer and 4 others replied that they had since abandoned plans to develop tests for genetic disorders. This left 14 respondents, including the 2 companies that were interested in tests but were not developing probes.

In response to the first questionnaire, 12 companies said they had completely rejected or abandoned the construction of human DNA probes. The second version of the follow-up questionnaire was sent to them, and 10 replied. (The four companies that replied to the first version that they had abandoned or rejected some but not all plans to develop probes were not sent the second version.)

Uncertainties in the commercial development of DNA-based tests

No company has yet demonstrated the profitability of DNA-based tests. Because of this, together with an uncertain future, it is not surprising that only a few companies have ventured into the area and others have explicitly rejected it. The diseases for which tests are available are generally rare, limiting the size of the market, particularly since the test-

Table 6.1 Response to First Survey of Biotechnology Companies

	Number of companies	Percentage
Total number of surveys mailed	118	100
Number of surveys completed (as of 1986)	85	72
Company response:		
Constructing human DNA probes	42[a]	49
Planning to construct probes within 5 years	8[a]	9
Had abandoned or rejected human DNA probe construction	12	14
None of the above	23	27

[a]Twenty-two of the 50 companies represented on these two rows reported using or planning to use human DNA probes for tests for genetic or chromosomal disorders. One of these 22 was using protein data bases to identify probes, and one was using probes in a clinical reference laboratory.

Table 6.2 Purpose of Developing Human DNA Probes among Companies Reporting Current or Future Construction of Human DNA Probes ($N = 50$)

Purpose of probe[a]	Number of companies	Percentage
Research	38	76
Diagnosis of human disease	33	66
Cancer	20	40
Single gene	16	32
Chromosomal	14	28
Immunologic	10	20
Other:		
Multifactorial	1	2
Paternity test	2	4
Protein production	26	52
Gene therapy	4	8
Other	3	6

[a]Some companies selected more than one application for the probe.

Table 6.3 Response to Follow-up Survey: Test Developers

	Number of companies	Percentage
Total number of surveys mailed	22	100
Number of surveys completed (as of 1987)	18	81
Companies		
Had abandoned test development	4	22
Were developing DNA-based tests	12	66
Had related research interests	2	11

ing for most of these diseases is restricted to families in which the disease has already occurred. In addition, DNA-based test technology is still cumbersome. Once the few pioneers demonstrate the commercial success of testing, other firms will enter the field.[34] Eight of the 10 "abandoners" said they would reconsider their decision under certain circumstances, including discovery of the genes responsible for predispositions to common disorders, technological advances that would allow direct testing of large populations or simultaneous tests for multiple diseases, and the success of other companies marketing genetic tests.

Return on investment. High development costs and small market size were the most frequent reasons given by the companies that had rejected or abandoned DNA-based test development. Although everyone in the population may be an appropriate target for genetic screening, health care providers and the public may be hard to convince. Moreover, once a person is tested to determine the presence of a disease-causing or susceptibility-conferring allele, there is no need ever to repeat the test (assuming the person retains a record of the test results). Most other routine medical tests, including those used for screening (such as "Pap" smears), are given many times to the same person. Two of the 4 companies that had abandoned test development between receipt of the first and second questionnaires also cited high development costs and small market size. Seven of the 8 "abandoners" that gave estimates in completing the second questionnaire placed sales of DNA probes, reagents, or kits in the United States in 1990 at less than $50 million. In contrast, only half of the test developers gave estimates that low; the others estimated between $100 million and $200 million in sales. The abandoners were also more conservative than developers in estimating laboratory revenues from genetic tests, and only 2 of the 10 abandoners agreed with the statement, "Within five years, the demand for genetic testing will outstrip current laboratory capabilities." On the other hand, 8 of the 14 developers agreed with the statement.

Despite the greater optimism of the developers, not one saw its sales of genetic test materials reaching $100 million by 1990. Nor did these companies consider genetic tests to be big money makers. Five respondents estimated that projected sales related to genetic tests would be less than 10 percent of total sales by 1990, and none placed them as high as 40 percent. An element of desperation may have led some of the companies to consider genetic testing. David Botstein, then a scientific adviser to Collaborative Research, Inc. (CRI), told me in 1985 that the company became interested in the diagnosis of human genetic disease "as a last resort." CRI anticipated that it could get into the marketing phase more quickly with tests for genetic disorders than with its other products.

Controversy: Prenatal diagnosis and abortion. Because genetic tests touch on issues of public concern, biotechnology companies may be wary of developing them. At Genentech I was told, "[We] don't want to be associated with prenatal diagnosis now; it's too controversial." Scientists at another company expressed concern that the antiabortion movement might organize a boycott against the company's other products. On the other hand, an article reviewing the commercial prospects for human genetic disease diagnosis commented: "Already popular with pregnant women, prenatal diagnosis is likely to become much more so when it is earlier, safer, and cheaper than it is today."[35]

Seven companies indicated on the first questionnaire that the controversy engendered by the construction of human DNA sequences led to their decision not to develop them. Five of the 10 abandoners agreed with the statement on the second questionnaire, "The anti-abortion movement has affected (or will affect) the rate of commercial development of genetic tests." Only 4 of the 14 test developers agreed. Developers also placed little importance on public opinion in selecting disorders for test development (table 6.4). (This question was not asked of abandoners.) Despite the importance given by some companies to having a treatment available for the disorders they selected for test development (table 6.4), only 1 of the 14 (9 percent) *agreed* with the statement, "Genetic tests for late-onset conditions (e.g., Huntington disease, Alzheimer disease) should *not* be available for purposes of prenatal diagnosis." This is consistent with the lack of importance companies attached to the age of onset of a disorder when considering test development (table 6.4). A slightly higher proportion of test developers (8 of 14) than abandoners (5 of 10) agreed with the statement, "Tests for genetic predisposition to a disease should not be made routinely available until there are clinical data clearly indicating that medical intervention or change in lifestyle

Table 6.4 Disease Characteristics Influencing Test Development ($N = 12$)

Disease characteristics	Number of companies by rank[a]			Mean Rank
	1–2	3–4	5–6	
Incidence/prevalence	10	1	0	1.3
Availability of treatment	5	5	1	2.9
Severity of disease	4	5	2	3.2
Cost of treatment	1	7	3	4.1
Age at onset of symptoms	1	2	8	4.5
Public opinion	1	2	8	5.0

[a]1 = most important; 6 = least important. One respondent did not rank the characteristics.

will benefit the susceptible individual." Those who disagreed may have believed that prenatal diagnosis was appropriate.

Although prenatal testing and carrier screening (see below) are important for commercial test development, biotechnology companies also emphasize the role of tests in improving the diagnosis or management of treatable conditions. For instance, Cetus representatives pointed out that a test to detect a susceptibility-conferring allele for insulin-dependent diabetes mellitus—a disease they are actively studying—could be used to screen asymptomatic children; those with the allele could then be monitored more closely (see chapters 5 and 7). Integrated Genetics' test for adult polycystic kidney disease is being used to screen asymptomatic relatives who are potential donors of kidneys to affected individuals; a relative who has the allele for this late-onset disorder but who does not yet manifest it would not be a good donor.

Interest in common disorders

The biotechnology companies that have entered the field of genetic testing almost all anticipate that tests for common disorders will not be long in coming. A brochure distributed by one company at the annual meeting of the American Society of Human Genetics in October 1987 included the following: "Research at Integrated Genetics and in other laboratories is expected to generate markers at an increasing pace for additional genetic diseases, as well as the pre-disposition to conditions with a genetic component, such as cardiovascular disease, neurological disorders and certain cancers."[36] A pamphlet distributed by another company, Collaborative Research, stated: "Over the long term, Collaborative Research intends to apply its DNA marker technology toward the analysis of multifactorial diseases with clear genetic components, and the identification of DNA markers associated with predispositions to certain diseases. The company supports the development of DNA marker tests which will provide prospective analysis of risk factors for such diseases with genetic components as diabetes, heart disease, certain cancers and psychiatric disorders such as manic depression."[37] Pursuant to this end, Collaborative Research developed a linkage map of the human genome.[38] The press release announcing this feat stated: "An ability to diagnose common diseases early in life or in utero taps a market estimated at several hundred million dollars a year in the United States, according to Dr. Orrie M. Friedman, Chairman of Collaborative."[39]

The recent localization, on specific chromosomes, of genes playing a major role in the causation of Alzheimer disease, bipolar affective disorder, colorectal cancer, and juvenile diabetes mellitus, which have been described in earlier chapters, justifies the companies' optimism. In fact, Integrated Genetics has also distributed a brochure describing the state of research on the Alzheimer gene, maintaining that "Integrated Genetics will continue to play a major role in the research and development of DNA markers and their diagnostic applications for Alzheimer disease and other inherited disorders."[40]

California Biotechnology, Inc., claims to have developed markers near the apolipoprotein genes on chromosome 11 that may be associated with an increased risk of coronary artery disease and others that may be associated with decreased risk. Phillipe Frossard, staff scientist with the company, told *Science* that the company is devising "a blood test that can tell who is susceptible to cardiovascular disease. By looking at a battery of markers, each of which provides some information on risk, he [Frossard] expects to have an accurate test that will cost, if used on a large scale, about $50. Information from this test, he believes, could be used by individuals 'for early prevention. They can control their diets, exercise, stop smoking, go on cholesterol-lowering diets, and use blood pressure—lowering drugs.'"[41] Frossard told me in November 1987 that his company was collaborating with investigators at several universities in a search for associations between specific RFLPs and enzyme variants, on the one hand, and atherosclerosis, hypertension, non-insulin-dependent diabetes, and neuropsychiatric disorders, on the other. Four thousand patients were being studied.[42]

In 1986, Focus Technologies was reported soon to be ready to use tests at the DNA and protein level to detect individuals at risk for common diseases. Nelson M. Schneider, then managing director of Focus, told the *Washington Post* that the company is "studying 187 markers that indicate the risk of getting 160 different diseases and . . . conducting cost-benefit analyses on which to use. A marker for an extremely rare disorder, or a marker that required complicated and expensive processing for a minor problem, would not be cost-effective."[43] The company declined to specify which markers it may use, but cited cardiovascular and pulmonary diseases as examples. The Equitable Life Assurance Society provided Focus with more than $1 million to develop the program. Although Focus contracted with the Chesapeake and Potomac Telephone Company to provide a multiple-risk profile on 1,000 of its employees on a voluntary, confidential basis, no genetic tests had been included in the program as of mid-1988. The results were to be given to the employees and, if they wish, to their respective personal physicians, but not to their employer.[44]

In their response to the second questionnaire, 9 of 11 test developers ranked incidence/prevalence of a disorder as the most important factor, and one ranked it next most important (table 6.4), in selecting a disorder for test development.

Orphan diseases

Persons with rare disorders have seldom had the benefit of scientific advances, because companies have been unwilling to bear the expense of developing and evaluating new diagnostic and therapeutic reagents for them. This applies to many genetic diseases as well. "Although identifiable genetic diseases in the aggregate probably burden up to five percent of the population, individually they are rare. The potential market for diagnosis is simply too small to be economically worthwhile in most genetic diseases."[45] Nine of the 12 companies developing genetic tests that replied to the second questionnaire are not developing, and do not plan to develop, tests for which fewer than 1 per 1,000 individuals are at risk.

In an effort to remedy the problem, in 1982 Congress passed the Orphan Disease Act (Public Law 97-219), which offers financial incentives to companies developing low-monetary yield but beneficial products. No appropriations have yet been made under the act, but the FDA has provided funds for the development of orphan disease products, including in vitro diagnostics.[46] Genetic test development has not received support under the FDA program, although therapies for rare genetic diseases have. Some biotechnology companies, including 2 of the 3 respondents to the second questionnaire, have obtained Small Business Innovative Research (SBIR) grants from NIH to develop their tests. Five of the 9 commercial developers that are not developing tests for rare disorders said they would consider doing so if they received public or foundation support.

The lack of suitable DNA-based tests for common disorders has led a few companies to offer tests for rare disorders. At least three companies have established commercial reference laboratories to perform tests for rare disorders such as cystic fibrosis, adult polycystic kidney disease, thalassemia, sickle cell anemia, factor IX deficiency (hemophilia B), retinoblastoma, and some disorders of sex development (using a probe of the Y chromosome). Tests for neurofibromatosis and Huntington disease were in the planning and pilot stages, respectively, at the end of 1987. Integrated Genetics and Collaborative Research also plan to store DNA samples (for future testing) for a nominal charge. By marketing laboratory services now, they will establish themselves as leaders in this new diagnostic field. This may position them well for the time when they sell DNA-based test probes or equipment, or when tests for more common disorders become available.

I doubt, however, that commercial reference laboratories whose services consist primarily of linkage studies for rare disorders will bring much of a return on investment. The tests depend on accurate diagnosis in family members. Moreover, the interpretation of results requires considerable time with the families. The few companies that have set up testing laboratories count on referring physicians for accurate diagnosis and for counseling (although they provide full interpretation of test results to the physicians). Rather than send specimens to the commercial laboratories, many nongeneticist physicians will prefer to send their patients to genetic centers that can perform clinical diagnostic and counseling functions as well as recombinant DNA analysis. Most recombinant DNA testing is being done now in university-affiliated laboratories, some of it at little or no cost to the patient. (The Cystic Fibrosis Foundation, which provides support to the medical centers that care for the majority of affected children in the United States, has helped establish a network of university-based laboratories that will accept specimens from these centers.) Companies like CRI and Integrated Genetics may be unable to attract many additional families.

It is true that CRI's success in finding RFLP markers throughout the human genome gives it "a unique and powerful resource for developing DNA diagnostic and analytic tests of highest quality."[47] Whether it continues to offer tests for the numerous rare diseases that will prove to be linked to one set or another of these markers once tests for common diseases are feasible is problematic.

The ability to gain a handle on more common diseases may diminish publicly supported research on rare, single-gene disorders. NIH staff told me that applications for such research are not plentiful and, particularly if they are clinically oriented (even when employing recombinant DNA technology), do not fare well in competitive review.[48] As biotechnologic advances permit testing for risks of common disease, university-based labs will not retain much interest in rare ones. Without additional support, these diseases may then be orphaned to an even greater extent than they are now.

Screening

Heterozygotes. The development of tests to directly detect the mutation or mutations responsible for relatively rare single-gene disorders like cystic fibrosis will permit screening for carriers in the general population. Although cystic fibrosis occurs only once in every two thousand births, the heterozygote frequency is approximately one in twenty. Four of the six companies I visited are working on cystic fibrosis (CF), with the development of a carrier screening test as their ultimate goal.

Integrated Genetics, Inc., reported to the Securities and Exchange Commission that it was "in the initial phase . . . of a multi-year program to develop a screening test which will permit identification of adult carriers of the cystic fibrosis gene. . . . The company believes that, due to the severe nature of the disease and the high frequency of the gene in the population, an effective screening test which would detect carriers of the gene would have very substantial demand."[49] The rationale for carrier testing is made gingerly. The brochure recently distributed by Integrated Genetics that describes testing for cystic fibrosis links carrier testing with prenatal diagnosis.[50] Although entitled *Prenatal Diagnosis and Carrier Detection for Inherited Disease*, the brochure does not describe prenatal diagnosis anywhere, and the word *abortion* is not mentioned.

Most recessive disorders are much less common than cystic fibrosis, and it is not clear how much commercial interest they would excite. Should it be possible, however, to develop an inexpensive test that would detect multiple rare disorders in the same specimen, interest might be kindled. Eleven of the 12 test developers that responded to the follow-up questionnaire are developing tests for single-gene disorders. All 12 developers are using, or plan to use, tests that detect mutations directly. (Six are currently using oligonucleotide probes, 2 are using denaturing gradient gels, and 2 are employing RNA-DNA heteroduplex formation.)

Common, late-onset disorders. Eventually, direct tests for mutations that result in common, late-onset diseases may become available, thereby permitting population-based screening. Before then, tests for polymorphisms very tightly linked to alleles predisposing to common disorders may be developed. The commercial value of tests for common disorders and predispositions may, however, be less than the hype suggests. The polymorphisms will not be specific, so the predictive value of a positive result will be low. Many of the these disorders are multifactorial in origin. Consequently, the mutations identified by tests may not always cause disease; expression may be influenced by genes at other loci and by environmental factors. Moreover, the specific mutations may account for only a fraction of all cases of a given disease. (This last factor is unlikely to deter the use of such tests, but it will reduce their validity.) Finally, the use that will be made of a positive result may greatly influence the demand for the test. If no treatment is available, or if the disorder is not severe enough for many people to choose prenatal diagnosis and abortion, the demand may be low.

Demand can be manipulated. For instance, in the brochure referred to above in which the words *prenatal diagnosis* appear in the title, cystic fibrosis is referred to as a "lethal" disorder. Because many patients with it live into their twenties, some would argue with this characterization. Yet such a characterization makes the case stronger for prenatal diagnosis.

Eight of 12 test developers responding to the survey indicated that they were developing tests for multifactorial (common) disorders.

Chromosomal abnormalities. DNA probes could well replace cytogenetic chromosome analysis (karyotyping; see chapter 5) for the detection of abnormalities in which less or more than 46 chromosomes are present. This will occur when chromosome analysis of fetal cells is performed in a much larger proportion of all pregnancies. At the present time, the most frequent use of chromosome analysis in clinical genetics is in older pregnant women (usually 35 years of age or older) who are at increased risk of having infants with Down syndrome (trisomy 21) and other trisomies. But they comprise only about 5 percent of all pregnancies. The finding that low maternal serum alpha-fetoprotein (MSAFP) concentration increases the risk of Down syndrome in pregnant women of all ages[51] has already expanded the use of chromosome analysis to younger pregnant women. Moreover, chromosome analysis of fetal cells is often performed on pregnant women with high MSAFPs, regardless of their age, who are at risk of having fetuses with neural tube defects and who require analysis of amniotic fluid to confirm the diagnosis.[52] Further increases in the number of pregnancies in which chromosome analysis is performed will occur when physicians develop the ability to obtain fetal cells from the maternal circulatory system early in pregnancy, thereby avoiding any danger to the fetus.

Although cytogenetic analysis (karyotyping) is able to meet the current volume of prenatal testing for chromosomal abnormalities, it is almost at its limits. According to Ann Willey of the New York State Birth Defects Institute, shortages of trained personnel exist, and the costs of the procedure are such that third-party payers will be unwilling to pay for the procedure should it be extended to other women who are not at as great a risk as those in whom karyotyping is currently performed. My discussions with cytogeneticists suggest that significant reductions in costs are not likely to result from further improvements in chromosome scanning. With additional but highly likely improvements in technology, tests based on DNA probes could meet the expanded volume much less expensively than karyotyping. The one drawback is that they will not detect many of the subtle but clinically significant changes that can be recognized by karyotyping.

Because of the current success of cytogenetic analyses, biotechnology companies are not as interested in DNA-based tests for detecting abnormalities in chromosome number as in screening for other types of disorders. Nevertheless, 5 of the 12 developers said they were working on tests for chromosomal disorders.

Simplifying the technology

Methods involving Southern blots, highly radioactive short-lived isotopes, and autoradiography are not appropriate for widespread testing and present obstacles to commercial development. It is not surprising, therefore, that 44 companies responding to the first questionnaire (53 percent)—including some companies that were developing probes against infectious agents—indicated they were attempting to simplify the technology for the detection of DNA sequences. At Integrated Genetics, I was told that eventually its tests would be so simple that "people could do it at home themselves if the interpretation was as simple as the test." Leonard Lerman, then director of diagnostics at the Genetics Institute, told me that the instructions for its tests (still to be developed) will be very simple, "fitting on one side of a 3 × 5 card." At Genentech, the one company I visited that was not actively engaged in developing tests for genetic diseases, Senior Director of Research Reinaldo Gomez told me that if the methods become "user friendly," the company may enter that area of research.[53]

In 1984, Cetus shareholders were told that the company was pursuing the "development of sensitive, accurate and easy-to-use diagnostic tests." One, which was "expected to reach the market in the near term," was "a sickle cell anemia genetic screening test."[54] When I visited Cetus in February 1985, scientists Henry Erlich and Norm Arnheim told me they would have a workable method in six months, although they declined to describe the method. The company, they said, was primarily interested in developing tests for infectious agents, but turned to human genetic disorders because sensitivity and the speed of the assay were less important considerations; even if Cetus failed to develop a method that could be applied to infectious as well as genetic diseases, the company could still market a genetic test. As it turned out, the method is remarkably sensitive and rapid. Cetus is now applying it to a test for the HIV virus that causes the acquired immune deficiency syndrome (AIDS).

Erlich and Arnheim kept to their timetable. By June 1985, Cetus scientists had submitted a description of the polymerase chain reaction (PCR; see chapter 4) for presentation at the American Society of Human Genetics' annual meeting. The full method was published the following December,[55] and its application to the prenatal diagnosis of sickle cell anemia was reported in 1987.[56] The method can yield results in a single day on DNA in cells obtained from a small amount of blood or from chorionic villi sampling without culturing. The polymerization of DNA from one molecule is sufficient to permit detection.[57] Purification of the DNA from the cells is not needed. RFLPs can be compared without the use of Southern blots or radioactive probes. The method also simplifies tests for the presence of deletions and known point mutations. It can also be used to sequence specific DNA segments, thereby doing away with the need to clone them.[58] The method has accelerated research on gene sequencing and the detection of mutations.

Protecting proprietary interests

By patenting inventions or processes of the type represented by Cetus's PCR, companies can protect their investments. Cetus has, in fact, patented the PCR process. Until the patent expires (in seventeen years in the United States), no other company can market the product. One market analyst has predicted that the Cetus Corporation's profits from the PCR machine will reach $200 million by 1990.[59]

Although competing instrumentation may be designed and awarded a patent, if the first company has a sufficient jump in marketing, the purchasers of its equipment—which represents a capital investment—will think twice before switching. Consumables, such as probes and kits, are much less secure; should a better probe come on the market, a testing laboratory will either exhaust its supply and then purchase the competing product or it will discard its remaining inventory at relatively little cost compared to that of scrapping capital equipment.

There are other reasons why probes for specific sequences or related enzymes or other reagents are unlikely to afford companies an exclusive lock on tests for specific disorders, despite their patentability. Although the Medical College of Georgia patented the use of a specific restriction enzyme for detecting sickle cell anemia, and gave an exclusive license to Molecular Diagnostics, Inc., it has not been able to prevent the development of competing tests. Cetus got around the patent by using a different restriction enzyme in developing its PCR test for sickle cell anemia. California Biotechnology, Inc., is patenting probes and RFLPs that may prove useful in tests for specific disorders. The company hopes to afford itself protection by seeking patents on probes that extend several kilobases on each side of the polymorphic site of interest. Whether it will succeed remains to be seen.[60]

Collaborative Research, Inc. (CRI), is counting on gaining an exclusive right to commercial tests for diseases linked to the many probes it has mapped. Dr. Orie Friedman, chairman and chief executive officer of CRI, told *Science*: "We have 54 markers on chromosome 7. We have mapped it in a way no chromosome has ever been mapped—we really own chromosome 7."[61] Friedman's statement came after CRI, in collaboration with Canadian, French, and Danish investigators, announced that it had found a marker linked to the cystic fibrosis gene.[62] In the initial announcements, CRI did not indicate that the marker was on chromosome 7. Although they may not have had this information, other investigators believed they were withholding it in order to retard the ability of their competitors to test markers they had on chromosome 7, thereby giving CRI and its collaborators more time to find additional markers. Within weeks, however, a group at the University of Utah, learning that the marker was on chromosome 7, discovered a much tighter linkage of the CF gene to a marker other than the one announced by Collaborative Research.[63] Another closely linked marker was then quickly reported from London.[64]

Unless Stanford University is awarded a patent on the use of linkage to make predictions (and, as agreed, grants an exclusive license to CRI), CRI cannot challenge the use of probes by other laboratories to provide clinical predictions of cystic fibrosis. If Stanford is awarded the patent, and CRI receives an exclusive license, the company could license to other companies and still have substantial earnings. CRI stated recently "that it will make its DNA probes and other data that comprise the map widely available to academic scientists."[65] Although the statement adds that it will do so "while protecting its proprietary rights," the use of CRI's probes will help other investigators find other markers and eventually a direct test for the disease-causing mutation or mutations. At that point, the Stanford patent would give CRI little advantage in tests for cystic fibrosis.

It must be borne in mind that the technology for genetic testing will not forever remain dependent on DNA probes. As genetic defects for various diseases are discovered, tests for alterations or a deficiency of the protein products—when they can be detected in readily accessible tissues at a developmental stage that makes prediction or diagnosis useful—will replace DNA tests. DNA-related patents will not protect against such tests. Companies that have invested in monoclonal antibodies, which could form the basis of protein-detection tests, could well be competing with those that have developed DNA probes.

Marketing arrangements

Most of the companies active in developing tests today are small and relatively new. Few of them plan large-scale manufacturing of the probes, test kits, or instruments they develop. Instead, they will sign agreements with other companies to do this. Genetics Institute has an arrangement with Allied Chemical to sell, and probably produce, reagents they develop. In 1986, Molecular Diagnostics, Inc., financed in part by Bayer, was negotiating with Ames—another Bayer subsidiary—to market its tests. Cetus has an agreement with Kodak (which is already marketing diagnostic machines) that will facilitate the sale of a simple, automated PCR machine for clinical use. Cetus also has an arrangement with Perkin-Elmer Corporation—an established manufacturer and distributor of research laboratory instruments—to market an automated PCR machine for research use. Genentech has formed a subsidiary with Baxter-Travenol for the marketing of diagnostics. The manufacturing of reagents and test kits depends, therefore, not only on the development of tests by the small companies but also on the perception of others that a profitable market exists. Judging from the alliances formed so far, this does not appear to be a problem.

Summary and Conclusions

Without basic research, conducted largely with public funds, today's biotechnology industry would amount to little. Although the discoveries have led to a host of practical applications—including genetic tests—further progress, particularly in understanding the pathogenesis of disease and how to prevent, interrupt, or reverse the harmful processes, will require additional research. Diminished government support, increased efforts on the part of universities to capitalize on the practical applications of research, and industry's increased interest in collaborating with university-based investigators could deflect current support for basic research into more practical channels, thereby diminishing the rate of future discoveries on which further breakthroughs depend. The growth of research and development within the commercial sector could also deplete the universities of skillful investigators and teachers who are needed to train continuing generations of scientists.

Plentiful public support for research and a university atmosphere unfettered by efforts to seek short-term commercial gain facilitated the discovery of recombinant DNA technology, which has many potential commercial applications. A small number of companies are channeling this information into the development of tests for genetic disorders. The fundamental knowledge needed for DNA-based genetic testing has been transferred! Genetic testing is at this time a commercial venture of considerable uncertainty. This is reflected by the finding that a number of companies specifically decided not to develop tests for human genetic disorders.

Nevertheless, with the exception of rare disorders, there is sufficient commercial interest in genetic diseases to assure the development of genetic tests. However, company efforts to maximize the return on their investments could pose a threat to the appropriate use of genetic tests. For example, companies may focus on tests for common disorders for which the benefits of testing are not always clear. Or they may promote carrier screening without making the implications of the test explicit—specifically, that abortion is one endpoint for individuals or couples predicted to be at risk.

Moreover, the commercialization of genetic tests could deny appropriate testing to certain groups. Tests for rare diseases may not be adequately developed. In that event, persons at risk for those diseases will be deprived of options that are available to those at risk for common disorders, for which predictive tests have been developed. Instead of the burden of disease or the availability of an effective intervention being the determinant of test development, return on investment could become the driving force. This, in turn, would lead to a second form of deprivation: tests that are priced out of the reach of some people. Although health insurance companies may eventually embrace genetic tests (with untoward consequences when they do), they are unlikely to reimburse for some of them until the technology becomes well established. In the meantime, people whose insurance does not cover testing—as well as the millions of people without health insurance—will be deprived of testing.

Concern about protecting their proprietary interests may have inhibited some companies from developing genetic tests, and resulted in excessive secrecy on the part of those that have. The companies that have entered the field are exploring different ways of protecting their position. Some companies are concentrating on simplifying and automating the technology, while others are developing probes for specific disorders. The protection afforded by patents seems greater for the former. At least one company is focusing on developing probes for many markers, which will facilitate the development of multiple tests. Should a patent be awarded on the use of RFLPs in linkage analysis, this company could control the commercial use of family-centered testing, which it is already providing through its reference laboratory. A few other companies have established reference laboratories for selling testing services. This may position them well with health care providers for the time when they do market a product. On the other hand, they may not compete favorably with university-based comprehensive genetic service centers that can provide diagnostic and counseling services as well as testing.

The use of genetic testing in ways that enhance or are inimical to the best interests of individuals and society depends on how the tests are transmitted from the biotechnology companies to consumers. I turn to this process of diffusion in chapter 7.

Technology Transmittance: From Commercial Development to the Widespread Use of Genetic Tests

With a few companies already providing the services, and others poised to market the test probes or instruments, genetic tests based on recombinant DNA technology are about to be transmitted to health care professionals and through them to the public, the ultimate users. Biotechnology companies that have established reference laboratories will market to health care professionals. (At present, they are not offering tests directly to patients.) Companies selling probes and instruments will market to commercial, hospital, and health department laboratories, and as the technology is simplified, to physicians for use in their office laboratories. (Home testing has even been mentioned!) Physicians will *offer* testing to their patients, or in some circumstances will obtain specimens without consent.

If the interests of manufacturers, health care providers, and the public were congruent, then transmittance could proceed without tension. Companies are generally in business to maximize profits, which means selling as many services or products as they can. Although it is ultimately in the companies' best interests to ensure the validity of the tests, and in the laboratories' best interests to ensure high quality, neither is likely to occur without governmental regulation.

Health care providers who have been adequately trained in genetics are in short supply. Consequently, there may be an insufficient number of health care providers to deliver genetic services to the public competently. A lack of knowledge of genetics as well as inadequate reimbursement for some genetic services may slow the adoption of new genetic tests, but the exigencies of practices and concerns about legal liability may speed adoption even when providers are not fully prepared to deal with the implications of genetic tests.

Before agreeing to be tested, consumers should seek to understand how the tests will lead to the prevention or amelioration of genetic diseases and what price will be exacted in medical complications (iatrogenesis), life style changes, or monetary costs (tests, medicines, special diets, etc.). When treatment is not available, potential users should weigh whether avoidance of the particular condition (through alternative reproductive strategies) is consonant with their moral values. To reach decisions that are in their best interests, consumers will need to have adequate information. This will depend on how much knowledge of genetics and disease they have before they are confronted with testing, and on how effectively information is communicated by health care providers before and after testing.

In this chapter, I will deal in turn with the following concerns: ensuring the validity and reliability of genetic tests; the magnitude of the rise in the use of such tests; the adequacy of professional resources to meet the increasing use; factors influencing the adoption of tests by health care providers; public knowledge and acceptance of genetic testing; and, finally, communicating information on tests and test results.

Ensuring Validity

Although tests at the DNA level may be more sensitive and specific than neoclassical tests at the gene-product level or beyond, false negatives and false positives are likely to occur. I dealt with these problems in chapter 5 and will only summarize them here.

Crossing over, erroneous clinical diagnoses, and nonpaternity reduce the validity of linkage studies. The presence of disease-causing mutations at loci other than the one being probed (genetic heterogeneity) reduces the sensitivity of linkage studies as well as direct tests for mutation. Tests designed to detect specific disease-causing mutations at a single locus will miss other mutations at that locus. Finally, mutations that cause disease in the families used to develop the test may not cause disease in all unrelated individuals (variable expressivity).

The validation of linkage studies involves testing a large number of unrelated families in which the disease has occurred. The validation of direct tests involves testing populations that include both affected and unaffected individuals. Large numbers of tested people will be needed, particularly for relatively uncommon disorders, and it may be necessary to follow individuals for some time after the test to determine whether it correctly predicted the absence or presence of the disease.

Pressures to employ genetic tests that have not been adequately validated have already been felt. James Gusella, who localized the gene related to Huntington disease to chromosome 4 in a small number of families, gave the probe to other investigators to see if the same linkage existed in additional families. Until such investigations established the validity of the test with greater confidence, however, he did not want to give the probe to physicians seeking to use it for clinical diagnosis. Gusella pointed out that in the absence of linkage, using his probe "would be no better than guesswork."[1] One group of clinicians to whom Gusella denied the probe complained:

> If Wasserman [sic] had published his test for syphilis, which was far from reliable, in a way which delayed its application, neurosyphilis might now be more common than Huntington's chorea. This infectious disease involved far more difficult problems in handling patients and their families; many individuals must have been distressed by investigations based on error and there were probably a few suicides. But the disease is now rare in Northern Europe. In no field of effective medicine can techniques be applied without casualties.[2]

The authors of this letter dismissed rather lightly erroneous results and even suicides. The historical record indicates that there were more than a few "casualties." Commenting on the Wassermann test, Walsh McDermott, late professor of medicine and public health at Cornell, wrote:

> Of all those people yielding positive reactions, only about one-half were actually syphilitic. But this "validation," so to speak, of the test, this characterization of its inadequacies, was only performed decades after large-scale public health campaigns (including laws governing premarital examinations) had brought thousands of people under treatment. . . . These four or five decades, during which thousands of patients who did not have syphilis were subjected to the shame and dangers of antisyphilitic therapy, are not from the medical era of bleedings and leeches, but from the modern era of interventionist technology.[3]

Moreover, even when the primary lesion of syphilis was present, the outcome was not always dire. Long-term follow-up now reveals that most people who contracted the primary lesions of syphilis earlier in this century, and who were not treated, did not develop the late, disabling stages of the disease.[4] The consequences of being a true positive were not always disastrous. (It will be interesting to learn whether the current tests for the HIV antibody are as accurate predictors of the acquired immune deficiency syndrome [AIDS] in the general population as they are currently claimed to be in high-risk populations of homosexual men and intravenous drug users.)

Although it is as yet unknown whether the variable expressivity of syphilis is genetic, tests for genetic susceptibility to multifactorial disorders also are likely to predict falsely the occurrence of severe disease.

Tests for single-gene disorders whose expressivity is not complete will yield false positives as well. A false positive in prenatal diagnosis could result in the abortion of an unaffected fetus. In those already born, it could result in unnecessary and perhaps unsafe treatment—perhaps for a lifetime—or living with needless dread that a disease will eventually appear.

Pregnant women whose elevated serum AFP levels prove to be falsely positive not only manifest considerable distress and mood changes while awaiting the results[5] but also experience residual anxiety.[6] Occasionally, despite the birth of a healthy baby, the parents persist in thinking that something is wrong.[7] This is also true in newborn screening. According to one study, after being told that repeat tests proved their infants' initial tests to be falsely positive, about one-fifth of parents had lingering concerns about their children's health.[8] Whether such concerns have permanent effects on these children or their parents has not been determined.

The importance of validity is also evident in considering the implications of false negative test results. Their occurrence may have greater deleterious effects than only the occurrence of avoidable or preventable disease. In newborn screening for PKU, for instance, health care providers may disregard the possibility of a false negative test result, with the consequence that when an infant presents with early signs of developmental delay, they disregard the possibility of PKU.[9] As a result, the diagnosis is frequently delayed for many years, causing the parents considerable anguish as their infant's retardation becomes more evident. After the diagnosis is made, the parents sometimes sue. This adds considerably to the costs of the screening program. Although it is doubtful that the outcome would be significantly improved by earlier diagnosis after the signs of retardation appeared, this may not be the case for other disorders. Usually the screening laboratory, not the manufacturer of reagents, is sued. However, if the manufacturer fails to provide accurate data on validity, or adequate instructions on how its product is to be used, it too could be liable. Manufacturers are seeking legislation that would reduce their liability for malfunctioning devices.

Regulating the marketing of genetic tests

Efforts to determine the validity of diagnostic tests have improved since the days of Wassermann, and we might expect that genetic tests will not be marketed until their validity has been established and is acceptably high. Satisfying this expectation depends largely on the actions of the Food and Drug Administration (FDA). Under 1976 amendments to the Food, Drug, and Cosmetic Act, FDA has the authority to regulate medical devices, which include reagents or kits intended for use in the diagnosis or prevention of disease.[10]

Premarket notification. The first step in securing FDA permission to market a device is the requirement that the manufacturer notify the agency—the "510(k) process" (named for the section of the amendments in which it was stipulated)—before introducing a device into interstate commerce.[11] Within 90 days, the FDA determines whether the device is substantially equivalent to one marketed prior to May 28, 1976. (Devices that were marketed before the date on which the amendments were enacted would not have had to go through the premarket approval process described below.) If deemed equivalent, the device can be marketed immediately. (The FDA can require manufacturers to supply evidence of the safety and effectiveness of some "preamendments" devices, but as of the end of 1986, such evidence had been required for only three devices.)[12]

Premarket approval. Designations of substantial equivalence are possible for some DNA-based genetic tests. However, when the FDA decides the testing device is not substantially equivalent, it automatically designates it a "Class III" device and thereby subjects it to the "premarket approval (PMA)" process. Class III devices are "life-sustaining or life supporting, are implanted in the body, or present potential unreasonable risk of illness or injury" (e.g., pacemakers and intraocular lenses).[13] Only about 5 percent of all testing devices are subject to Class III regulation.[14] The only Class III genetic test is the kit for maternal serum alpha-fetoprotein determination.

Manufacturers can petition for the reclassification of a device as either "Class I" or "Class II." Class I devices are so inherently safe and effective that regulation entails only "general controls," which include annual registration of the manufacturer and the device, and adherence to good manufacturing practices. Tongue depressors fall into Class I. Class II devices are those whose safety and effectiveness cannot be reasonably assured through general controls alone but for which enough information is at hand to establish "performance standards." (The FDA has not yet established such standards for any Class II device.) Genetic tests for abnormal hemoglobins and alpha-1-antitrypsin deficiency, phenylalanine test systems (for PKU), and chromosome culture kits have been designated Class II devices.[15] A manufacturer could petition for reclassification of a DNA-based test, deemed by the FDA not to be substantially equivalent, on the grounds that non-DNA-based genetic tests were in Class II. If the FDA accepted the reclassification, it might be satisfied with data showing that the probe accurately detects the *mutation or mutations* it is designed to detect. This, of course, does not address the validity of the test in accurately predicting the absence or presence of *disease*. When performance standards for Class II genetic tests are formulated, they could provide guidance on this point.

If the manufacturer does not petition for reclassification, or if its petition is denied, it must provide reasonable assurance that the device is safe and effective. Because there is not likely to be another test that provides the same diagnostic information as the new one (if there was, substantial equivalence could be demonstrated), the manufacturer will have to present information on the sensitivity or specificity of the test not in terms of another test but in terms of the disease itself. The FDA has no guidelines by which to determine acceptable levels of sensitivity and specificity. Moreover, because these levels will vary with the uses of the test and also with the prevalence of the condition being tested, guidelines—if they are established—should deal with each disorder separately.

When data are unavailable to prove that a device that poses a significant risk is in fact safe and effective, a manufacturer can apply to the FDA for an investigational device exemption (IDE).[16] IDEs can be requested before premarket 510(k) notification. Upon the completion of clinical investigations under an IDE, the manufacturer can use the data in support of a 510(k) notification or a PMA application.

As noted earlier, the collection of data on validity may take considerable time and involve the testing of many people. The FDA can approve the marketing of the test on an interim basis provided the manufacturer has an approved IDE.[17] In such instances, potential users of the test may attribute greater merit to the test than is warranted unless they are warned that the data on validity are incomplete.

The FDA is required to process a PMA application within 180 days of its receipt but can "stop the clock" if additional information is required of the manufacturer. Consequently, most applications for premarket approval take more than six months to process. It is therefore advantageous to be able prove that a proposed device is equivalent to an approved device through the premarket notification process.

According to the General Accounting Office (GAO), the 1985 draft of an FDA task force report on PMAs concluded that there were not enough FDA staff physicians to evaluate industry assertions, that data requirements for deciding safety and effectiveness were inconsistent, and that guidelines were lacking for describing the data required for the approval of devices in various generic groups.[18]

Substantial equivalence. Fewer than 2 percent of 510(k) notifications are found to be not substantially equivalent. As the GAO report commented, "The premarketing notification process is potentially vulnerable because of the subjective criteria manufacturers are allowed for their 510(k) submissions, the vague definition of 'substantial equivalence,' and problems of staffing resources at FDA."[19]

Because tests based on recombinant DNA methods are a significant departure from previous technology, it might seem that they could not be substantially equivalent to preamendments devices. The FDA takes the view, however, that methodology per se does not affect substantial equivalence. Thus the first eleven DNA probes of which the FDA was notified by the 510(k) process—all for infectious diseases—were deemed substantially equivalent to preamendments tests. That determination was made, according to FDA Commissioner Frank Young, on the basis of "intended use and performance."[20] According to FDA regulations, performance characteristics include "accuracy, precision, specificity, and sensitivity."[21]

The FDA could find DNA-based genetic tests for sickle cell anemia and cystic fibrosis to be substantially equivalent to preamendments tests based on hemoglobin electrophoresis and sweat chloride concentration, respectively. The same is true for tests for other disorders for which tests already exist. A critical issue is the intended use stated by the manufacturer. Neither hemoglobin electrophoresis nor the sweat chloride test can be used for prenatal diagnosis, and the latter cannot be used for detecting carriers. Although DNA-based tests for mutations can accomplish both, manufacturers could claim that the DNA-based tests are being marketed only for the uses served by the existing tests. Once marketed, purchasers could use the tests for new purposes. They might do so with impunity in view of the limited capacity of the FDA to detect misuse (see below). The FDA could prevent this by recognizing that the intended use of DNA-based genetic tests almost always extends beyond existing tests and cannot, therefore, be deemed substantially equivalent. If, instead, the FDA finds such tests to be substantially equivalent, it would place them in the same class as the preexisting tests. (As I mentioned earlier, hemoglobin electrophoresis is in Class II; the sweat chloride test has not yet been classified.) This would compound the problem since there are as yet no performance standards for Class II devices.

Commissioner Young recognized that "evaluating the . . . performance [of DNA-based genetic tests] in the absence of other confirmatory tests will present a challenge. A relevant database on particular probes and diseases may best be developed through clinical investigations performed under an Investigational Device Exemption from the FDA."[22] It is interesting to note that the commissioner did not say that the PMA process was the only way for evaluation when no confirmatory tests were available.

Challenges in regulating genetic tests

The safe and effective use of genetic tests, including those that are DNA based, often depends on physicians' abilities. As long as tests are used primarily by genetic specialists, this will not pose much of a problem. But widespread use by other health care providers, as will soon be the case, could create difficulties in two areas in particular.

The first is the use of RFLP probes for linkage to specific disease-causing alleles. The ability of the linkage method to predict disease in any one person depends not only on the results in relatives but also on the accuracy of diagnosis in those cases. How is the FDA to ensure that correct diagnoses will be made?

The second relates to the phenomena of genetic heterogeneity, variable expressivity, and, in the case of linkage studies, recombination. New DNA-based tests will seldom predict with certainty that a disease will occur in the future. How is the FDA to ensure that the probabilistic nature of the findings is adequately communicated to those who are tested?

The 1976 amendments to the Food, Drug, and Cosmetic Act permit the FDA to restrict the sale, distribution, and use of a medical device because of its potential for harm or because of the collateral measures necessary for its use. Despite the urging by a number of professional and consumer groups that the sale of MSAFP kits be restricted in order to reduce misinterpretation of a positive test result and the possible abortion of unaffected fetuses, the FDA withdrew a proposed rule that would have limited the sale of kits to laboratories or centers that could, among other things, ensure adequate follow-up.[23] In discussing DNA probes, Commissioner Young stated: "The FDA also cannot decide for practitioners when a test is appropriate, and under what circumstances any particular test should be used. These are judgments that must be made for individual cases. FDA does not have now or should not have a direct regulatory role in the practice of a physician."[24] When physicians' lack of understanding presents a major obstacle to the effective *and safe* use of a new technology, the choices are to withhold use of the technology, ignore the hazards, or limit use of the technology to those who understand it. Commissioner Young apparently rejected the last option, and seemed eager to encourage test development.

Postmarket surveillance

In line with "good manufacturing practices," the FDA expects manufacturers to keep records of complaints about marketed devices and to review them for possible investigation. Examination of these records is supposed to be part of the FDA's biannual inspection of manufacturing facilities and operations. The FDA also maintains a voluntary problem-reporting system primarily through health care professionals. At the end of 1984, a mandatory medical-device reporting rule went into effect. It requires manufacturers to report to the FDA when they receive or become aware of information that one of their marketed devices has caused serious injury or death or has malfunctioned in a way that makes such adverse outcomes more likely. (It is doubtful that the failure of a genetic test to predict future disease correctly would be covered.)

The GAO evaluated the extent of the underreporting of problems related to ten medical devices, including implants, drug dispensers, and one in vitro monitoring device, but excluding diagnostics. Two hundred randomly selected hospitals were asked if they had a problem with one of the ten devices. Thus a maximum of 2,000 problems could have been reported. From the hospitals, the GAO obtained data on 1,175 device-related problems. About 37 percent of those reporting problems said that the problems could have caused serious injury or death. Only 593 (51 percent) of all the problems were made known to any organization outside the hospitals. Most were reported to manufacturers. Fewer than 1 percent of the problems were reported directly to the FDA.[25] It is probable that the percentage reported by practitioners outside of hospitals would be even lower. Given this dismal record, the FDA would be hard pressed to detect misuse or to determine the validity of genetic tests by current postmarketing surveillance procedures.

As I have already pointed out, the collection of adequate data to validate genetic tests may take a considerable period. IDEs could be used for a protracted period, but it is possible that the laboratories performing the tests under them would be of higher quality than those that offered testing after marketing. It is also possible that the population tested under an IDE would not be representative of the population using the test after marketing. For all these reasons, some form of postmarketing surveillance seems advisable. A number of methods for epidemiologic surveillance have recently been described.[26]

Circumventing the FDA approval process

I have already discussed how a manufacturer's success in getting the FDA to deem a new product substantially equivalent to one already on the market may greatly reduce the time and effort needed to get a new device marketed. There are at least two other ways that this can be accomplished with even less interference by the FDA.

The first entails labeling the kit, probe, or reagent "for investigational use only; the performance characteristics of this product have not been established," or something similar. The FDA does not have to be notified about the use of a product labeled in this way so long as it does not pose a "significant risk."[27] Federal regulations include in the definition of a "significant risk device" one that is "of substantial importance in diagnosing . . . disease, or otherwise preventing impairment of human health . . . [but that] presents a potential for serious risk to the health, safety, or welfare of a subject."[28] However, the determination of whether the particular device meets this definition is up to the manufacturer, which must gain the concurrence of an Institutional Review Board. The manufacturer is also expected to keep records regarding the "investigation," and not to sell the device at a profit. An FDA official pointed out to me that a manufacturer could expand the cost of the device to include a substantial return. He also noted that it is highly unlikely that the FDA has the capability of determining whether a manufacturer maintains adequate records, or would even be aware that sales were proceeding unless "someone blew the whistle."

In our survey of biotechnology companies (see chapter 6), 3 of 12 test developers reported that they were making genetic tests/probes available in such "investigational" kits. Two others planned to do so within five years.

It is doubtful that physicians without training in genetics or general medical laboratories would purchase such probes or kits unless they were enlisted to participate in a formally defined investigation of the safety and effectiveness of a test. On the other hand, geneticists (primarily in university-based laboratories) are accustomed to purchasing research products. These specialists satisfy most of the current demand for testing, considering the relatively few disorders for which probes are available. As probes for additional diseases are developed, the demand could increase markedly. At that point, marketing probes for "investigational use only" will not suffice.

The second means of circumvention will be possible even when many probes become available. Instead of marketing the kits or probes they manufacture, biotechnology companies could establish their own reference laboratories and provide a service instead of a product. The FDA does not bear responsibility for regulating laboratories in which genetic testing devices are used. Although there are regulations governing laboratories that provide services, these vary from state to state and are often not very stringent. Moreover, university laboratories that are engaged in research but that also perform some genetic testing are often not approved for providing clinical services by the relevant regulatory body. (As the volume of their services expands and they collect fees from third-party payers, they will have to be licensed to provide these services.)[29]

The establishment of commercial reference laboratories offers some means of circumvention, but I doubt that it will be important in the total scheme of providing genetic tests. As I mentioned in chapter 6, such labs will be unable to compete with university genetic centers that provide clinical as well as laboratory services. More important, as the technology is simplified, companies will find greater returns in marketing kits or probes to hospitals, independent commercial laboratories that perform multiple tests, and eventually to physicians for use in their office laboratories. When that occurs, the question of ensuring the reliability of tests in multiple-test laboratories will assume great importance.

Ensuring Reliability

When a genetic test goes through the FDA premarket approval process, the evidence on validity is usually obtained in well-designed field trials. The submitted data, therefore, reflect efficacy, or how the test performs under ideal conditions, rather than effectiveness, or performance under routine conditions. With many laboratories performing genetic tests after they are approved and marketed, effectiveness will be quite different from efficacy. For a number of costly procedures, the Health Care Financing Administration (HCFA), which provides Medicare reimbursement, has requested assessments of effectiveness even after the FDA has approved devices on the basis of efficacy.[30] Effectiveness is influenced by more than the laboratory. Specimens must be collected, labeled properly, and sent to the laboratory; after the specimen is analyzed the results must be returned in a timely manner to the health care provider.

Quality control of laboratories

Four to six billion laboratory tests are performed a year in some 46,000 laboratories. About half of the tests are performed in hospital laboratories, 25–30 percent in independent labs. Most of the remainder are performed in physicians' office laboratories, but the proportion of all tests performed in office laboratories is increasing rapidly.[31]

There is no uniform procedure for ensuring the quality of clinical testing through licensing. "Only about half of the states have enacted laboratory regulation, and most if it is feeble."[32] Physicians' office laboratories are regulated in only thirteen states.[33]

Many states accept the Joint Commission on Accreditation of Health Care Organizations' inspections of hospital laboratories. The Joint Commission rarely decertifies a laboratory based on its findings; decertification would require revocation of the accreditation of the entire hospital.[34] Some laboratories voluntarily participate in the quality-assurance programs of the College of American Pathologists (CAP). Although the results are returned to the participants, action is seldom taken against laboratories that do badly. "Ours is not a regulatory program," a CAP physician told the *Wall Street Journal*.[35] (States can require participation in CAP programs, and a few of them ask to see the results.)

Under the Clinical Laboratory Improvement Act (CLIA) of 1967, the Centers for Disease Control (CDC) has purview of laboratories that receive specimens from other states. As a result of recent changes, CDC relies more on education to ensure quality than on the evaluation of test performance. It has maintained a proficiency-testing program for laboratories that perform newborn screening. There is evidence that the performance of newborn screening laboratories has improved as a result of the quality-assurance program at CDC.[36]

HCFA periodically inspects laboratories serving large numbers of Medicare patients and has also assumed responsibility for inspecting labs that receive out-of-state specimens. Although it has stopped laboratories from doing certain tests on interstate specimens, it continues to reimburse the labs for running these tests on Medicare patients within the state.[37] When clinical laboratories are licensed, the responsible licensing agencies do not require them to demonstrate proficiency on every procedure. HCFA officials have said that failure to demonstrate proficiency on a single procedure does not warrant regulatory action.[38]

Surveys done on screening procedures often demonstrate a lack of proficiency. In 1985 CAP found that almost half of 5,000 laboratories performing cholesterol analyses failed to come within 5 percent of the "true" cholesterol concentration; 15 percent of them were unacceptably off.[39] Cervical cancer screening (Pap test) labs have sometimes failed to detect precancerous lesions; this has resulted in the death of at least one person.[40]

An examination of laboratory experience with newborn screening illustrates the need for quality-assurance programs in genetic testing. In a survey of health departments, my colleagues and I found a more than twentyfold difference in the ratio of false to true positives for newborn PKU tests. This difference could not be explained by genetic differences in the populations being tested or in the cutpoints used in testing. The most plausible explanation was the variable ability of laboratories to perform and interpret the tests.[41]

A CDC survey of health departments conducted in 1983 found that 43 infants with PKU and 33 with congenital hypothyroidism had been missed in routine screening.[42] For both disorders, the missed cases represented approximately 1 percent of the affected infants discovered by screening. Because health departments are not aware of all missed cases, the finding underestimates the problem. Over half of all the oversights

(56 percent) were attributed to faulty laboratory procedures. Twenty-nine percent of the missed newborn screening cases resulted in some legal action, including claims of up to $20 million. Many of the cases were still pending in 1986, but settlements of up to $3 million have been reported.[43] In 1985 the American Bar Association concluded "that the best way to avoid lawsuits . . . [is] to assure that newborn screening programs follow clear guidelines for quality assurance."[44]

Only New York State requires cytogenetics laboratories to participate in its proficiency-testing program, and no state yet has procedures in place to assure the proficiency of laboratories that will perform DNA-based genetic tests. The Middle Atlantic Region Human Genetics Network has received a federal grant to develop a proficiency-testing program for laboratories performing DNA-based tests.[45] Centralized proficiency programs do exist for other genetic tests. The Foundation for Blood Research in Scarborough Maine runs a proficiency-testing program for alpha-fetoprotein tests. Michael Kaback established one for laboratories performing Tay-Sachs screening. Participation in these programs is voluntary.

The quality of the testing process

Although, as already mentioned, more than half of all the missed cases in the CDC survey of newborn screening programs were due to laboratory errors, an additional 16 percent were due to avoidable "prelaboratory" errors such as the failure of specimens to reach the laboratory or the failure to request another specimen when the first was unsatisfactory. An additional 20 percent resulted from "postlaboratory" errors, such as the failure of the physician or hospital to send a repeat specimen after the first was reported to be abnormal, or the failure of the hospital or physician to locate the patient.[46] False negatives in newborn screening were almost three times more likely to occur in programs handling fewer than 50,000 specimens a year than in programs handling more.[47] According to the survey, the smaller programs were more likely to involve private and hospital laboratories, the larger ones state and regional laboratories.

Using a computerized surveillance system that tracks the entire screening process, the Oregon newborn screening program found that 58 percent of newborn screening specimens were submitted incorrectly (excluding babies who never were tested).[48] More than 16 percent of specimens took over five days to reach the laboratory; such delays could jeopardize the outcome for infants with some of the disorders for which testing is performed.

The Anticipated Volume of Genetic Tests

Tables 7.1 and 7.2 present estimates of the volume of genetic screening once DNA-based tests are marketed for certain disorders. The specific disorders listed are for illustrative purposes; tests for other disorders may

Table 7.1 Estimated Annual Volume of Screening for Heterozygotes and Chromosome Abnormalities after DNA-Based Tests Are Marketed

Target population and condition	Number of tests	Number of positive heterozygotes[a]	Number of affected fetuses
Young women[b]			
Cystic fibrosis	750,000	37,500	
Sickle cell anemia	152,000	12,160	
Hemophilia	940,000	94	
Duchenne muscular dystrophy	940,000	188	
Totals	2,782,000	49,942	
Male partners of heterozygotes			
Cystic fibrosis	37,500	1,875	
Sickle cell anemia	12,160	970	
Totals	49,660	2,845	
Pregnant women[c]			
Chromosome abnormalities	2,407,000		4,332

[a]Assumes perfect sensitivity and specificity.

[b]The number of women screened is equivalent to 25 percent of women giving birth in 1985. Source: National Center for Health Statistics. Advance report of final natality statistics, 1985. Hyattsville, Md.: National Center for Health Statistics, 1987; DHHS publication no (PHS) 87-1120. (Mo Vit Stat Rep 1987;36[4 suppl]). This source also indicates the percentage of all births that were first-borns and the percentage of pregnant women coming for care in the first three months; data are presented by race. The estimates take into consideration that women are screened only before the birth of their first child (about 40 percent of all live births are first-borns), that only women who come for care during their first pregnancy before the fourth month (about 80 percent) will be screened, and that 20 percent of women satisfying these two criteria will refuse screening. The estimate for cystic fibrosis is limited to white women, while that for sickle cell anemia is limited to blacks. The number of positives is based on the known carrier frequencies.

[c]Number of pregnant women coming for care in the first two months of pregnancy in 1985. Source: same as for note b. The number of positives is based on the expected frequency of severe chromosome abnormalities. Source: Kalter H, Warkany J. Congenital malformations: etiologic factors and their role in prevention. N Engl J Med 1983;308:424–431, 491–97.

Table 7.2 Estimated Annual Volume of Screening for Common Genetic Predispositions after DNA-Based Tests Are Marketed

Target population and condition	Number of tests	Number positive
Infants[a]		
Insulin-dependent diabetes	3.8 million	190,000
Coronary artery disease	3.4 million	170,000
Children 10–14 years[b]		
Lung cancer	2.7 million	170,000
Adults 15–29 years		
Breast cancer[c]	2.1 million (females)	105,000
Bipolar affective disorder[d]	2.1 million	105,000
Alzheimer disease	2.1 million	105,000
Totals	16.2 million	810,000

[a]In view of the high frequency of false positives, and the absence of additional tests to distinguish true from false positives, an estimated 10 percent of parents of newborns will refuse screening for these disorders.

[b]An estimated 15 percent of children between the ages of 10 and 14 years will be screened each year. Therefore, by the time a child reaches the age of 15, he or she will have a 75 percent chance of being tested. The remainder will either not have come for care in those years or will not have been tested because of their or their parents' refusal.

[c]Women between the ages of 15 and 29 years are screened at the time of their first visit to a health care provider. It is assumed that all women in this age bracket will make at least one such visit. The estimate assumes that all women will accept testing.

[d]Men and women between the ages of 15 and 29 years are screened at the time of their first visit to a health care provider. It is assumed that all persons in this age bracket will make one such visit. In view of the uncertain benefits of screening, 50 percent refuse testing.

be marketed instead of or in addition to those shown. (The reader is referred to chapter 5 for additional information about some of the disorders chosen.) Although family-based linkage studies may involve greater inputs of professional time per family, they are ignored because their volume is dwarfed by screening. For the same reason, prenatal diagnosis in couples at risk also is excluded.

The estimates are conservatively biased—that is, they tend to minimize the number screened for any condition in any year. With the exception of screening for chromosomal abnormalities, which is offered to a woman every time she becomes pregnant, no person will be screened more than once for a given carrier state or predisposition. This will be possible if the persons tested are given and retain test results or if those providing care subsequent to the time the test was performed have access to the result. The estimates do not include people who have passed the age group or life stage (e.g., pregnancy) at which testing is targeted but who may still derive benefit from screening. This includes older siblings of those detected by screening. The numbers of such people will be large in the first few years of screening, but will soon dwindle as all those who want screening obtain it at the target time. The estimates shown here were made from recent population data[49] without any adjustment for upward or downward trends. For single-gene and chromosomal disorders, tests are assumed to be of perfect sensitivity and specificity. (Because a lower specificity will have a greater effect on the number of positive results than will a lower sensitivity of the same proportion, this assumption minimizes the number of positive results.)

Screening for heterozygotes for autosomal recessive and X-linked disorders

The estimates reflect the screening of women before or during their first pregnancy, and the subsequent testing of the male partners of those who prove to be heterozygotes for autosomal recessive disorders. As table 7.1 shows, heterozygote screening will result in almost three million tests, and about 50,000 positive results. Most tests will be offered by obstetricians or other primary-care physicians and will not involve geneticists. (The number of tests is ten times the total number of clients currently served at genetic centers.) These physicians may well refer people with positive results to geneticists. The referral of all such women would represent a less than 20 percent increase of clients coming to genetic centers; if only women who were heterozygotes for the autosomal recessive disorders whose spouses were also carriers were referred, the increase would be considerably smaller. In either case, the anticipated number could probably be absorbed by the current supply of genetic specialists plus those in training.

Screening for chromosomal abnormalities

Chromosome analyses of all pregnant women coming for care in the first three months will be feasible when a safe and simple procedure for obtaining fetal cells is developed. With 20 percent of pregnant women refusing to be tested, 2.7 million women would be tested annually, of whom more than 4,300 would be positive (table 7.1). Tests will be offered primarily by obstetricians, but geneticists could be called on to counsel women with positive results. There probably will be a sufficient number to do this.

Screening for genetic susceptibilities

Familial forms of the disorders shown in table 7.2 will affect between 1 and 0.1 percent of the population tested who survive to the age at which the disorders manifest. I have arbitrarily assumed that the markers occur in 5 percent of the healthy population, giving predictive values of positive test results between 20 percent and 2 percent.[50]

Screening for susceptibilities should occur prior to the age at which irreversible damage occurs and at a time when the interventions will yield maximum benefit. For insulin-dependent diabetes, with onset sometimes in childhood, and for hyperlipidemic forms of coronary artery disease (CAD), for which early intervention may prove most beneficial, newborn screening would be appropriate. Screening for the genetic predisposition to develop lung cancer from smoking could be delayed until later childhood. At that point, those with positive results could be counseled as to the higher-than-average risks of their smoking. (Whether knowledge of their susceptibility will enhance the effectiveness of anti-smoking advice remains unknown, however.)

For breast cancer, for which the principal test is monitoring (mammography) for early signs of neoplasia, screening could be deferred until young adulthood. Although current recommendations are that all women over the age of 50 receive mammography annually, in view of the higher risk of familial breast cancer in young women,[51] monitoring at age 30 in those with genetic susceptibilities would have a relatively high yield of positive results.

For bipolar affective disorder and Alzheimer disease, identification before early adulthood is unlikely to have any benefit. There is no evidence that current therapy for bipolar affective disorder would be any more effective if started before symptoms appeared. There is no established effective therapy for Alzheimer disease. Identification in early adulthood will still give individuals at risk the opportunity to avoid the conception or birth of an affected child. Because screening will identify asymptomatic individuals who might not want to know that they might develop the disease, refusal rates are likely to be high.

Human Resources for Providing Genetic Services

Inadequacies in validating genetic tests before they are marketed, and in ensuring the quality of laboratories performing them after they are, will certainly not retard the diffusion of genetic testing, and might even accelerate it. In this section, I examine the quantitative and qualitative adequacy of human resources to deal with the anticipated expansion of genetic testing and attendant services.

Professionals with special training in genetics

With the exception of screening tests for a few disorders, most genetic tests are provided by genetic specialists. Moreover, many nongeneticist physicians who are involved in screening—for instance, pediatricians with newborn screening and obstetricians with alpha-fetoprotein screening or chromosome analysis—refer patients with positive test results to genetic centers.

Most genetic specialists (63 percent) are located within university-affiliated medical centers and are pediatricians (table 7.3). Only 9 percent of the university-affiliated programs are housed within departments of medicine, yet a considerable amount of future genetic testing is likely to involve adults. The number of genetic specialists forming their own groups or joining health maintenance organizations is probably increasing.

Data in a study conducted in the late 1970s[52] suggested that the average center saw about 500 outpatients per year. Probably most centers now see between 1,000 and 2,000 clients per year. The increase is due to greater demand, especially for prenatal diagnosis (which is the reason for the majority of visits), and some response on the supply side, including growth

Table 7.3 Clinical Genetic Service Programs by Location[a]

Program and location	Number	Percent
University-based programs		
Department of Pediatrics	74	36
Department of Obstetrics	13	6
Departments of Pediatrics and Obstetrics	12	6
Department of Genetics	15	7
Department of Medicine[b]	12	6
Other departments	4	2
Children's hospitals	24	12
Private hospitals	32	16
Public health facilities, regional centers	12	6
Health maintenance organizations	6	3
Totals	204	100

[a]Data from Clinical genetic service center directory listings, USDHHS, 1985. Directory of Medical Genetics Services.

[b]Five centers listing genetics program within a department of medicine also had services available through another department such as pediatrics, obstetrics, or preventive medicine.

in service staff size, greater use of group counseling, and videotapes to describe techniques such as amniocentesis. The approximately 200 clinical genetic service centers throughout the United States[53] serve approximately 300,000 people annually. This number is small compared to visits to other specialists, who receive many more referrals from other providers.

Although genetics centers are directed by physicians, many employ master's level–trained genetic associates, nurses, and social workers,[54] who provide much of the patient contact, including interviewing and counseling.

Availability. As of the end of 1987, a total of only 1,342 professionals were certified in at least one of the five subspecialties of the American Board of Medical Genetics; 1,131 of them were certified in a discipline that enables them to provide direct patient care. This sum is comprised of approximately 500 physicians, 500 master's level counselors, and 100 Ph.D.'s.[55] Approximately 30 percent of the providers of genetic services may not be certified[56] (including about 200 nurses and a much smaller number of social workers),[57] boosting the total of providers to about 1,800 at the very most. With 300,000 people per year coming to genetic centers, this represents an average load of fewer than 200 clients per provider per year. There is probably a large deviation from the mean, as these professionals differ markedly in the proportion of time they spend providing genetic services. Even taking this into consideration, one might argue that the ratio of providers to clients is so small that the supply is more than adequate. The lengthy time spent counseling weakens this argument, however. A recent study in one genetics center documented that the time spent by physicians and counselors varied between one and three hours for each new family and between 28 and 101 minutes for each returning family.[58] If an average of three hours is spent for each new client (at an initial and a follow-up visit), with three full days devoted to outpatient clinics per week, each provider could see about 300 new clients per year. Although this suggests that some centers could see more patients without adding staff, several centers report unfilled positions for clinical (M.D., Ph.D.) geneticists and counselors. They anticipate a doubling or tripling of unfilled slots in the next five years as demand increases out of proportion to supply.[59]

The current training of medical geneticists and counselors. The current training of medical geneticists and counselors will not satisfy the anticipated increase in demand. Only about fifty physicians complete fellowship training in genetics each year. The nine principal programs that offer master's degrees in genetic counseling graduate only about sixty students per year. In neither category did the number increase appreciably between 1984 and 1987.[60] Taking into consideration the retirement of older geneticists (and the failure of some others to enter clinical practice), the net growth in the number of specialized providers of genetic services is probably no more than one hundred per year. At current training rates, it will take at least ten years for the number of specialists to double.

The role of health care providers without special training in genetics

As table 7.2 shows, the anticipated volume of tests performed and the number of people with positive results is enormous, far exceeding the capacity of geneticists either to inform prior to testing or to counsel afterward. At its current rate of growth, the specialty of medical genetics will be unable to deal with the potential referrals that will result from an expansion of genetic testing, let alone provide the tests. As the demand for genetic services increases, undoubtedly more physicians will enter the specialty. (I doubt, however, that their numbers will be sufficient to offer and provide tests to the target populations shown in table 7.2, even though doing so could be highly remunerative.)

The volume of tests will also strain the capacity of nongeneticists to provide them. Considerable time will be needed to explain the reasons why the tests should be performed and to counsel those with positive results. One counseling session per year for infants and children with positive test results would equal approximately the total number of office visits of children under the age of 15 that have been devoted to medical counseling, although it would represent less than 0.5 percent of all visits made by children under that age to physicians' offices. One counseling visit per year for each adult with positive test results would represent about 3 percent of all medical counseling office visits by those between 15 and 64 years of age.[61]

Commercial test developers recognize that nongeneticist health care providers will be using genetic tests. Although 11 of the 14 companies with an interest in genetic tests that responded to the survey described in chapter 6 rated genetic clinics as important or very important test sites, 10 rated health departments, 9 rated prepaid health groups, and 7 rated private primary-care medical facilities as important or very important test sites. The companies' interest in health departments is not surprising. Newborn screening tests and, to a lesser extent, maternal serum AFP screening, have been performed in health department laboratories. Moreover, the involvement of health departments has often resulted from legislative or regulatory mandates requiring either that screening be offered or that tests be performed on the target group. This, of course, ensures the largest volume of tests. Almost all genetic screening programs mandated or supervised by health departments refer persons with positive test results to their personal physicians, most of whom are private or hospital based. The involvement of a large number of primary-care physicians in genetic testing is, therefore, unavoidable.

Nongeneticist health care providers are probably as competent as geneticists in informing people prior to testing about the medical indications for testing (e.g., more frequent monitoring, therapy, or life style changes), and in suggesting or instituting these interventions in those with positive results. They will have greater difficulty explaining the chance of false positives or the genetic aspects, such as the risks of having affected offspring. For bipolar affective disorder and Alzheimer disease, the genetic aspects are extremely important. Many physicians do not recognize the role of genetic testing. They are unfamiliar with genetic concepts, and with tests of low predictive value. These factors may slow their adoption of genetic tests, as may the shortage of personnel who can assist them in providing the tests.

Appreciating genetic tests. Lack of physician enthusiasm for genetic tests is evident. Although a representative sample of primary-care physicians surveyed in 1974 favored screening for particular traits or conditions, about 40 percent preferred that such screening be conducted by community-organized campaigns rather than as part of general medical practice.[62] In this survey and one conducted four years later,[63] about one-quarter of responding physicians doubted that screening newborns for PKU was beneficial. Few physicians refer patients for genetic screening.[64] People who come for Tay-Sachs carrier screening obtain more information about screening from the media, brochures, and religious and lay groups than from physicians.[65] Obstetricians have been slow to adopt maternal serum AFP screening.[66] Low utilization rates of prenatal diagnosis in the United States[67] can be attributed to women not being offered it rather than to their refusing it.[68]

Nor have physicians been enthusiastic about adopting other types of screening or preventive procedures. In a 1984 survey of 1,000 primary-care providers, the percentage of physicians who reported that their practices satisfied American Cancer Society guidelines was 11 percent for mammography, 18 percent for proctoscopy, 48 percent for stool blood-sampling, and 75 percent for Papinocolau cervical smears.[69] Many pediatricians have not yet incorporated counseling on such known risk factors as diet, smoking, weight, and substance abuse into their practices.[70] Only 20–30 percent of these physicians believe they are likely to be effective in assisting children and adolescents to modify their life styles and thereby avoid the risk of cardiovascular disease as adults.

The initially slow adoption of new technologies is not unusual.[71] As I will discuss in the next section, incentives and pressures can accelerate adoption. However, unless physicians have an adequate understanding of how to use the technology, misuse may result.

Understanding genetics. Genetics has not been emphasized in U.S. medical schools. In 1974, three-quarters of a sample of board-certified pediatricians, obstetricians/gynecologists, and family physicians reported no genetics courses in their medical school training.[72] Less than 2 percent believed that physicians in general were competent to provide such counseling. As of 1985, 20 percent of U.S. medical schools were still without genetics courses.[73] Moreover, scant attention is paid to common, multifactorial disorders in the genetics courses that do exist—just 12 percent of genetics curricula cover them, according to a 1978 survey.[74] In the late 1970s, only 3 percent of the questions on the National Board examinations, which are taken by most medical-school graduates to obtain their licenses, dealt with human genetics. (Having had a course in genetics was a significant predictor of correct responses to these questions.)[75]

Genetics topics are seldom covered in continuing education programs. Their ability to improve physicians' knowledge or to alter performance is equivocal at best.[76] My colleagues and I failed to find any difference in knowledge of maternal serum AFP screening between obstetricians who received educational interventions and a comparable group who did not.[77] (Knowledge was higher among the small group of physicians who adopted screening after the educational interventions but before they started to test.)

Understanding test results. Physicians have difficulty interpreting the results of laboratory tests when some uncertainty is attached to the results.[78] In the area of genetic testing, only 50 percent of pediatricians and family practitioners chose the correct answer, "1 in 20," as the likelihood that a newborn with a moderate elevation of blood phenylalanine (8 mg/dl) upon screening for PKU would actually develop the disease. The other choices were "virtually certain" or "1 in 20,000."[79] The 24 percent who picked "virtually certain" might have started infants who did not have the disease on the recommended special diet, possibly causing them serious damage. In the study of obstetricians' knowledge of AFP testing for neural tube defects already mentioned, we found that only 22 percent of physicians who had received information on the subject (including the predictive value of a positive result) knew that the chance of a neural tube defect's being present was less than 5 percent when the screening test was positive.[80] Some of those selecting "80 to 90 percent" (the highest percentage given in the multiple-choice question) might have recommended proceeding directly to abortion after the abnormal screening test result was obtained. Until physicians have a better understanding of the high fallibility of tests applied to apparently healthy populations and of the need for confirmatory studies, considerable harm may result from testing.

Reasoning about test results seems to deteriorate during medical school. I posed the following question in writing to medical students and physicians at the Johns Hopkins School of Medicine: "If a test to detect a disease that occurs in one of 1,000 people is falsely positive in 5 percent of unaffected people, what is the chance that a person found to have a positive result actually has the disease?" Eighty-four percent of first-year students ($n = 76$), 73 percent of third-year students ($n = 94$), and 49 percent of interns and residents ($n = 110$) selected the correct answer, "2 percent."[81] The downward trend was highly significant ($p < 0.001$). Most of those giving incorrect answers greatly overestimated the predictive value of the test.

One explanation for this frequent rate of error, drawn from work in cognitive psychology,[82] is that experience can distort the assessment of probabilities. In contrast to first-year students, third-year students and, to an even greater extent, house officers are immersed in a hospital setting in which tests are used to confirm the suspicion of disease. The probability that a disease will occur in only 1 of 1,000 people runs counter to the latter groups' experience. It is the low prevalence of the disease that causes the test's predictive value to be so low.

To remove the difference in clinical experience, I formulated a question unrelated to medicine: "If automobile inspection to detect a serious fault that occurs in one of 1,000 cars also fails 5 percent of automobiles without the fault, what is the chance that a car that fails inspection actually has the serious fault?" The correct answer here, too, is 2 percent. Either this question or the one on testing for disease was asked of practicing physicians returning to Johns Hopkins for continuing education courses in pediatrics or medicine ($n = 272$) and of the next two incoming classes of medical students ($n = 203$). Compared to the practicing physicians, a significantly higher proportion of students answered both questions correctly. However, a higher proportion of practicing physicians answered the automobile question correctly than gave the correct answer to the disease question (59 percent versus 48 percent, $p = .05$). Thus the decline in reasoning ability may be influenced by physicians' preoccupation with sick patients. They may be better able to use tests to determine which disease a person has rather than to determine whether or not a disease will occur.

In addition to understanding genetics and test results, physicians must be able to communicate information related to genetics and results if genetic testing is to be used appropriately. Because effective communication depends not only on how information is transmitted but also on how it is received, I will defer consideration of this important topic until after I have examined the public's understanding of genetics and risks.

Nonphysician health care providers. As I have already noted, master's level–trained genetic counselors, nurses, and social workers are important team members in genetics clinics. Could they also perform the same role in assisting nongeneticist physicians? Of the three groups, master's-level genetics associates have the most training in genetics. Licensure and third-party reimbursement policies require that the vast majority work with geneticists. Nevertheless, a few are working at health maintenance organizations.[83] Some modification of the training of these genetics associates will be needed to enable them to assume more confidently a role in assisting nongeneticists in providing new genetic tests and related services. Physician geneticists may resist such changes, however, because they weaken their dominance of the counselors and may reduce the number of referrals of other physicians to them.

Although genetics is addressed in nursing textbooks, and genetics texts have been written by nurses for nurses,[84] only an average of 10 hours are devoted to genetics in nurses training that culminates in a baccalaureate degree.[85] A 1979 study found that only 4.2 percent of senior students and practicing nurses had adequate knowledge of commonly encountered genetic disorders.[86] Exposure to genetics course work appears to have affected nursing practice. Pediatric nurse practitioners who had taken a genetics course were more likely than others to make a referral to a genetics clinic regardless of the proximity of the facility.[87]

In a 1984 survey to which 55 of 88 graduate schools of social work responded, 22 percent had some genetics in their curriculum and 60 percent reported field placements that involved students with genetic content and practice. Nearly two-thirds of the schools agreed that there was too little genetics in their curriculum and that the lack of faculty "expertise" was an obstacle to further curriculum development.[88]

Governmental support for genetics education

Without significant changes in the curricula used to train nonphysician providers of genetic services, there seems little chance that they will be able to work with nongeneticist physicians in providing genetic services. The Bureau of Maternal and Child Health and Resources Development of the U.S. Department of Health and Human Services has provided support to develop modules on genetics for integration into social work foundation courses. With the bureau's support, 11 continuing education courses in 1986–87 directed primarily at nursing school faculty members reached about 500 health care professionals.[89] The bureau has not, however, supported the training of genetic counselors,[90] nor has it supported efforts to improve the teaching of genetics in medical schools. Through grants to regional genetics networks, it has provided support to some continuing professional education programs for physicians.

Factors Influencing Physicians to Adopt Genetic Tests

A lack of understanding of genetics and test use will slow the adoption of tests by many physicians, but will not stop it. Companies marketing tests will target their advertising to nongeneticist physicians as well as to geneticists. Such advertising is already an important source of physician awareness of medical innovations, even though awareness is not necessarily accompanied by full understanding.[91] Although physicians with greater awareness and understanding may be the first to adopt tests, other factors will also influence adoption once tests are simple enough to be marketed to general physicians. I deal with two of these factors—method of reimbursement and fear of liability—in this section, and a third—consumer acceptance—in the following sections.

The method of reimbursement

Fee-for-service payment. Under traditional fee-for-service payment arrangements, physicians have little incentive to consider costs in ordering tests and other procedures. As long as physicians can collect the bills—and the amount paid to them is commensurate with their time and effort—their enthusiasm for genetic tests may be great, regardless of the benefits or potential cost savings. At the present time, however, fewer than half of Blue Cross/Blue Shield plans responding to a recent survey reimburse for carrier screening tests. On the other hand, over 85 percent cover maternal serum AFP tests and amniotic fluid chromosome and AFP studies.[92] Genetic counseling, which is covered by less than 60 percent of the Blue Cross/Blue Shield plans,[93] is often not reimbursed at a rate commensurate with the physician input involved. As insurers recognize that long-term savings accrue from testing (see chapter 8), the number of third-party payers reimbursing for genetic services will increase, as may the amounts for services that are currently underreimbursed.

Prepayment. As with other insurers, the owners and operators of prepaid plans (health maintenance organizations, or HMOs) are unwilling to pay for services that are not cost saving. Sometimes genetic tests will fit the bill, but not always. Tests that predict disease in the distant future may not be profitable to the plan, because benefits (savings) will not be realized for many years. By then, the client may no longer be a subscriber to the plan. HMOs may, however, find it cost saving to offer carrier screening and tests for fetal chromosomal abnormalities. Parents who decide on the basis of the tests to avoid the conception or birth of an infant whose care will be costly will save the HMO money; unless the test is for a very rare disorder and the unit cost of the test is very high, the cost of testing is unlikely to exceed the cost of caring for an affected infant.

Although genetic tests are not currently used to deny enrollment in group policies, they could be used to deny enrollment to individuals. It might also be possible for HMOs to negotiate exclusion criteria with group subscribers. HMOs could also use genetic tests as part of a marketing strategy to attract younger persons who are concerned about their long-term health and receptive to a plan that offers individually tailored preventive health care packages.

Legal liability

Personal physicians have been sued for not ensuring that a satisfactory newborn screening test was performed on one of their infant patients. Many of these cases have been settled out of court, with physicians, or more usually their malpractice insurance company, agreeing to contribute to a settlement.[94] Obstetricians who failed to advise women at risk for prenatally diagnosable conditions of the availability of amniocentesis have been the targets of successful litigation.[95] Even if tests are not widely enough used to be considered "standard care," as long as the tests are available the suits may be successful. The growing consistency with which the courts have recognized negligence in failing to offer genetic testing for reproductive purposes may rapidly lead physicians to offer such tests.

Aware of the danger of malpractice litigation, the American College of Obstetrics and Gynecology (ACOG) advised its members that it is "imperative that every prenatal patient be advised of the availability of [the maternal serum AFP] test."[96] In our study of MSAFP screening, the vast majority of physicians told us that when their professional society recommends screening, they will adopt it.[97] It should be noted that ACOG told its members to "advise" patients of the test's availability, not automatically to perform it.

Genetic Testing and the Public

Unless testing is to be mandated or performed without informed consent—possibilities that I examine in the next chapter—the rate of transmittance of genetic tests will ultimately depend on consumer awareness, access, and acceptance. For those who are aware and have access, the ability of health care professionals to communicate information will influence not only acceptance but the decisions those who are tested make following the report of the results.

Knowledge and awareness

Although lengthy articles on genetic testing have appeared in popular magazines such as *Time* and *Newsweek* and in several newspapers, and television documentaries on the topic have been aired, a large proportion of the public has probably not been reached. Almost two-thirds of those polled by Louis Harris recently for the Office of Technology Assessment said that they do not regularly read a science section of the newspaper.[98] A very small part of television viewing time is spent on public-interest programs. Voluntary organizations such as the March of Dimes and the Cystic Fibrosis Foundation provide information about genetic diseases to the public, but the emphasis has not been on genetic testing.

Governmental efforts. Under the National Sickle Cell Anemia, Cooley Anemia, Tay-Sachs, and Genetic Diseases Act of 1976 (Public Law 94-278), an effort to "develop information and [dispense] educational materials to persons providing health care, to teachers and students, and to the public in general in order to rapidly make available the latest advances in the testing, diagnosis, counseling and treatment of individuals respecting genetic disease" has only partially succeeded. The National Center for Education in Maternal and Child Health (NCEMCH) has amassed a wealth of materials on genetic disorders and genetic services. It has not succeeded in distributing them widely, however. According to 1986–87 data supplied to the Office of Technology Assessment by NCEMCH, only about 50 requests for genetic information from the entire country are processed per month. Students make nearly one-third of these requests, followed by health providers (26 percent) and consumers (17 percent). In a six-month period covered by the data, only 46 consumers—most of them parents or parents-to-be—requested materials. I doubt that requests are so few because the public is well informed. A much more likely explanation is that NCEMCH has not established adequate channels through which to distribute its materials.

Genetics in the schools. With the failure to reach many people who have finished their schooling, attention logically turns to the formal educational system. Unfortunately, the schools have not rapidly incorporated advances in human genetics into the curriculum. A recent examination of the eight most frequently used high-school biology texts,[99] which all were copyrighted after 1980, failed to turn up any mention of the use of recombinant DNA technology for the detection of heterozygotes and homozygotes for any genetic disease, even though the method was first reported in 1978.[100]

Although the new textbooks devote more attention to human genetic disorders than did the older editions, this treatment is restricted almost exclusively to scientific issues. Information about the personal and societal implications of screening, counseling, treatment, and prevention of genetic disorders is sparse. For example, although each of the eight books covers amniocentesis, only one addresses the difficult choices that a pregnant woman faces in deciding whether or not to use it. One of the texts discusses neonatal screening for phenylketonuria, but none addresses screening for heterozygotes or for late-onset disorders, all of which will soon be available. Only three of the eight texts mention cystic fibrosis, despite the frequency of the disorder and the number of at-risk matings that will be identified as gene probes become more informative.

The laws of probability as they pertain to the inheritance of single-gene disorders are discussed without exception, but no consideration is given to the uncertain nature of test results or to problems of sensitivity, specificity, and predictive value. How people make decisions when there are uncertainties attached to the choices is not covered.

One explanation for the poor coverage of human genetics in high-school biology texts is the increase in the number of challenges being made to educational materials on religious grounds.[101] Textbook publishers are reluctant to risk criticism and economic reprisals from groups that protest the inclusion of such topics as evolution and prenatal diagnosis. This is particularly so when these groups are influential in states that represent a large share of the market.

With governmental and private support, the Biological Sciences Curriculum Study organization has developed ancillary materials for classroom use that deal with applications of recombinant DNA in medicine, including genetic testing. Ethical and policy, as well as scientific, issues are covered. These materials have reached fewer than 15 percent of the 2.25 million high-school students enrolled in biology classes.[102]

Poor teacher preparation is another factor contributing to the sorry state of genetics education. Many teachers completed their own training before recombinant DNA techniques were developed. With more lucrative careers beckoning, too few newly trained graduates are being drawn to high-school teaching. Many teachers are uncomfortable teaching topics in the science classroom that will invariably raise questions about personal decision making. Although many states require continuing education, few teachers have had the opportunity to attend formal courses or workshops that would bring them up to date in genetics.[103]

Awareness of tests for specific disorders. Despite the inadequate knowledge of the public, many people are aware of genetic tests. Virtually all newborns are screened for PKU, although parents may not always be aware that their infants have been tested and may not appreciate the genetic nature of the disorder. For diseases concentrated in ethnic or racial groups (sickle cell anemia, Tay-Sachs, thalassemia), community-based efforts to increase awareness have been fairly successful. For instance, in a campaign in the New Orleans Jewish community to encourage testing for Tay-Sachs carriers, only 13 percent of nonparticipants had not heard of the screening program.[104]

Most diseases for which genetic testing will be possible will not be concentrated in cohesive communities, however, and awareness of their availability may not be as high. In a survey of women of advanced maternal age who recently had a baby without undergoing amniocentesis, 25 percent had never heard of the test, 20 percent reported their physician did not recommend the test, 30 percent had not had the test because they did not perceive their pregnancies as being at increased risk, and 21 percent opposed abortion.[105] This confirms a point made earlier, that generalist physicians have not been strong advocates of genetic testing.

Most relatives of persons affected with genetic disorders are aware of genetic tests, but some are not. In the latter case, the disease or its genetic origin is concealed by members of the family, or health providers fail to deal with the genetic component of the disorder. Patients with multifactorial disorders and even some with single-gene ones (e.g., hemophilia, sickle cell anemia, and cystic fibrosis) are not usually referred to genetics clinics. In these instances, the extent to which primary-care physicians or nongeneticist specialists discuss risks is unknown, but probably is not great. A survey in Veterans' Administration hospitals revealed that despite claims that genetic information was available to families of patients with Huntington disease, fewer than 1 percent of the 78 hospitals studied had a formal policy regarding the provision of genetic counseling. Moreover, in some cases the information was provided by untrained personnel and was inaccurate.[106]

Access

Family linkage studies can cost $1,000. Screening tests generally cost much less. In neither case have third-party payers consistently reimbursed for these tests. The cost of chorionic villi sampling or amniocentesis, particularly when karyotyping is performed, exceeds $500, and if the fetus is affected and the family chooses abortion, another hefty expense is incurred. In some states, the costs of testing are covered for women on Medicaid, but the costs of aborting an affected fetus are not. This is also the case for federal employees and their dependents who are covered through employee group insurance plans. Because of the absence of third-party coverage for abortion, some women are deterred from obtaining prenatal diagnosis.

Referring to the lack of coverage by Blue Cross/Blue Shield plans for carrier screening tests and genetic counseling, the authors of a recent Blue Cross and Blue Shield Association report commented that "lack of coverage, resulting in out of pocket payments [by] individuals, may discourage many from seeking appropriate genetic services."[107]

Strategies to avoid the conception of an affected offspring are very expensive; reimbursement policies when the indications are genetic have not been established. Artificial insemination by a donor can cost as much as $2,000 and in vitro fertilization and surrogate motherhood considerably more. Couples who oppose abortion may well initiate genetic testing only if they can afford these procedures or if they wish to adopt, which also can be costly.

Problems of access undoubtedly contribute to the overrepresentation of well-educated, upper-income women in genetic clinics[108] and in prenatal screening programs.[109] Although federal support has led a number of university-based medical centers to establish satellite units, people in rural areas remain underserved. This may result from a lack of referrals by local public health nurses and physicians as well as a lack of access to genetic services. The dearth of minority geneticists and genetic counselors also may deter members of minorities from seeking these services.

Acceptance

In the Harris poll conducted for the Office of Technology Assessment, 83 percent of respondents said that before having children they would take a test that would tell them "whether or not it is likely their children would inherit a fatal genetic disease."[110] Sixty-nine percent said they wanted tests that could detect a genetic disease "in the fetus during the early stages of pregnancy," and 66 percent said they wanted to take a test to determine if they themselves were likely to develop a fatal disease later in life.[111]

A number of studies have examined the attitudes or practices of various groups that are more directly confronted with decisions regarding genetic tests. The level of acceptance is likely to be influenced by whether prevention or amelioration rather than avoidance is possible, the severity of the disorder, and the presence of a family history.

The possibility of prevention or amelioration. Parents are quite receptive to having their infants screened for diseases that will impair development but for which preventive interventions are available. In Maryland, where informed consent is required for newborn screening, more than 99.95 percent of mothers accept it.[112] Because there has been little experience with screening in infancy or childhood for late-onset diseases, I can only speculate that the level of acceptance of such screening will be lower, particularly when the interventions interfere with normal child-rearing (such as long-term administration of medicine, highly restrictive diets, and limitations of activity). As treated children grow older, they may reject the treatments accepted on their behalf by their parents. Screening for genetic predispositions among adults may attract those who have already taken steps to lower their risk. Those who come for screening for risk factors for heart disease, for instance, may be the ones who have already changed their diet to reduce their cholesterol levels.[113]

Avoidance only. When no postnatal interventions are effective, avoidance becomes the major option. Some people who reject avoidance options will still want to know their risk of having an affected fetus, but the largest proportion of those who accept testing will undoubtedly be those who accept avoidance.

Despite the vehemence of the antiabortion campaign in the United States, the level of acceptance of abortion in the general population is quite high. In a national survey conducted in 1980, 83 percent of respondents favored legal abortion for reason of defect.[114] In a study of 490 pregnant women conducted by my colleagues and myself in Maryland, 75 percent of the women said they would have an abortion if there was a very good chance their child would be born seriously mentally retarded, and 59 percent said they would have an abortion if there was a very good chance their child would have a serious physical handicap.[115] About half of the women were Catholic. Religious affiliation per se did not influence the attitude, but women who attended religious services less often and did not believe in life after death or that the Bible was the literal word of God were more likely to view abortion as justified. Commenting on the thalassemia program in Sardinia, Cao et al. pointed out that "even a medium-developed, prevalently rural, Catholic population accepts elective abortion as a method to prevent the birth of a child affected with a fatal recessive disorder."[116]

The rate of acceptance of abortion for birth defects is reflected in a comparable rate of acceptance of prenatal diagnosis, although as might be expected from the different attitudes of women toward mental retardation and physical defects, the rates vary depending on the severity of the condition, a point I will return to shortly. If chorionic villi sampling is proved comparable to amniocentesis in safety, its availability may well increase the acceptance of prenatal diagnosis because it can be performed earlier in pregnancy than amniocentesis. If it becomes possible to make prenatal diagnoses on fetal cells obtained from the mother's blood, acceptance should increase further because the test is noninvasive of the fetus. Women who are unalterably opposed to abortion may use this test to help themselves prepare for the birth of an affected infant.

Little is known about the acceptance of options to avoid the conception of infants at risk for genetic disorders. Undoubtedly some couples will prefer avoidance of conception over abortion for moral or religious reasons.

In one sickle cell screening program in Orchemenos, Greece, undertaken before prenatal diagnosis was possible (so not mating with another carrier was the only means of avoidance), 23 percent of the inhabitants were found to have the sickle cell trait. Follow-up revealed that the number of infants with sickle cell anemia born to parents who had been screened was not lower than that expected on the basis of random matings. In two of the four matings that resulted in the birth of an affected infant, the women concealed their carrier status from their partners. In the other two, the partners proceeded with the marriage knowing the risks of having affected offspring.[117] In a survey conducted prior to the discovery of the probe for Huntington disease, 69 percent of males 45 years of age or younger and 40 percent of males over the age of 45 who had a 50 percent chance of being affected said they would be willing for their wives to be artificially inseminated by donor sperm to avoid the risk of having affected offspring.[118] It will be interesting to see how many choose this option now that testing is available.

Carrier screening. Screening programs for carriers of Tay-Sachs, sickle cell, and thalassemia have been undertaken largely because no postnatal interventions are possible for these diseases. Acceptance of Tay-Sachs screening has been studied most extensively.

Despite intensive publicity, only about one-quarter of young Jewish adults avail themselves of Tay-Sachs carrier screening.[119] Opposition to abortion does not appear to be a major factor.[120] A consistent finding has been that those who came for screening had more education and more knowledge of the disease than those who did not come.[121] Expectations of what medicine can accomplish in the way of treatment and cures may partially explain the low acceptance rates. In a baseline survey of Jews of reproductive age, most of whom were married, Massarik and Kaback found that 75 percent held the erroneous belief that genetic disease is curable, and 93 percent thought that it is always (12 percent) or sometimes (81 percent) treatable. The authors commented that the finding

> reveals an exceptionally widespread faith in the capability of the physician to intervene in alleviation of genetic disorders. . . . It is as though people might be saying, "After all, genetic disease is just another disease." Given this formulation, respondents are inclined to assume implicitly a usual sequence of events that may be paraphrased by the patient's statement "I don't feel well," followed by "I need a doctor," which in turn leads to a series of steps calling for medical diagnosis, treatment, and the reestablishment of well being.[122]

According to the health-belief model, proposed to explain health-seeking behavior,[123] the acceptance of Tay-Sachs carrier screening should depend on a health motivation (the wish to have healthy children), the perceived susceptibility (the chance of being a carrier), the perceived severity (the impact of being a carrier on one's reproductive plans), the perceived benefit of taking action (carrier couples can use prenatal diagnosis and selective abortion), and the perceived absence of barriers (screening in the community at no or low cost). In the studies cited, the findings were often at variance with the model. Many young adults wanting to have children did not avail themselves of screening; the risks of being a carrier were frequently underestimated by those coming for screening (discussed further below), and those who perceived the impact to be less severe were more often the ones who came for screening. I an. unaware of studies of acceptance rates for sickle cell screening. In a study of black women, about half who attended health department family planning or prenatal clinics were screened; informed consent was obtained in most but not all cases, so *voluntary* acceptance rates may have been somewhat lower.[124] Fewer than 10 percent of reproductive-age adults in ethnic groups at high risk for thalassemia came for carrier screening for that disorder in Montreal.[125] In the Greek Cypriot community in Great Britain, approximately half of the couples estimated to be at risk for thalassemia have been identified through screening.[126] In villages in largely Catholic Sardinia, between 23 and 62 percent of the total population between the ages of 15 and 44 years came for screening.[127] It may be that in southern Europe, where carriers are more likely to mate with each other than are their counterparts in North America, the greater incidence of the disease accounts for a higher rate of acceptance of screening than has been found in North America.

The acceptance rates in community-based, voluntary carrier screening programs in the United States and Canada are fairly low. The higher estimates that I used earlier in this chapter to project the need for health care providers were based on the assumption that if carrier screening and other forms of genetic testing are provided as part of regular medical care, acceptance rates will be higher. This is discussed further in chapter 8.

Evidence is accumulating on the acceptance of genetic tests to detect fatal, late-onset disorders. According to one report, of 346 at-risk individuals who were informed of the availability of linkage studies for Huntington disease, only 47 (14 percent) have requested testing.[128] In another study, however, performed after the linkage method was published but before testing was available, 87 of 131 respondents (66 percent) said they would want the test.[129] Fifteen of the 31 who wanted more children said they would use prenatal diagnosis to detect the disorder; another 5 were unsure. Religious affiliation influenced the choices of all 131. Respondents to a survey of those at risk for adult polycystic kidney disease also expressed this ambivalence. Although some favored it for family-planning purposes, others opposed it because if they were found to be at risk, this would inhibit them from having children.[130]

Factors influencing the acceptance of testing

The certainty of the test. For untreatable multifactorial disorders for which tests cannot predict the occurrence of disease with certainty, the highest risk conveyed by a positive test result might not be high enough for many individuals to consider using the test to avoid either the conception or the birth of affected offspring. In our study of women's attitudes toward maternal serum AFP screening for neural tube defects, only 2 percent of women said they would have an abortion if the chance of the fetus's being affected was one out of four. The percentage increased to 14 percent if the chance was one out of two, to 34 percent if it was three out of four, to 58 percent if it was ninety-five out of one hundred, and to 91 percent when there was no uncertainty about the fetus's being affected.[131]

The severity of the disorder. There are several dimensions to severity: magnitude and nature of the disability, pain, age of the patient at onset, and duration. Severity is likely to play a greater role in influencing a person's acceptance of testing when preventive or ameliorative intervention is not possible. For then the question arises, "Does this disorder warrant avoidance?" And avoidance raises difficult moral choices. Among early-onset disorders there is already some evidence that the magnitude of the disability influences the acceptance of testing as well as avoidance. As I have already pointed out, the risk of mental retardation is more likely to lead to acceptance of abortion than is the risk of severe physical handicap. Among the conditions associated with developmental delay, acceptance varies, although cultural factors as well as differences in severity may account for this variation. The acceptance of prenatal diagnosis for Down syndrome, primarily by older pregnant women without a past history, varies between 60 percent and 80 percent,[132] but for Tay-Sachs about 90 percent of couples identified by screening choose it. Among physical defects, prenatal diagnosis appears to be more widely accepted for thalassemia than for sickle cell anemia;[133] survival is generally longer in person's with the latter disorder. Although prenatal testing for late-onset disorders like Huntington disease is just beginning to be offered, the surveys already cited indicate that its acceptance is lower than that for early-onset conditions.

Whether the proportion of pregnant women favoring avoidance options will change as additional tests become available remains to be seen. The availability of the tests themselves may reduce the tolerance for severity, particularly when many couples are intent on limiting the size of their families. Discussing the rising tide of malpractice cases in his specialty, one obstetrician commented: "When you deliver a baby today parents expect it to come out perfectly. Unfortunately, it doesn't always turn out that way. Twenty years ago, it was considered an act of God. Today, there are no more acts of God. They expect you should have been able to do something."[134] Genetic disorders explain some of those "acts of God." Genetic tests and their sequelae may be the "something" that can be done.

The family history. Parents with a living child with a serious genetic disorder face a serious dilemma in deciding whether to have more children. On the one hand, they may be unable to cope emotionally or financially with having another child. On the other, they are concerned about the effect their reproductive plans will have on the living child. If they stop having children or use prenatal diagnosis and abort affected fetuses, the earlier child could interpret their decision to mean that he or she, too, should never have been born. Many couples derive strength and satisfaction from helping their children overcome many of the adversities of serious disability.

The proportion of parents of children with cystic fibrosis who favor abortion to avoid serious untreatable disease in their offspring—51 percent[135]—is considerably less than that of pregnant women in general (see above). Although 75 percent of couples who already have a child with cystic fibrosis and are still considering having additional children say they will use prenatal diagnosis,[136] at least 40 percent of such couples have in the past undertaken pregnancies—knowing the risks—without prenatal diagnosis.[137] It will be interesting to see how many couples with affected children choose prenatal diagnosis for cystic fibrosis and Duchenne muscular dystrophy now that these tests are available.

Siblings of children with autosomal recessive diseases, who have a 50 percent chance of being carriers, appear eager to use prenatal diagnosis when they begin families of their own. There is apparently considerable interest among the siblings of cystic fibrosis patients in learning whether in fact they are carriers.

Parents who themselves have an avoidable disability also face a dilemma. As one woman with spina bifida wrote, "Could I choose to abort a baby with my own disability? . . . But then . . . could I choose to continue the life of someone possibly destined to endure some of the same treatments I had experienced?"[138]

Organizations for the handicapped—including some genetic disease foundations—have expressed ambivalence about prenatal diagnosis, partly for the reasons just described. They also fear that in promoting prenatal diagnosis they will portray a distorted picture of the seriousness and hopelessness of a given disease.

Communicating information on genetic tests and test results

If the decision to have genetic tests is to be consonant with personal values, individuals must have a clear understanding of the implications of the tests both before they are tested and after they receive the results.

Pretest information. People who have had contact with a relative affected by the disease for which testing is available will often have some knowledge of the severity of the disease, though not always of the risks of recurrence. Yet most people who consider genetic screening actually know very little about any aspect of the disease.

One way of ensuring that this information is provided is through informed consent. Such consent is almost always obtained prior to linkage studies, but this is far from the case in screening. In most states, the screening of newborns is conducted without obtaining parental consent.[139] The parents of an infant with a positive test result first hear about the testing when they are informed of the result. According to a sickle cell screening survey conducted in Maryland in 1981, 38 percent of hospitals, clinics, local health departments, and other organizations providing screening did not obtain informed consent. Only 30 percent of the organizations provided printed prescreening educational materials. Most respondents said they provided information orally.[140]

When informed consent is sought, the disclosure statement should contain information on the nature of the disease, the test, and the implications of both positive and negative results. I have seen brochures on prenatal diagnosis for pregnant women that fail to mention that abortion is an option when test results are positive. In the consent process, understanding is influenced by the readability of the consent statement, the time and manner in which it is delivered, and the opportunity the subject has to deliberate before reaching a decision.[141] The amount of time women have to think about amniocentesis, following the presentation of information, influences the rate of acceptance of the procedure.[142]

Although consent is obtained before amniocentesis is performed, the physicians who refer women for counseling prior to the procedure do not always explain what the test is about. According to one study, 10 percent of women coming for amniocentesis reported that their local doctor had not explained the procedure; 12 percent said the doctor had not explained what the test would show. This study also found that 54 percent of women coming for prenatal diagnosis learned about the procedure from a nonphysician source. The geneticists who conducted this survey in the mid-1970s concluded, "The experience would be improved . . . if the referring physicians were to explain the procedure and what the test could show."[143] More recently, a sociologist, Barbara Katz Rothman, noted:

> While observing [prenatal counseling] sessions, a number of times I got the distinct impression that the client had no idea what this was about. . . . For example, right near the end of a session . . . the father finally asked, "So, tell me, what if you do find something? What can you do about it?" And another woman . . . asked toward the end of a session, "I'm just so curious—if something is wrong, what could I do at this point?" In both cases the counselors (two different counselors, with quite different styles) gave the answer that the choices were between continuing and terminating the pregnancy. But the information was not given until it was requested.[144]

In Dr. Rothman's view, "Counselors will probably spend very little time helping people decide to have the [prenatal diagnostic] tests. . . . Decision-making counseling occurs with a diagnosis."[145]

Communicating results. Screening programs do not communicate test results if they are negative. This is almost always the case in newborn screening, and sometimes in maternal serum AFP screening as well. In one AFP program, women with negative results who had been told the outcome of the test were considerably less anxious than women who had been told that unless they were notified, they could assume the confirmatory test was normal. The authors of the report comment, "This indicates that the 'no news is good news' principle is a bad one and one in which patients pay, in terms of anxiety, a high price for an administrative economy."[146]

Even when the results of newborn screening tests are positive, physicians may be reluctant to tell parents until they have confirmation. In one study, more than half of the parents surveyed reported that they were not told that the first test was abnormal when informed that a repeat test was needed. Either they were not given a reason or they were told that repeat testing was routine, that a mistake had been made on the first test, or that the specimen had been lost.[147]

Individuals who have positive test results do not always have a clear understanding of the disorder for which they have been tested (particularly in screening programs, where most people do not present a family history), including the severity and risks of occurrence. In a Seattle sickle cell screening program, the parents of children identified as having the sickle cell trait were told the difference between trait and disease. Nevertheless, "Forty-three percent of the carrier group parents and 71 % of the control group parents (of non-carrier children) considered sickle cell trait to be a *disease*. Specifically, these parents thought the carrier required frequent medical care that ranged from undefined 'treatment' to blood transfusion. . . . Roughly half of both the carrier (49%) and control (51%) group parents thought that some restrictions should be placed on the physical activities of sickle trait carriers."[148] In a survey of university students regarding Tay-Sachs testing, 30 percent of those who were tested, compared to 41 percent of those who were not, had a low "index of knowledge" of Tay-Sachs disease and how it was transmitted from one generation to the next.[149] In that study and in a survey of young married Jewish couples, almost one-third of those who accepted screening said their reproductive plans would be affected if *one* mate was found to be a carrier. Yet for this recessive disorder, both mates have to be carriers to place their offspring at risk. Only 16 percent of the young Jewish couples recognized that their risk of being a carrier was one in thirty or greater.[150] After the results of a Montreal high-school screening program for thalassemia were reported to the participants, only 33 percent of carriers and 18 percent of noncarriers had correct knowledge of the Mendelian probabilities of having an affected child.[151]

Communicating risk is not a simple task. As part of the Maryland study on AFP testing described earlier, 190 pregnant women were asked, "What does 1 out of 1000 mean to you?" They were given three choices:

"less than 1 percent," "10 percent," or " greater than 10 percent." Over
one-quarter could not give the correct answer; one-fifth of the women
said it meant "10 percent"; and 6 percent said it meant "greater than 10
percent."[152] Half of the women were told that the risk of a serious birth
defect was 4 in 100, while the other half were advised that it was 40 in
1,000. Seventy-four percent of the first group translated this correctly to 4
percent, but only 41 percent of the second group did ($p < 0.01$). The ability
to answer correctly influenced women's interpretation of the probability
of a neural tube defect, which, they were told, occurred in 1 in 1,000 pregnancies. Of those who gave the correct percentage equivalent of 1 in
1,000, 16 percent said the defect occurred "often or occasionally," as opposed to "rarely or very rarely." On the other hand, of those who overestimated the percentage, 31 percent said the defect occurred "often or
occasionally."

Recognition of the difficulty of communicating risks also comes from
studies of genetic counseling. According to an analysis of nine studies on
counseling published since 1970, "Many parents of children with a genetic disorder have an inadequate understanding of the genetic implications of the disease, even after one or more genetic counseling sessions."[153] In a large, multicenter survey of counseling conducted in the
United States in the late 1970s, more than half of the 87 percent of people
who came with inaccurate knowledge of risk still had an inaccurate
knowledge of it after counseling, and of the 13 percent who came with
accurate knowledge, one-sixth had inaccurate knowledge afterward.[154]

Genetic counselors tend to perceive risks as higher than clients perceive them,[155] and also higher than counselors did in the early 1970s.[156]
Whether the counselor's perception of the risk confronted by a client influenced the client's perception of whether that risk was "high" or "low"
was not reported in the multicenter study; but the study did report the
finding that those clients who perceived their numerical risk as higher
than that of others at the same risk were more likely to have discussed
with the counselor the question of having another child.[157]

The way risks are posed also influences choices.[158] The decision to
have a genetic test may be different if the risk is put as a 25 percent
chance of having an affected child rather than a 75 percent chance of having a normal child. Telling people that a particular trait (e.g., smoking, or
a susceptibility-conferring genotype) increases the chance of death by
some multiple of the risk to people without the trait may have a greater
influence on people when the absolute risks are small (e.g., 1 in 1,000
compared to 1 in 10,000 in others) than telling them the absolute risk.[159]
Putting risk in personal terms—as is done in health risk appraisals in
which people are told their own risk of dying by a certain age compared to

the risk of others—may improve the chance that people will take action, but evidence is lacking that this is very effective, particularly in young adults.[160] People who are resistant to modifying a single risk factor may recognize that they will still be exposed to a large number of risk factors that can do them in prematurely.

Communicating other information. Although numerical risk is an important factor in the decisions people reach following testing, it is not the only factor. Experience from genetic counseling suggests that people put greater weight on their ability to cope than on precise numerical risks.[161] Yet counselors do not often deal with many of the factors that influence coping.[162] In only 42 percent of the counseling sessions analyzed in the above-mentioned multicenter study was the counselor aware of what the client most wanted to discuss.[163] Counselors were more likely to be aware when the risks to potential offspring were lower. The authors suggest that when the risk is higher "it may tend to dominate the counselor's definition of the client's situation. . . . Helping the client understand the 'bad news' perhaps blinds the counselor to the fact that the client may wish to discuss something else, say prognosis of a living affected child."

Anticipating the untoward effects of testing. Almost half of the individuals identified as carriers in Tay-Sachs screening programs said they were worried when they first learned of the results.[164] In one eight-year follow-up, 19 percent reported they were still worried.[165] It has also been reported that some individuals with negative results stigmatize those with positive results and have feelings of superiority. In a high-school Tay-Sachs screening program, about 10 percent of noncarriers said they would not mate with a carrier. Moreover, 10 percent of noncarriers had an "improved self-image" (only one of forty-five carriers did) on learning their screening test results.[166] These fears and perceptions reflect knowledge deficiencies, which may in turn have resulted from inadequate communication.

Early in this chapter, I mentioned the anxiety associated with false positive test results. The anxiety associated with true positive results may be even greater. According to one study, abortion of a wanted child following positive prenatal diagnosis was associated with depression in 92 percent of women and 82 percent of their mates.[167] Whether there are lasting effects on these women and their marriages, future reproductive plans, or children has not been studied. Frequently, support and follow-up from geneticists and counselors is negligible.

Advancing the time of the diagnosis of untreatable disorders by predictive genetic testing may have harmful side effects. Usually, the clinical diagnosis of Duchenne muscular dystrophy is not made until after the age of 2 years. Detection of this disease by newborn screening might interfere with the bonding between a child and his parents.

Early identification of children at risk for adult-onset disease also has its problems. In a study of families in which one parent had hyperlipoproteinemic heart disease, children 2–19 years of age were tested for hyperlipidemia; they or their parents were informed of the results. Males with positive test results had significantly higher scores on attributes of impulsive hyperactive behavior than their unaffected brothers.[168] This is more likely due to labeling than to the disease itself. Bergman and Stamm have documented the unnecessary restrictions placed on children whose parents are told that their children have heart murmurs. Many of these children are subsequently diagnosed as not having cardiac pathology, yet for years their activities were severely restricted.[169] Questions have been raised about the propriety of reducing fat intake in young children,[170] but some pediatricians are already testing children at high risk, presumably because of their family history.[171] Definitive studies on the effectiveness of early dietary or drug interventions will not be available for many years. How parents and labeled children cope with these uncertainties is an important area for study.

That the harmful consequences of screening may exceed the beneficial ones was recently reported in a randomized controlled trial of an ongoing, routine developmental screening program. Preschool children were randomized to one of three groups: (1) those to whom the developmental screening test was given, whose parents were informed of the results, and who were referred for treatment due to positive test results; (2) those to whom the test was administered and who had positive results, but whose parents were not informed of the results and for whom no action was taken; or (3) those to whom the test was not given. Although the children with positive results in the first two groups had a higher rate of school problems than those with negative test results, the children with positive results who received interventions had no fewer problems and scored no better on intellectual and school achievement tests than those who did not receive the interventions. However, 68 percent of the parents of those with positive results in the first group, who knew the results, said they were worried about the child's schoolwork, compared to 35 percent of the parents who did not know the results.[172] If genetic tests for dyslexia or other specific learning disabilities are used before interventions are proven effective, labeling and parental worry may be the major consequences.

The anxiety generated by identifying young adults as at risk for late-onset disease may be enormous, particularly when the risks prior to testing were unknown by the person or were not very high (as in multifactorial disorders), and when the predictive value of a positive result is less than certainty. Will the daily functioning of people identified as at risk for cancer be impaired by excessive worry? Will positive tests for bipolar affective disorder become a self-fulfilling prophecy as those labeled as at risk, or their close relatives and friends, overreact to every change in mood? How much concern will forgetting a name cause a person who has been identified as susceptible to Alzheimer disease?

It is true that for dominant disorders like Huntington disease a negative test result will alleviate anxiety for those with a 50 percent chance of having the disease. But what about those with a positive test result? Of the 87 people at risk for Huntington disease in one of the surveys mentioned earlier who said they would want to be tested, 13 said they might commit suicide if their result was positive.[173]

Summary and Conclusions

Early in this chapter, I quoted some physicians who were willing to write off "a few suicides" for the benefits of widespread testing for venereal disease. I have closed with a description of the real danger of suicide from the introduction of genetic testing for late-onset disorders.

Suicide is not the only danger. Anxiety over the risks of future disease and personal (as well as political) conflict over the use of abortion to avoid the birth of affected progeny will occur as well. Most tests will give false positive results that, unless quickly proven to be false, will lead to unnecessary and sometimes dangerous interventions. When test results predict future disease, more harm than benefit may result, particularly when the predictive value is low, when the effectiveness of intervention has not been demonstrated, and when the magnitude of anxiety has not been anticipated. Labeling people as affected—whether they are or not—can have devastating results.

Fewer people will suffer harm from genetic testing if the dangers are averted before the new technology is widely transmitted. It is in the early stages of transmittance of DNA-based tests that the dangers are greatest.

First of all, the necessary regulatory mechanisms have not been adapted to the unusual aspects of these tests—namely, the need (in linkage studies) to test relatives, the frequent absence of confirmatory tests, and the use of tests to predict disease far into the future or even in the next generation. Yet manufacturers will continue to press for the marketing of tests, and the FDA may grant approval without considering all of the ramifications.

Second, the number of health care professionals needed to perform testing and related services is insufficient and current training is inadequate to ensure that many health care providers understand the limitations of the tests and communicate information about them in their patients' or clients' best interests. Yet financial and medicolegal pressures may force providers to perform the tests.

Third, many people are unaware of the importance of genetics and genetic tests to them personally, in terms of understanding how genes are transmitted and how genetic tests may confront them with difficult decisions. Yet people tend to accept testing after receiving minimal information. The extent to which testing is accepted varies according to the availability of a postnatal intervention, the nature of the disorder, the certainty afforded by the test, and other factors. The relatively low level of acceptance of carrier screening may be attributable to the community setting in which many of the programs are conducted. Acceptance might be more widespread if such testing was provided as part of routine medical care, but there might also be inherent resistance to such screening, leading to attempts to compel it (a topic I will consider in chapter 8).

At least one other problem discussed in this chapter affects the safety and effectiveness not only of genetic tests but of other tests as well: the quality of the laboratories performing the tests. As genetic tests become easier to perform, the number of laboratories in which they are processed will increase. I do not think it will be too long before some genetic tests are performed in physicians' office laboratories, now the fastest growing site of clinical testing. Unfortunately, quality control of hospital and commercial laboratories is inadequate in most states and virtually nonexistent for physicians' office laboratories in many.

As I will discuss in chapter 9, there are solutions to these problems. A thornier problem is how to increase the likelihood that persons coming for tests understand the implications and make decisions that are consonant with their own values. Unfortunately, much of the research in this area has been undertaken to maximize participation in programs rather than to assure understanding and autonomous decision making. We also have little understanding of the long-term consequences of identifying people as at risk for future disease or of having affected offspring.

If individual autonomy is to be preserved in genetic testing—as I believe it should be—an effective program must be developed that will enable people to choose the course of action that seems appropriate to them in view of their risk and, in the case of carrier and prenatal testing, their family goals. This is one of the commonly accepted objectives of genetic counseling.[174] To achieve it for testing, people must gain familiarity with the condition for which testing is proposed, be aware of the test's limitations, recognize the options available to them, and be able to choose freely among those options without pressure or penalty.

In this chapter I have touched on how autonomy can be unintentionally undermined by the ways in which risks are presented, by disparities in the perception of risk between health care providers and clients, and by a lack of awareness of clients' concerns. In chapter 8, I turn to ways in which autonomy can be intentionally undermined to satisfy the interests of persons other than those being tested.

Chapter 8

Testing: In Whose Best Interest?

In the previous chapter, I described the individuals who are candidates for genetic testing as the beneficiaries of the new DNA-based technology and the ones to decide whether or not to be tested. In this chapter, I deal with situations in which the decisions regarding testing or the release of test results are not left up to these individuals, at least not entirely, and may not be in their best interests. Such situations arise when the health care provider decides for the client, when tests are used in adoption or alternative reproductive procedures, when insurance companies use tests to exclude people from coverage and employers use them to deny employment, and, finally, when communities exert pressure on individuals to be screened. Each of these situations poses a potential conflict between the individual in whom testing is proposed and those who favor testing.

Do Doctors Know Best? Redressing the Physician-Patient Relationship

In the "old days," people sought medical care only when they were sick. Diagnostic tests were rudimentary, and tests predictive of future disease or of disease in one's offspring were nonexistent. Few effective drugs and surgical procedures were available, and the choice was whether to take the treatment at hand or not be treated at all. Medicine has changed drastically. Today, physicians not only treat disease but also have the tools to predict its future likelihood, which is something that not all patients expect or want. Genetic tests—among the newest additions to the armamentarium—provide information on aspects of life and reproduction for which physicians' advice was seldom sought in the past. Reproductive choices and decisions about life style are becoming increasingly medicalized. Yet some people would rather take their chances of having a child with a genetic disorder or of dying prematurely than have information on risks pressed on them.

The new biomedical technologies—among them, genetic tests—enhance the dominance of physicians over patients. Without inquiring too closely, physicians sometimes assume that their patients perceive the same need for tests as they do. At other times, they feel justified or even compelled to perform tests without informing their patients. The patient's trust in the physician—the basis of the physician-patient relationship—may be misplaced.

The knowledge a physician gains about his or her patients these days through the use of sophisticated tests is enormous. Even back in the nineteenth century, Nathaniel Hawthorne warned that under the powers of the skillful physician "will the soul of the sufferer be dissolved, and flow forth in a dark, but transparent stream, bringing all its mysteries into the daylight."[1] Today the mysteries of body fluids and genes are revealed as well. This information is often of interest to relatives, insurers and employers, and even the state, but revealing that information can undermine the physician-patient relationship.

Testing without informed consent

Obstetricians often perform tests on pregnant women without providing any explanation or obtaining consent. They justify not doing so by maintaining that they do not want to alarm women unnecessarily, since the tests will be normal in the vast majority of cases. This is a form of "therapeutic privilege," which permits physicians to withhold information from patients when providing it might have adverse health consequences. In a recent assessment of obstetricians' attitudes toward AFP screening for neural tube defects, 55 percent of the physicians surveyed were opposed to informed consent for the procedure.[2] My colleagues and I found little justification for their opposition. We found that women who were informed about maternal serum AFP testing were no more anxious than women who were not informed.[3]

Although physicians tend to overuse "therapeutic privilege,"[4] it might be legitimately invoked in deciding not to *offer* a test for a severe, untreatable disease to a patient at risk if the health care provider has good reason to fear that a positive result would cause the patient to take some drastic action, such as committing suicide. It is less likely that the physician would be considered justified in *performing* the test without first informing the client, and then revealing the result only if it was negative. Of course, if the patient knows the test is available, he or she may request that it be performed. Burke and Motulsky suggest that rather than unilaterally deciding not to offer testing when it may not be in the person's best interest, providers should discuss the implications with the patient and family and help them decide whether to proceed with testing. As they point out, "A full work-up of genetic disease may sometimes not be indicated."[5]

Another argument used against the informed-consent process is that it does not increase a person's understanding of a given procedure but takes a lot of time. Two studies conducted in Maryland have indicated significant increases in knowledge as a result of written disclosure prior to genetic screening. The costs in terms of health-professional time expended on both disclosure processes were negligible. In the first study, mothers were given a simple disclosure statement about newborn screening for phenylketonuria (PKU) and other metabolic disorders. One group of mothers was given a 29-point test of their knowledge prior to receiving the written disclosure; the other group was given the test after they had received the disclosure and signed the consent statement. Mothers in the first group scored significantly lower on the test than did those in the second group.[6]

In the second study, pregnant women's knowledge about maternal serum alpha-fetoprotein (MSAFP) screening for fetal neural tube defects was compared in two groups: those who had received a brochure about the procedure and either were waiting for the test or had already consented and had the test, and those who had not received the brochure. The knowledge of women in the first group about this type of screening was significantly greater than that of those in the second.[7]

Despite the increments in knowledge in both studies, many women's knowledge of the information in the disclosure statement remained incomplete, though they certainly were better prepared to make an informed decision after they had read the disclosure than before. It is interesting to note, however, that 60 percent of the women who consented to AFP screening reported that they had not discussed the test with their physician.

Medicolegal concerns may cause physicians to circumvent the informed-consent process. As one genetic counselor observed, some women come for prenatal diagnosis "because their doctors said they have to have it whether they want it or not."[8] The physician's fear of being sued by a woman who refuses testing and then has a baby with a detectable defect is probably greater than his or her worry about not informing a woman before drawing blood for prenatal prediction.[9] The courts have not yet ruled that a woman who would have refused testing (because, for instance, she opposed abortion) but who was not given the opportunity and was then told the result was positive has a basis for action.

When informed consent is needed

The legal basis for informed consent was enunciated by Justice Cardozo in 1914: "Every human being of adult years and sound mind has a right to determine what shall be done with his own body, and a surgeon who performs an operation without his patient's consent commits an assault for which he is liable in damages."[10] But consent is not needed for every "laying on of hands." The traditional basis for informed consent has been that disclosure is necessary only for those procedures for which it is customary. This basis is now giving way to requiring disclosure when a reasonable person would want to know. A few courts have gone even further and ruled in favor of plaintiffs who maintained they would not have undertaken the procedure if they had had full disclosure.[11] My colleagues and I found that about half of a representative sample of Maryland women who had just had babies favored informed consent for PKU screening, and 80 percent wanted to be informed prior to testing, even when the test was required and they did not have the right to refuse testing.[12] Given this finding, it is hard to argue that reasonable people would not want the opportunity to consent to, or refuse, any form of genetic testing.

Disclosing test results

A patient's personal physician undertakes genetic tests primarily for the benefit of the patient. Patients may be reluctant to convey test results to relatives (out of fear of being stigmatized or blamed for bad news or because they do not appreciate the risks to others) or to insurers or employers or prospective employers (for obvious reasons). Through discussion, the physician may be able to remove some, but certainly not all, of these concerns. Situations arise in which the patient refuses to permit the disclosure of information. Do laws and court rulings protect patient-physician confidentiality, or do they give physicians the right to disclose or perhaps even confer a duty to do so?

Most states have laws that penalize physicians for disclosing information in judicial proceedings or to third parties under most circumstances.[13] The basis for protecting confidentiality in patient-physician relationships is to ensure that the patient will not be deterred from seeking care out of fear that some finding will be disclosed to others. For instance, requiring that the results of testing for AIDS be made known might deter some people from being tested. Likewise, if stigmatization or refusal of insurance or employment resulted from a person's being a carrier of genetic disease, some people might refuse genetic testing.

Confidentiality can be breached when the patient is likely to cause direct harm to others by transmitting an infectious disease, performing a violent act, or endangering fellow workers or the public.

Disclosing to a spouse. Several court decisions state that a physician has a duty to warn either the patient or his family if there is a possibility that those living in the house with the patient might contract the disease by reason of its infectious nature.[14] Genetic disorders are not infectious but they are transmissible. If a person is a heterozygote for a genetic disease, he or she cannot transmit the disease-causing allele to any living person but can transmit it to offspring. Lori Andrews, a lawyer who has thoroughly studied the legal aspects of medical genetics, believes that "clearly there is a moral duty *on the part of the spouse* to disclose. However, it may not rise to the level of a legal right *on the part of the physician* to make such disclosure over the patient's protest."[15]

Cases regarding the communication of genetic information have apparently not been decided. Some court decisions involving disclosure of mental or intellectual findings on a patient to a spouse or fiancé(e) suggest that physicians have no legal right to disclose (*Schaffer v. Spicer*), while others suggest that they may, depending on the likelihood and extent of harm to the other party (*Berry v. Moench*).[16] Disclosure to a spouse has been upheld even when it threatened the marital relationship.[17]

A legal requirement for physicians to disclose genetic test results to a spouse might be advocated by those who maintain that the unborn have a "right" to be born free of avoidable disease, or by those who consider it a duty of prospective parents to keep future costs of care to a minimum by avoiding the birth of infants with costly but avoidable conditions. I will return to these arguments later in the chapter.

Disclosing to other relatives or a fiancé(e). Knowledge that a person carries a disease-causing allele may also be important to relatives who are at risk for the disease (if it is a dominant disorder) or of transmitting it to their offspring. Those who possess susceptibility-conferring alleles—for instance, a susceptibility to harmful reactions from certain drugs—may have relatives similarly at risk.

Texas law permits the disclosure of confidential information if the physician determines that physical injury to the patient or to others is imminent. In 1976, a California court ruled in the *Tarasoff* case that a psychiatrist has a legal obligation to warn a specific person whose life is endangered by the psychiatrist's patient.[18] Such precedents could have relevance to testing for alleles that confer a susceptibility to violent behavior toward oneself (e.g., bipolar affective disorder) or toward one's fiancé(e), spouse, or prospective children. Although the probability of harm may be increased by possessing a susceptibility-conferring allele, there is no assurance that the person will engage in violent behavior. This is quite a bit different from the *Tarasoff* case, in which a direct threat was made and subsequently carried out.

In 1983, the President's Commission for the Study of Ethical Problems in Medicine and Biomedical and Behavioral Research suggested that physicians may release genetic information to relatives without the patient's or client's consent provided certain conditions are met: (1) reasonable efforts to elicit voluntary consent to disclosure have failed; (2) there is a high probability both that harm will occur if the information is withheld and that the disclosed information could be used to avert harm; (3) the harm that identifiable individuals would suffer is serious; and (4) appropriate precautions are taken to ensure that only the genetic information needed for diagnosis and/or treatment of the disease in question is disclosed.[19]

A different view was taken in 1975 by the Committee for the Study of Inborn Errors of Metabolism of the National Academy of Sciences, which held that "under current law, genetic screeners would be ill advised to contact relatives without the screenee's explicit consent."[20] The Committee noted that the situation could be changed by requiring people coming for testing to agree in advance of the test to the release of pertinent information to relatives, or by having state legislatures enact statutes permitting or requiring professionals to disclose the information to relatives without consent of the person being tested. It added, however:

> Neither course of action is justified. . . . It is true that, in some individual cases, there is likely to be medical benefit from nonconsented disclosure to relatives. But there are broader social reasons that argue against pursuing these individual medical benefits in this way. Genetic screeners who contact possibly affected relatives are, of course, pressing unsolicited information on them. It is likely, in a significant number of cases, that these relatives will not want such information and will not be prepared (for ethical or emotional reasons) to benefit from it. Though relying on the consent of the initial patient screened does not guarantee that any relative contacted will welcome the genetic information, the possibility of benefit is at least increased when someone with personal knowledge of the relative has made the initial judgment that this information will be more useful than harmful.[21]

Lori Andrews has warned of the practical implications of establishing a precedent of warning relatives: "Exercising a right to disclose may ultimately set a standard creating a duty to disclose. The ramifications of such a duty could be awesome. Consider the burdens of tracking down all the close relatives in an instance of genetic disease."[22]

If the public's understanding of genetics increases concomitantly, fewer patients will feel stigmatized for having a genetic defect, and there will be very few situations in which the patient will not consent to disclosure to relatives. Moreover, as genetic testing becomes widespread, the likelihood that relatives will undergo testing independent of the patient who does not want the results communicated will increase. When such testing occurs, there is even less reason to breach confidentiality.

Disclosing to unrelated third parties. Generally a patient's consent is required before his or her personal physician releases medical information to third parties. Sometimes the patient may be unaware of the consequences of disclosing information in the record. It has been suggested that physicians discuss with their patients the implications of releasing information to third parties.[23] Physicians themselves may not realize the consequences, as I learned through personal experience. With the permission of a child's parents, I communicated to their son's school that the child had to have a special diet because he had PKU. Although it should have been apparent to his teachers that the child was functioning normally, he was placed in classes for the learning disabled. The school authorities knew that PKU was associated with mental retardation, but not that early dietary treatment could prevent it. Simply stating that the special diet was medically indicated would have sufficed.

For their part, parents will not always appreciate the wide dissemination of test results that indicate their child is at increased risk for a specific learning disability. Although such results may lead to a placement that will help the child attain a better outcome, they may also be used to stigmatize the child or to subject him or her to interventions that are not of proven value.

Many companies employ or contract with physicians to perform preemployment physicals, but the prospective employee is sometimes requested to have his or her physician supply the information. The physician's record may contain information that is not germane to the employee's ability to perform the job but that may still be used to deny employment. Physicians unwittingly provide information on employees when the employer requires that insurance reimbursement forms be processed within the company. (When an employer or insurance company employs its own health professionals to obtain medical information from workers or applicants, the traditional patient-physician relationship, and hence a duty of confidentiality, does not exist. Nevertheless, the company's physician frequently tells the employer only whether the person is fit to work or not [or is fit with certain restrictions], without divulging the reasons for the decision. Some courts have ruled that a third party's physician has no duty to disclose findings to the applicant, but others have given the opposite ruling.)[24]

When a statement from one's personal physician is required in order to obtain insurance, if the applicant does not consent to its release, he or she will not be insured. Physicians are liable if they supply fraudulent information. Once a person is insured, a personal physician's disclosure of information to third parties without the patient's consent depends on whether there is a public interest in disclosure. In a case in which a pediatrician did not tell the parents that their baby was born with a heart defect (and they then purchased life insurance), the father sued when the doctor told an insurance investigator, without the parents' consent, after the baby had died. The court ruled that once the father filed a claim, nondisclosure was no longer in the "public interest"[25] On the basis of the information provided by the pediatrician, the company refused to pay. In another case, however, the policyholders who filed a claim refused to consent to the insurance company's interviewing their physician. Recognizing the basis for confidentiality, the court held that the refusal should not prejudice the insurance claim.[26] There is, therefore, some ambiguity in defining the public interest.

In chapter 5, I briefly discussed the use of genetic tests in criminal proceedings. A basic tenet of the laws of confidentiality is that physicians cannot testify about a patient unless the patient waives confidentiality or the patient's condition is at issue, but courts can order testimony. Most courts have been highly protective of the confidentiality of medical records that are introduced in judicial proceedings, insisting that only relevant information be presented and ensuring that the disclosure remains within the courtroom.[27] Nevertheless, the "public interest" argument might be used to expand the release of genetic information in such cases.

Genetic tests are not an essential part of medical care, however, and if physicians are obliged to release results to third parties by expanding the scope of the "public interest," some people will forgo the personal benefits of knowing their future risks in order to protect their insurability, employability, or innocence.

Extension of the physician-patient relationship to other health care providers and DNA banks

The Hippocratic oath taken by physicians binds them to confidentiality. Other health care providers, such as genetic counselors, do not formally take such oaths. Nevertheless, in some states the confidentiality laws extend to other health care providers as well as to physicians, and in some cases the courts have extended the duty of confidentiality to cover people assisting physicians.[28]

Some university and commercial laboratories are already offering to store DNA for use in the future. Such DNA may be of great importance to the diagnosis of family members of an affected person via linkage studies. DNA is also the best "fingerprint" for a person's identity. A person's DNA could be used to determine paternity. With further advances in technology, it might not be too difficult to search through all the DNA in a donor bank to find the best match for someone in need of an organ transplant or, in the case of law enforcement agencies, to find a match with DNA obtained at the scene of a crime. It may also be of use to researchers. However, donors may object to the use of banked DNA for purposes other than the diagnoses or predictions for which they have expressly given consent. The same conflict between the patient's best interest and an overriding "public interest" arises here as in the release of genetic test results, but in the case of donor banks, the conflict can be more far-reaching. Referring to the banking of cell samples, the 1983 President's Commission commented: "It may be impossible at the time the material is placed in the system to know all the information that new tests might someday reveal."[29]

The Use of Genetic Tests in Adoption and Alternative Reproductive Procedures

Before a couple adopts a child, it may want to know whether the child is at risk for a genetic condition. Couples using sperm or ovum donation to avoid a recessive disease will want to know that the donor is not a carrier of an allele for the same disease. (That this occurs was indicated in a report of two siblings who died of a rare, autosomal recessive disorder, familial histiocytosis. Both were sired by sperm from the same donor.[30] In a 1985 survey of ten sperm banks, five were aware of births of children with genetic impairments.[31]) Couples will want to know that a woman who serves as a surrogate mother or who will transfer an embryo after being inseminated by the husband's sperm is not a carrier of the same disease-causing allele as the husband. Recipients will also want to know about other potentially deleterious genetic traits in the donor. In all of these cases, the genetic information, which could be obtained by testing, is obtained not for the primary benefit of the person being tested but for the adopting or receiving couple.

Adoption

At least thirteen states in this country have laws requiring that "genetic information" be obtained from biological parents and made available to adoptive parents.[32] As genetic tests become more widespread, they could be used instead of family histories to provide this information. At least ten states do not require genetic information.

Genetic information is usually made available without revealing the identity of the biological parents to the adoptive ones. It would therefore seem that there was little chance for any of the parties to be harmed. But what if the adoptive parents, or adoption agencies, wanted information on the risks of late-onset disorders, disorders that would not be likely to manifest in a biological parent at the time the parents placed the child for adoption? Testing the parents might reveal to them a propensity that they would prefer not to know about, although it might lead them to avoid having another affected child. Moreover, knowing that the adoptee was at risk for future disease might deter prospective parents from adopting.

These problems are not completely solved by testing the prospective adoptee rather than the biological parents. Again, if the test is positive, some parents will not adopt the child. Discovering that the child has a positive test result places one of the biological parents at risk. They might prefer not having the information.

In states in which genetic information need not be provided to adoptive parents, a parent whose adopted child manifests a detectable genetic disease might have a cognizable claim to damages for the extra costs of raising a child with the disorder. This threat of liability might increase the pressure on parents and adoption agencies to provide more complete genetic profiles of babies who are up for adoption, which in turn might increase the incidence of rejecting infants because of their genetic propensities.

Sperm and egg donors: Surrogate mothers

The American Fertility Society[33] and the American Association of Tissue Banks[34] have proposed guidelines for screening donors and rejecting those who demonstrate a significant risk of transmitting disease-causing or susceptibility-conferring genotypes or infectious agents, those who are carriers for the same disease-causing allele for a recessive disorder as one of the partners seeking donation, and those who are at increased risk of having offspring with chromosomal abnormalities. The guidelines could apply as well to women who agree to embryo transfer or surrogate motherhood following artificial insemination. Laws in Idaho and Oregon prohibit men who know they have a genetic defect from being sperm donors. These laws do not, however, provide for the genetic testing of potential donors. A new law in Ohio, as well as proposed statutes in Michigan and an ordinance in Washington, D.C., would require the genetic screening of donors.[35]

As long as there is a chance that the offspring of an alternative reproductive procedure will have a serious disease, such testing seems justified. In most cases, the contributor of the gamete is not a donor in the sense that he or she is making a gift, but rather is a "vendor" with something to sell. The buyer has more reason to beware in this transaction than in many others. It is not so easy to justify barring a "vendor" when he or she is the carrier of an allele for an autosomal recessive genetic disease for which the recipient parent is not; using such "vendors" would have a negligible effect on the gene pool. According to two surveys, a large proportion of sperm donors are willing to have information about themselves transmitted to the recipients, provided their identity is not revealed.[36]

The testing of donors (or vendors) is ordinarily undertaken for the benefit of recipients, but the question also arises as to whether donors should be informed of the results or referred for counseling. The tests may indicate that other offspring will be at risk. Some clinics follow a disclosure policy,[37] but other authorities have opposed it.[38] Some suggest discussing the issue with the donor beforehand.[39] In two Australian studies, virtually all donors wanted to know the reasons why their sperm were rejected.[40] Another study reported that donors did not feel stigmatized as a result of being rejected.[41] The duty to inform a donor might depend on whether there was a patient-physician relationship between the donor and the physician collecting the egg or sperm. This is almost certainly the case in ovum donation, but might be argued in sperm donation.

The Use of Genetic Tests by Insurance Companies

For a person to be sold an *individual* health or life insurance policy (at specified premium and conditions), the insurance company must determine what risk the person has of suffering an insured event: death in the case of life insurance; sickness, disability, or hospitalization in the case of health insurance. Medical information, which could include genetic test results, is used by insurers to determine whether an individual's risk exceeds that expected for other persons of the same age. Premiums are commensurate with risks. When the risks are too high, insurance will not be sold.

People who have *group* insurance do not usually have to provide medical information once they are in the group. The amount the group pays for insurance, however, is based on the risks of insured events experienced by people like those in the group. Consequently, if a group wants to keep its rate down, it will admit only people at low risk to the group. It determines risk by obtaining medical information at the time of admission to the group. About 65 percent of all people in the United States receive their health insurance through their employers.[42] Later in this chapter, I will discuss how employers who provide group coverage might use genetic tests on job applicants to exclude people who are likely to increase the cost of their insurance benefits. In this section, I will focus on individual insurance.

Slightly more Americans have individual life insurance than have group policies,[43] but many more have group health insurance than have individual policies.[44] About 50 percent of all "individual" health policies are written to cover family members as well. Individual insurance is purchased by those who are not eligible for group insurance, including employees of small companies that do not provide group insurance as a benefit, the self-employed, single parents whose insurance may be supported by a divorce settlement, students, new entrants into the labor force (who must work for a period before they become eligible), the unemployed, and those who want to supplement their group coverage.

The use of medical information

Information on an individual's medical history (and family members' histories when they are covered as well) is required on the forms that applicants are expected to complete themselves. If the response suggests that the applicant is at increased risk for a disease, or if the applicant is in a certain age or occupational category, additional information may be requested. This can be obtained from the personal physician, with the applicant's permission. Usually the physician is reimbursed for providing the information. Occasionally the applicant's physician may be asked to repeat a test or supply additional information.

Increasingly, instead of a physician's statement, insurers request that an examination be performed by registered nurses or physicians' assistants who are employed by multistate companies subject to state licensing. Blood and urine collected by paramedics are sent to central laboratories for further testing. Applicants are not told what specific tests will be performed (except when a test for AIDS is requested). Two of the laboratories used by most insurance companies (Home Office Reference Laboratory and Gibraltar Laboratory) are themselves subsidiaries of insurance companies. These laboratories perform a wide range of tests and report the results to the companies. Through their use of paramedics and centralized laboratories, insurance companies have considerable control over the type of medical information collected. Certainly they could perform genetic screening as such tests become available.

Underwriting. The use of medical and other information in determining an individual's insurability is known as "underwriting." The underwriter for a company may decide that a person is uninsurable, that a higher rate should be charged commensurate with increased risk, or that certain conditions should be excluded from coverage. The following list gives examples of genetic or gene-influenced conditions for which insurance companies have unconditionally denied medical or disability insurance or have granted conditional coverage:

Unconditional denial
Sickle cell anemia
Aplastic anemia
Angina pectoris
Arteriosclerosis
Huntington chorea
Insulin-dependent
   diabetes
Down syndrome
Polycycstic kidney
Muscular dystrophy

Conditional denial
Ankylosing spondylitis (within
   5 years)
Rheumatoid arthritis (active, or inactive less than two years)
Autism (under 21 years of age)
Spina bifida (unoperated or within
   one year of operation)
Duodenal or gastric ulcer (multiple
   attacks within past year)
Narcolepsy (within 2 years of last
   episode)

Antiselection. People who know that they are at increased risk for disease may well seek to purchase more insurance than they ordinarily would in order to protect themselves or their family against the anticipated event. This includes people who are covered through group insurance.[45] If the insurance company does not have knowledge of their increased risk, it will sell insurance to such people at the standard premium and without exclusions. As the anticipated events occur, the insurance company will pay out in claims a higher proportion of its premiums than it expected. It will, consequently, lose money or have to increase the premium. Increasing the premium means that fewer people will be able to buy insurance. To avoid this "antiselection," the insurance company protects itself in three ways.

First, if a preexisting condition is discovered by the insurance company within two years after the policy is sold, the policy can be canceled or rewritten. Preexisting conditions are those that have impaired the applicant's health to some degree. But what if the "preexisting" condition is a genetic test result that indicates the applicant will develop disease? It seems quite likely that if underwriters discovered such a result, they could cancel the policy. Whether their cancellation would be upheld in court might depend on the predictive value of the test in question. It seems unlikely that the discovery that a new family policyholder had previously been identified through genetic testing to be a carrier for a disease that places his or her offspring at risk (regardless of whether the spouse is a carrier as well) would permit the company to alter or cancel the policy. Being a heterozygote is not a condition in the usual medical sense. Moreover, in this instance the maximum chance that an offspring will be affected is 25 percent.

Second, the underwriter will determine if other insurance companies have information on the applicant that it does not have. More than 700 insurance companies belong to the Medical Information Bureau (now called MIB, Inc.) to guard against fraud and to make available to one another significant medical findings and test results on some applicants for health and life insurance. This process is explained to applicants, and their authorization of the insurance company to use MIB is part of their completed application for coverage. An underwriter's discovery that the current application does not contain all the information that appears in the MIB file alerts the underwriter to the possibility of untrue answers and usually leads to a request for more information. If the latter supports the information contained in the MIB file, the applicant may be refused insurance.

An official of MIB, Inc., stated recently that MIB did not "currently collect or store genetic data. . . . This does not mean to say, however, that should a highly accurate predictive test be developed the insurance industry would not give serious consideration to using the results in the underwriting process."[46]

Third, the insurance company will use predictive tests, or request results if they have been performed elsewhere, to avoid antiselection. It is important to note that once one insurance company adopts such tests for underwriting, others must follow suit. By excluding people on the basis of the test, a company can lower its standard premium and gain a competitive advantage. Individuals who test positive will turn to companies that do not use the test and will succeed in getting insurance at the old standard premium. But as they suffer events at greater than the expected rate, they will cost the company more money. To avoid this chain of events, all companies are likely to adopt predictive tests once one does so. The other side of the coin of excluding people at risk is that more people not at risk may be able to afford insurance at the lower standard premium.

As I mentioned in chapter 7, insurance companies today not only are not requiring the few genetic tests that are available but also sometimes are not reimbursing for them. They are beginning to recognize, however, that failure to reimburse for genetic tests and counseling provided by genetic services could "result in increased, long term medical costs associated with many of the diseases detected during genetic screening and laboratory tests."[47] As this recognition dawns, companies may begin to require genetic test results for some disorders as a condition of insurability.

The use of predictive genetic tests

Genetic tests that predict the occurrence of a disease that, if it were present at the time of application, would render the person uninsurable (or not insurable at the standard premium) might be used to deny or limit insurance. For instance, life insurance for a person with clinically diagnosed bipolar affective disorder is now written at approximately twice the standard rate. With the use of a predictive test, asymptomatic people found by the test to be at risk, even if currently insured at the standard rate, will have to pay a higher premium. Similar situations would hold for medical insurance for the conditions listed on page 195 (and also for life insurance for conditions that result in premature death). It is true that where traditionally a family history of a late-onset dominant disorder has been used to deny insurance to *all* of the asymptomatic offspring at risk (as is often the case for children of a person with Huntington disease), genetic tests now will permit half of those offspring to obtain insurance. But as genetic tests are developed for more conditions and for use in the general population, people who are now able to get insurance at standard premiums will be denied coverage. Overall, genetic tests will result in fewer people being insured.

Tests that predict the risk of having children with certain diseases might also be used to deny or limit family coverage to couples in whom both partners are carriers of the alleles for an autosomal recessive disorder. In family policies, unborn as well as born children are automatically covered until at least their eighteenth year. The use of predictive genetic tests would entail a change in current policy, for tests are seldom requested now for healthy applicants of reproductive age. A number of the disorders listed on page 195 can be diagnosed prenatally and are not insurable. These include sickle cell anemia, spina bifida, Down syndrome, Huntington disease, and muscular dystrophy. It is possible that companies will decide to grant family policies with the rider that only children without these defects are eligible for coverage. This would put pressure on persons at risk to avoid the conception or birth of affected offspring.

Social Security provides some protection to surviving spouses of covered persons and to the disabled. Consequently, there is a cushion of sorts for people who are denied life or disability insurance on the basis of genetic test results. For people under the age of 65 who are denied medical or hospitalization insurance because of genetic test results (and are ineligible for Medicare), a major out-of-pocket health crisis could drive them into poverty.

Criteria for choosing genetic tests

Before electing to use predictive tests in underwriting, insurance companies will require that the tests (and the diseases they predict) satisfy a number of criteria.

Timeliness. Diseases that will manifest or result in death soon after a policy is written are of greater interest than diseases that will appear later. The former are more costly in claims compared to premiums already paid. Moreover, in those instances there is less of a chance that an unrelated condition will appear in the interim. Most people obtain individual insurance before the age of 45, so tests for diseases that appear in middle life are of greatest concern to underwriters.

Cost. Insurers are unlikely to pay for expensive tests. Cost reductions can be anticipated as the technology for DNA-based tests becomes simplified. The time it takes to obtain test results is another component of costs to which insurers are sensitive. If a company insists on tests that its competitors do not require, and these add time to processing an individual's application, the company's competitive position will be adversely affected. The addition of many new tests or the routine genetic testing of applicants of reproductive age would entail significant costs that could be justified only by the savings they would lead to through reduced future claims.

Reliability. Poor reliability increases the likelihood that people subject to the test will be mislabeled. Insurance companies have no assurance of the reliability of test results reported by applicants' personal physicians. The use of central laboratories gives insurers greater confidence in the test results, provided these laboratories institute stringent quality assurance procedures or are required to do so by state or federal laws (see chapter 7).

Specificity and predictive value. Applicants for insurance who are denied coverage because of positive test results but who never develop the disease represent losses of low-risk customers to insurers. The use of tests of low specificity, regardless of the frequency of the disorder, and tests of high specificity for rare conditions can result in the needless loss of applicants. For instance, using a perfectly sensitive test with a specificity of 0.990 to detect a disease that has a prevalence of 1 in 1,000 will result in ten false positives for every true positive. Whether such a test is worth using will depend on whether the claims payments anticipated from the one true positive are greater than the dollars lost by excluding ten false positives and by performing the test.

Sensitivity. The chance that a test will fail to detect people with a disease makes that test less attractive to insurers. Nevertheless, every person at risk for developing the disease who is excluded from standard coverage as a result of the test saves the company claims payouts. If this anticipated saving is greater than the costs of the test—even if there are false negatives—insurers should be interested in adopting the test. Nevertheless, a highly specific predictive test (e.g., for low-density lipoprotein (LDL) receptor defects predicting coronary artery disease) might be preferred over a less specific one of somewhat greater sensitivity (e.g., cholesterol determinations) because it will result in the denial of insurance to fewer people.

Limiting the use or impact of genetic tests by insurance companies

With the exception of self-insured companies, which are regulated by the federal government under the Employee Retirement Income Security Act (ERISA—see below), insurance companies are regulated by the individual states within whose jurisdiction they operate. Consequently, it is the states that can prevent rate discrimination based on test results or that can bar the use of tests. In the early 1970s some insurance companies charged blacks with the sickle cell trait higher rates, even though they were not at a significantly greater risk for any disease or for a shortened life span than blacks who did not have the trait.[48] This unfair discrimination apparently has ended, in some cases as a result of state action. If an insurance company could show that the disease predicted by a test did increase its claims, state insurance commissioners would probably rule that higher premiums were justified.

In situations in which positive genetic test results do justify increased premiums on the basis of the principle "premium rates commensurate with risks," barring the use of tests is an alternative. Several states and the District of Columbia have prohibited or limited the use of tests for risk of AIDS for insurance purposes.[49] Another law in the District of Columbia prohibits discrimination against carriers of metabolic (genetic) disorders. One problem with this approach is that companies may stop doing business in states or jurisdictions that impose such restrictions, particularly if the fraction of their business that would be lost is small.

A New Jersey statute calls for consultation between the Department of Health and the Commissioner of Insurance to identify arbitrary and unreasonable discrimination against people with hereditary disorders and their families in insurance coverage. Maryland law empowers the state's Commission on Hereditary Disorders to investigate, and make recommendations to end, unjustified discrimination that might result from the identification of a person as a carrier of a genetic disorder.[50] It should be noted that in both New Jersey and Maryland, "reasonable" discrimination—that is, discrimination based on true increases in risk—might be tolerated. It is not permissible to use race in setting premiums, although risks differ between races. Some states do not permit sex to be used either. The result is that the race or sex at lower risk pays a higher premium than it would if these factors were used in rate setting, but society has made a judgment that social equity is more important.

If genetic tests are not barred, more people will join the 37 million who are already without any form of health insurance. Fifteen states have attempted to provide coverage to people who cannot get private insurance, by establishing special funds to cover people who are at high risk.[51] Some people with genetic diseases who do not qualify for private health insurance have already joined these high-risk pools. In some states, insurance companies are required to pay into these pools, but self-insured employers are exempt from having to pay because they are regulated by federal statute (ERISA). As a result of inadequate funding, the premiums are high and individuals often must pay coinsurance costs and deductibles.

Genetic Testing by Employers

In the early 1980s, a preplacement or preemployment examination was used in 88 percent of companies with over 500 workers, in 56 percent of companies with 100–499 workers, and 27 percent of firms with fewer than 100 workers.[52] Standards in the Occupational Safety and Health Act of 1970 regarding examinations of certain workers state: "The examination shall include the personal history of the employee, family and occupational background, including genetic and environmental factors."[53] In a memo dated 22 August 1980, the Occupational Safety and Health Administration (OSHA) indicated that the standards do not require genetic testing of any employee, nor do they require the exclusion of otherwise qualified employees on the basis of genetic testing.[54] Nothing in the memo, however, prohibits genetic testing. Although only a few companies include genetic tests in their examinations, the picture could change as tests become more widely available.

The reasons why employers use genetic tests

Both government and private employers use a variety of tests on prospective and current employees. These include tests for drugs and the risk of AIDS, back X-rays, polygraph tests, and tests for cigarette smoking.[55] Their reasons for doing so include concerns about the person's ability to perform the job; the safety of coworkers, the public, or the employer's property; workers' compensation costs; and insurance and pension costs. Genetic tests could be used for virtually all of these purposes. Some employers have also encouraged voluntary, confidential testing of employees as part of health promotion or wellness programs. Genetic tests could be included in such programs, too. I described one biotechnology company's interest in such testing in chapter 6.

Job performance and safety. Genetic disorders that are not evident at the time of hiring but whose occurrence is predicted by genetic tests could interfere with job performance and safety. An apparently healthy airline pilot at risk for one of the gene-influenced forms of heart disease could suffer a heart attack in flight, endangering all on board. Some persons with retinitis pigmentosa insidiously lose their sight in adult life, beginning with night blindness and resulting in their impaired ability to perform jobs requiring visual acuity. Manic-depressive disorder or Huntington disease could influence on-the-job performance as well as absenteeism.

Worker's compensation and liability claims. Workers found by genetic tests to have susceptibilities to workplace exposure not only may exhibit greater absenteeism as a result of their susceptibility but also may make a larger than usual number of claims under workers' compensation laws. Claims for a disease resulting from workplace exposure, but in which a susceptibility (genetic or otherwise) played a role, would probably qualify for workers' compensation.[56] Because the amount an employer pays for workers' compensation insurance is determined by the past compensation record of the employer, employers might use genetic tests to detect and exclude those with genetic predispositions. I was recently told of an individual with a congenital physical handicap (spina bifida) who was given a job only after he waived his right to make worker's compensation claims. Yet he would be at greater risk for an on-the-job accident because of his disability.[57]

A small amount of testing in the workplace has already been reported.

A survey conducted for the Congressional Office of Technology Assessment (OTA) in 1982 found that seventeen large companies were testing or had tested employees for sickle cell anemia, glucose-6-phosphate dehydrogenase deficiency, or alpha-1-antitrypsin deficiency.[58] Following the discovery of an at-risk employee, the most frequent action taken by a company was to inform the person of a potential problem. Five companies transferred the at-risk employees, three asked them to use a personal protection device, and two suggested that the employees obtain other jobs.

At one Du Pont Company plant, employees found to be sickle cell trait carriers who had hemoglobin concentrations of less than 14 g/dl were restricted from handling certain chemicals.[59] Because screening was not performed for other genetic conditions that might also result in hemoglobin concentrations below 14 g/dl (such a value *might* indicate borderline anemia), and because persons with sickle cell trait might well have hemoglobin concentrations below the cutpoint for reasons entirely unrelated to their sickle cell status, the procedure was clearly discriminatory. In addition to screening employees already on the job, as in this case, Du Pont also screened black job applicants for sickle cell trait. Dr. Bruce Karrh, corporate medical director of Du Pont, told a congressional subcommittee in 1981 that the program was voluntary and was for the employees' "education and edification," but he admitted that the company had no education or counseling program. Moreover, Du Pont officials and federal regulatory agencies had access to the test results without employee consent.[60]

For many years, the United States Air Force Academy screened applicants for sickle cell trait and denied them entry because of alleged dangers to carriers. The policy has been reversed.[61] However, the recent report of an increased risk of sudden, unexplained death of those with sickle cell trait during extremely strenuous basic military training[62] may rekindle discrimination against those with the trait.

It is doubtful that current tests can detect predispositions to harm from workplace exposures with sufficient accuracy to justify the testing or removal of susceptible workers. The OTA report concluded "that the data were not extensive enough to draw any conclusions on the correlation between given genetic traits and risk for disease." In view of the genetic variations in response to chemicals and drugs that are already known (see chapter 3), and the capabilities of recombinant DNA technology to locate and identify susceptibility-conferring genotypes, it is only a matter of time before additional tests will be developed. Even then, however, it is likely that for many chemicals a continuous gradient of susceptibility will be found instead of a situation in which one group of people is highly susceptible while everyone else is resistant. When there are several different variant alleles, each conferring a different degree of susceptibility, drawing a line between "susceptible" and "resistant" will be arbitrary.

Some physical and chemical agents encountered in the workplace (or elsewhere—e.g., cigarette smoke) will have multiple toxic effects. Persons genetically less susceptible to the harmful effect for which screening is performed may be more susceptible to other effects, for which screening is not available. Reducing ambient levels of toxic substances in the workplace will be to the advantage of all workers. Screening for genetic susceptibilities will not.

Women who suffer work-related illnesses are limited to filing claims under workers' compensation, but their liveborn children who have suffered damage in utero can sue for personal damages. Fear of such liability suits, the settlement of which may be much more costly than a compensation claim, is one of the reasons why a number of companies refuse to employ women in jobs that pose reproductive hazards.[63] Women have won lawsuits because these policies discriminated against them unfairly: the substances may pose reproductive hazards to men as well. Such an argument might not be supportable if employers excluded women who, on the basis of genetic tests, were predisposed to having infants with birth defects as a result of workplace exposures during pregnancy.

If and when genetic testing for a susceptibility became standard practice, an employer who did not perform the test might be liable for failure to detect an employee's propensity to suffer a work-related condition.[64] The Federal Employers' Liability Act (FELA) permits interstate railroad employees to bring actions for negligence against their employers in federal or state courts. Consequently, employers who "fail to give a pre-employment back X-ray and as a result of that unnecessarily expose the particular employee to a hazard that he would have avoided had [the employer] given him the X-ray . . . are open to unlimited liability under the . . . Act in the event the employee is in fact injured."[65] Such suits, however, have apparently not been brought.[66]

Insurance and pensions. Insurance costs are the largest single component of employee benefits, which constitute 37 percent of total payroll costs.[67] Employers of large numbers of workers usually pay at least part of the costs of health insurance for their workers through group plans. As I mentioned earlier, enrollment in group insurance plans does not usually require medical information.[68] Consequently, individuals within the group who do not qualify for individual insurance are still covered. The inclusion of such individuals increases the costs of insurance to employers.[69] Although these costs could be passed on to consumers in terms of higher prices, from the point of view of competition with other companies (and to maximize profit) an alternative policy would be to keep the costs as low as possible. This is accomplished by requiring medical information, which could include genetic test results, at the time of hiring. Either workers found to be at risk for high utilization of insurance benefits could be refused employment or the particular disease for which they are at risk could be excluded from coverage on the basis of their susceptibility.

Increasingly, large firms are "self-insuring"; rather than paying the group premiums to insurance companies, they are paying claims directly, either by administering the plan themselves or by hiring third-party administrators. In 1985 more than one-fourth of workers receiving employee health benefits were covered under self-insured plans, more than double the proportion in 1980.[70] Employers that self-insure may use tests and other information that some states deny to insurance companies.[71] Thus employers that self-insure can use tests, such as those for antibodies to the AIDS virus, that insurance companies are prohibited from using in some states.

Only one-third of employers with fewer than ten employees provide group health insurance. With such a small number of workers, an extra expense incurred by one employee could not be covered by the total payments for the group unless such payments were very high. Small companies may, however, pay part of the costs of their employees' individual insurance.[72] When employers pay at least part of the health insurance premium for individual insurance for their employees, they also have incentive to deny employment to those who are unlikely to qualify for insurance at the standard rate. They may find it too costly, however, to set up their own medical examination program.

Proposed federal legislation requiring employers to provide health insurance for their workers is intended to reduce the number of people without such insurance. Unless, however, rigid controls are set on the medical information used to screen potential employees, such legislation might result in the exclusion of people at high risk for future disease. Faced with having to extend coverage, employers might have a greater incentive to screen out high-risk workers to keep their insurance costs down.

Having a work force free of latent or potential disease will reduce health insurance costs, but it will not reduce pension costs if these workers live longer. (In general, the costs to employers of group life insurance are relatively insignificant compared to pension costs.) Theoretically, pension costs could be reduced by hiring workers in whom genetic or other tests revealed a high probability of death at around age 65 from, for instance, coronary heart disease. So too would hiring smokers, who have a greater chance of dying prematurely. Pension expenditures loom farther in the future than expenditures for medical insurance, and consequently they may not be of immediate concern to current management.[73]

Sharing medical information

Just as insurance companies protect against antiselection by sharing information, so do some employers. Companies have been reported to circulate lists of employees who have filed work-injury lawsuits.[74] Reports that workers have filed more than one such suit might reveal workers who have genetic or other susceptibilities and who might file gain. Such injuries, of course, may have occurred through no fault of the worker. A more direct way of sharing information about susceptibilities would be to share records on genetic test results. But because employers do not have to provide reasons for not hiring, job applicants with susceptibilities identified by preemployment genetic tests may never know why they have difficulty securing employment.

The Occupational Safety and Health Act permits employees in certain industries to have access to some of their records, but this does not apply to job applicants or to workers in nonregulated industries. A survey of the Fortune 500 companies indicated that 83 percent of the respondents denied workers access to their employee records.[75] The percentage may decrease as more states pass worker right-to-know laws, but these laws may not permit workers to examine their entire medical record. Right-to-know laws are often limited to informing workers of their exposure to specific toxic substances.

The criteria for choosing genetic tests

Before adding genetic tests to the existing battery of information collected in preplacement examinations, employers will consider the costs of new tests in relation to the benefits to be derived from them. Many of the considerations discussed for insurance companies would apply to employers too, with one important difference. In the presence of an abundant supply of labor, employers will be less concerned about screening out potential workers with (false) positive test results who would never develop the disease.

The money employers save by refusing to hire workers on the basis of genetic tests may well increase societal costs. If all employers drawing from a given labor market use tests for common predispositions, workers with positive results will find themselves excluded from most jobs. Government programs may eventually pick up the unemployment and health benefits costs for these individuals.

Limitations on the use of predictive genetic tests by employers

The Fourth Amendment protection against "unreasonable searches and seizures" may insulate federal and state employees from compulsory testing, but certain tests, such as for drug usage, have been deemed reasonable and are currently under judicial review. The relationship between private employers and employees, which is based on principles of contract, is beyond the reach of the Bill of Rights. However, private firms engaged in interstate commerce are subject to federal regulation. A number of federal and state statutes provide workers in the public and private sectors with some protection against discrimination based on predictive testing.

Title VII of the Civil Rights Act. This section of the law prohibits discrimination in the hiring, discharge, or terms of employment on the basis of race, color, religion, sex, or national origin. Refusal to hire those at risk for diseases that are more prevalent in certain groups covered by the Act, such as sickle cell anemia or thalassemia, could be a violation. Policies whose intent is not discriminatory but whose consequences are would be in violation (disparate impact). Thus the Equal Employment Opportunity Commission ruled that an employer violated Title VII by refusing to hire a black woman because she had sickle cell anemia, a disease found predominantly among blacks. The employer argued that it would reject all applicants with sickle cell anemia, regardless of race.[76]

In disparate-impact cases, discriminatory practices are permissible if they are based on "business necessity" or "job relatedness." The business necessity of denying employment arises from the need to maintain a safe and efficient operation of the business when there is no acceptable alternative. Under job relatedness, persons can be denied employment only when they cannot perform the job for which they are being evaluated. For instance, individuals found to have a genetic susceptibility to a workplace exposure might be legitimately refused employment or discharged under Title VII. It is doubtful that higher insurance costs per se, which result from having a racially related genetic condition, would qualify as a business necessity or job-related exclusion under Title VII or other legislation discussed here.[77] Section 704(a) of Title VII might permit an employee to refuse to submit to a genetic test that was perceived to be discriminatory.

Federal and state laws to protect the handicapped. Title VII of the Civil Rights Act does not prohibit denying employment to those at risk for diseases that are not associated with specific groups protected by the Act. Such individuals might, however, be protected under the Rehabilitation

Act of 1973, which affords protection to handicapped employees of the federal government and of federal contractors and other recipients of federal funds. Under the Act, the handicap must be "substantial," but it need not be apparent at the time of job placement. Individuals "regarded" as being impaired because they are believed likely to become so in the future are protected by the Act.[78]

Thus far, the courts have ruled only in cases in which the risk of future impairment was based on disease that had been clinically manifest in the past but was in remission at the time of the disputed decision regarding hiring or continued employment. In *School Board of Nassau Co. v. Arline*,[79] the United States Supreme Court explicitly refused to rule on whether the Act covered a person who had never had symptoms of a disease but who had a positive test indicating that the disease might develop. Most experts believe, however, that the Court would extend protection of the Act to asymptomatic carriers. In general, the courts have been more supportive of employer actions taken against workers because of the workers' possible threat to the safety of others than of actions taken because the workers' behavior or illness threatens their own health.[80]

Most states have passed laws extending protection of the handicapped to jobs that are not covered by federal law. They vary considerably in terms of who they would protect. At one extreme, North Carolina and Illinois limit protection to those with physical and mental conditions that interfere with the performance of major life functions.[81] Unless job applicants or employees can demonstrate such a condition to be present, they are not protected. Such laws would not afford protection to those found at risk for future disease by genetic testing. At the other extreme, courts in the state of Washington have maintained that any condition that prevents normal function in some way is a potential handicap and that people with such conditions are protected by the state's law. Moreover, discrimination is permissible only when the individual cannot perform the specific job.[82]

A Maryland law states that "an employer may not require an applicant to answer any questions, written or oral, pertaining to any physical, psychological, or psychiatric illness, disability, handicap or treatment which does not bear a direct, material, and timely relationship to the applicant's fitness or capacity to properly perform the activities or responsibilities of the desired position."[83] The law permits a medical evaluation, but only "for the purpose of assessing an applicant's ability to perform a job." Persons denied employment because a genetic test result indicated an increased risk of future disease would be considered to have a protected handicap unless the disease had "a direct, material, and timely relationship" to the applicant's ability to perform the job.

Court decisions in states in which job relatedness of the handicap must be shown in order for discrimination to be permitted suggest that positive genetic test results will have to have a high predictive value before they can be used to deny employment.[84] Tests that predict disorders whose expressivity is not certain may not qualify. It has not been determined how high a test's predictive value must be. In addition, discrimination will be permitted only when no reasonable accommodation by the employer will permit the handicapped individual to perform the necessary job functions. When genetic tests are used to detect persons susceptible to harmful reactions from chemical or physical agents in the workplace, the question of what constitutes reasonable accommodation must be considered.

Under the Occupational Safety and Health Act, the secretary of labor must set exposures to potentially toxic substances at levels at which "no employee" will suffer ill effects even when exposed for an entire working lifetime, but the additional language that permissible exposure levels (PELs) must be established to the "extent feasible" makes it doubtful that the most sensitive workers will be protected.[85] Screening to detect hypersusceptible workers who would suffer harm at exposures below the PELs and denying them jobs involving such exposures would be one way of "protecting" such workers from harm.

State laws prohibiting tests for specific conditions. Florida, Louisiana, New Jersey, and North Carolina prohibit discrimination in employment based on sickle cell trait.[86] The New Jersey statute also prohibits employment discrimination based on an individual's "atypical hereditary cellular or blood trait." This is defined to include hemoglobin C trait, thalassemia trait, Tay-Sachs trait, cystic fibrosis trait, as well as sickle cell trait. Presumably, discrimination against homozygotes with these disorders is permissible under these laws.

The Employee Retirement Income Security Act. Under section 510 of the Employee Retirement Income Security Act (ERISA), an employer cannot discharge an employee for the purpose of reducing health insurance or other benefit costs. Section 510 does not apply to job applicants, so it affords no protection against unlimited predictive testing of them. This contrasts with the statutes dealing with the handicapped, which cover both hiring and promotion.

Collective bargaining agreements. Labor unions could play a role in determining the use of predictive testing through collective-bargaining negotiations. In fulfillment of its duty to serve the interest of all its workers, a union would be expected to oppose predictive testing that discriminated against employees. It is under no obligation, however, to negotiate in the area of medical examinations. When the hiring of high-risk individuals jeopardizes the safety or welfare of the majority of workers, unions might not wish to oppose testing that would result in the exclusion of high-risk workers. On the other hand, when tests are used solely to lower employer costs, unions would be more inclined to oppose them.

Although unions can choose to negotiate the matter of preemployment medical examinations, in most contracts new employees can be fired during a probation period without union involvement. Unions have played a role in limiting employers' access to the results of medical examinations and tests in voluntary employee health-promoting programs. Even if unions are vigorous in opposing predictive tests, a declining proportion of U.S. workers will be covered by collective-bargaining agreements. Fewer than 25 percent of all nonagricultural workers belonged to unions in 1980, compared to 31 percent in 1970.[87] The percentage is even lower now.

Genetic Testing in the "Public Interest"

Some people object to virtually every use of genetic tests. Their objections are based on moral or religious beliefs (which do not permit any action, such as avoidance, should a positive result be found), on an acceptance of pain and suffering (which others would reject), on a fear of discrimination or reprisal, on a right to privacy, on a reluctance to "mend one's ways" in order to stay healthy or live longer, or on ignorance. The last reason can (and should) be overcome, but when it is, people still refuse testing for all of the other reasons.

At the other extreme, some people argue that to refuse genetic testing is not in the public interest. To them, personal autonomy is not sacrosanct. Their arguments fall into two categories, utility and compassion.

The utilitarian argument

Utilitarians argue that if people at risk for genetic diseases can be identified, actions can be taken that will lead to the greater good for the greater number. Refusing insurance to high-risk people means lower premiums for others. Refusing employment to workers with genetic susceptibilities means lower production costs and perhaps lower prices. Carrier testing, prenatal diagnosis, and abortion of affected fetuses reduces the burden on medical resources, thereby lowering the costs of medical care for all who share in its payment (whether through public or private channels).

In his presidential address to the American Association for the Advancement of Science in 1970, the prominent geneticist Bentley Glass summed up the utilitarian position: "In an overpopulated world it can no longer be affirmed that the right of the man and woman to reproduce as they see fit is inviolate. . . . No parents will . . . have the right to burden society with a malformed or mentally incompetent child. Just as every child must have the right to full educational opportunity and a sound nutrition, so every child has the inalienable right to a sound heritage."[88] Glass spoke at the dawn of the era of carrier screening and prenatal diagnosis. He was well aware of this as he spoke: "Unlimited access to state-regulated abortion will combine with the now perfected techniques of determining chromosome abnormalities in the developing fetus to rid us of the several percentages of all births that today represent uncontrollable defects such as mongolism (Down's syndrome) and sex deviants such as the XYY type. Genetic clinics will be constructed to which, before long, as many as 100 different recessive hereditary defects can be detected in the carriers, who may be warned against or prohibited from having offspring."[89]

Biotechnology companies that develop tests will profit from the widest possible use of genetic testing. At the companies I visited, I repeatedly heard the argument that society should not be compelled to pay for genetic disorders if testing could, through early detection, reduce their burden. It is not surprising that most of the companies with an interest in tests predicted an increased use of testing by insurers and employers by the year 2000 (table 8.1).

Table 8.1 Predictions of Biotechnology Companies with Interests in Genetic Tests on Uses and Implications of Tests by the Year 2000

Occurrence by the year 2000	Number of companies	
	Likely	Unlikely
Mandatory genetic testing	8	5
Employers use genetic tests to:		
Screen job applicants	6	6
Exclude susceptible workers	10	2
Insurance companies use genetic tests to evaluate applicants	8	4
Increased use of abortion services	9	4
Stigmatization of individuals carrying deleterious genes	4	7
Eugenic applications of genetic tests	3	9

Determining whether genetic testing is cost saving

Before promoting widespread testing, the utilitarians will need to demonstrate two things: that the savings from testing exceed the costs, and that testing is the most efficient (or cost-effective) way of reducing the costs. If public funds are to be expended, the question will be asked whether the program is affordable (even if cost effective) and whether resources could better be used to accomplish other objectives. I have touched on some of the issues of the cost of testing to insurers and employers. Much of what I consider now will be used by those groups in deciding whether testing is cost saving to them. It will also be used to determine whether community- or statewide genetic testing is justified.

Savings. Without genetic testing and appropriate follow-up, affected individuals (either in the generation screened or in the next generation in the case of carrier screening) will manifest illness. Averting the costs of this illness constitutes the gross savings of testing. The costs of this illness can be estimated in terms of dollars or years of life lost. Dollar costs can be broken down into direct costs of caring for the illness and indirect costs, in which loss from the productive work force figures prominently. There are problems in measuring both components. In estimating direct costs, little consideration is given to the likelihood that someone who is saved from an illness by genetic testing will develop some other illness or injury that also will entail costs. Neglecting this factor tends to exaggerate the savings. In measuring productivity, not every affected individual will have the same potential earning power. Nor is productivity widely accepted as an appropriate way to measure the value of a life.

Measuring years of life lost (which translates into years of life gained if testing is undertaken) gets around some of these problems, but quality of life must be taken into consideration. Testing may result in increased years of life, but when survivors are retarded or restricted in their activity, some adjustment should be made. It becomes very difficult to take into consideration the costs to the parents in aborting a wanted pregnancy.

Using years of life lost rather than dollar costs can give very different results. A disease that results in very early death—for example, maple syrup urine disease—would be very costly in terms of years of life lost. Because death comes rapidly to an affected infant, however, the lifetime costs of medical care would be relatively small in the absence of early detection.

A problem also arises in deciding what value to give the affected fetus when abortion is one of the planned outcomes of genetic testing, for then there is no gain in years of life. However, without prenatal diagnosis some couples would not undertake a pregnancy if they knew they were at risk.

The extra years of life of having a healthy baby (when the results of prenatal diagnosis are negative) could be measured against having no baby at all.

Costs. The costs of the testing program must be subtracted from the gross savings (if they are measured in dollars) to give net savings. Another way of calculating the relation of savings to costs is to divide savings ("benefits") by costs to give a benefit:cost ratio. If the savings are defined in terms of years of life gained, then a ratio of the costs per year of life gained can be calculated. When prenatal diagnosis and abortion are being assessed, the costs per abortion of affected fetuses in those desiring this outcome could be measured.[90]

In assessing costs, the collection and analysis of specimens and the reporting of results have to be included. Once a program is in place for collecting specimens for one test, it will add on relatively little to use that same specimen for tests for additional disorders. The interventions that follow the identification of someone at risk for genetic disease or for such disease in one's offspring, beginning with confirmation of the positive test result, also must be counted. The costs of a lifetime of treatment (following early identification) could be greater than the averted costs, particularly when death—in the absence of testing—occurred early in life.[91] The frequency of treatment failure (due, for instance, to noncompliance) and of harmful reactions to treatment should be estimated and the resultant costs added to the costs of testing. Erroneous test results also contribute. The costs of false negatives include diagnosing and managing the missed cases and also, on occasion, defending and settling malpractice suits.[92] The costs of false positives include follow-up and treating some cases needlessly with some chance of doing harm.[93] Thus the sensitivity and specificity of the test have an important bearing on costs and benefits and the decision to test as a matter of policy.

Cost savings from genetic testing. Econometric studies of newborn screening for PKU, prenatal AFP screening, and prenatal testing of pregnancies in older pregnant women for chromosomal abnormalities have found the programs to be cost beneficial.[94] The authors of a recent British study concluded that "prevention of a small number of births" resulting from DNA-based prenatal diagnosis of infants at risk for cystic fibrosis, hemophilia, and muscular dystrophy, and in couples identified by carrier screening to be at risk of having offspring with beta thalassemia and sickle cell anemia, "would result in savings—an unusual situation for a new development in the NHS (National Health Service)," and that this savings justified the establishment of regional DNA-based screening laboratories.[95]

There is a difference, however, between the cost savings from neonatal screening for PKU and those from prenatal diagnosis. The former depend on an inexpensive means of preventing retardation after birth, thereby lowering the need for special education or institutionalization.[96] The benefits of carrier screening and prenatal diagnosis reflect the *absence* rather than the presence of an effective means of preventing disability in those born with a genetic disorder. Current care for cystic fibrosis, Duchenne muscular dystrophy, and thalassemia is supportive rather than curative or even ameliorative. Because these conditions are not usually rapidly fatal, the special care is needed over many years and is costly.

With further advances in technology, which seem likely, DNA-based tests for multiple disorders will be possible on one specimen. Once the specimen is collected, therefore, the costs of additional tests will be relatively small. (It is highly unlikely, however, that the point will ever be reached at which some disease-causing or susceptibility-conferring allele will be found in every pregnancy. Even if fifty conditions, each with a frequency of 1 in 1,000, were tested for simultaneously, 95 percent of the tested fetuses would be unaffected. When a couple is at risk for a dominant disorder, they still have a 50 percent chance of having a normal child; for X-linked and recessive disorders, that chance is 75 percent.) For many disorders, tests will be developed before definitive therapies are discovered, and increased emphasis could be placed on avoidance strategies.

Although I am unaware of econometric analyses of genetic screening for common, late-onset disorders such as Alzheimer disease, the large number of persons affected (even if only a fraction of them have a detectable genetic basis for the disease) and the costly, protracted care they require would make prenatal diagnosis and abortion cost-saving measures. It is true that because the costs are so far in the future, the savings in current dollars would be less than those for diseases in which onset occurs earlier. Savings might also be realized from the prenatal detection and abortion of those predisposed to breast or other forms of cancer with low cure rates. Although prenatally diagnosable causes of blindness, deafness, mental retardation, or congenital malformation account for only a minority of those afflicted with these handicaps, eliminating them by abortion would reduce their burden to society.

The hidden assumption in such arguments is that the people who are born free of these detectable disorders will incur fewer health care costs in their lifetime. If they were all to live to a ripe old age and then quickly and quietly die without imposing a burden on society, the argument might have some merit. But there is no evidence that that will happen; new diseases will arise to plague humankind as we change our environment and our behavior. In the short run, it seems likely, even with expanded testing, that the money saved by reducing the cost of caring for one illness will quickly be spent in caring for another.[97]

The cost savings of genetic screening to identify a high-risk group within the population that can then be monitored for early signs of disease remain to be determined. The predictive value and sensitivity of the monitoring test as well as the screening test, and the benefits of early intervention when early signs are detected, all need to be established.

The excess of benefits over costs for any program is highly dependent on the proportion of the target population that complies with the program. If couples at risk refuse testing, infants requiring expensive care will be born; the cost of their care will be greater than the money saved by screening fewer people. I have estimated that prenatal AFP screening for neural tube defects would cease to be cost effective if fewer than 40 percent of pregnant women were screened.[98] A recent analysis of thalassemia screening showed that benefits barely exceed costs when half of the target population is screened.[99]

Alternative approaches. Identifying those with genetic susceptibilities may not be the only approach to reducing the burden of genetic diseases. Particularly when exposure to an environmental agent is known to enhance genetic susceptibility, or when dietary modification can reduce susceptibility, and when the disorders are fairly common, interventions that affect the entire population may result in greater cost savings than genetic testing.

Assuming that lowering cholesterol in childhood is effective in reducing the risk of coronary heart disease, Berwick et al. examined three alternative childhood interventions to achieve this goal: public education, selective screening, and mass screening.[100] A mass-media educational campaign to reduce everyone's dietary lipids was the most cost effective approach to reducing coronary disease, but it was also the most expensive. Testing the ten-year-old offspring of parents who had suffered a myocardial infarction for hypercholesterolemia and then treating those identified (assuming that prolonged dietary therapy works) was estimated to be less cost effective than the mass-media approach and to save fewer lives. It was, however, considerably less expensive than the mass-media campaign when applied to populations of identical size. Universal screening of ten year olds for hypercholesterolemia was the least cost effective approach, and was intermediate in total costs between the other two approaches. It was, therefore, less desirable than either of the other options from the standpoint of both the benefit:cost ratio and the total cost. This analysis suggests that for dominant disorders with low mutation rates, limiting genetic testing to those with a family history may be more efficient than population-wide screening.

Resistance will be encountered to approaches that disregard differences in risk, such as efforts to reduce the amount of saturated fat and cholesterol in the American diet or to increase taxes on cigarettes or alcohol. Some people will object to the restriction of freedom imposed by these efforts. Companies whose manufacturing practices involve the use of toxic substances have claimed that efforts to reduce the exposure of all workers to levels that ensure a safe workplace for everyone are too costly. They might well prefer to screen out workers who are the most susceptible. Genetic screening then shifts the blame from the perpetrator to the victim. It is interesting to note that the cost to industry of reducing the exposure of workers to the toxic substances vinyl chloride and beryllium proved much lower than the companies had originally projected.[101]

Affordability and competitive uses. The cholesterol example indicates a dilemma that sometimes faces policy makers: the most cost effective program is too expensive to undertake. In such a case, is a less cost effective but cheaper policy adopted, or is the entire project dropped, with public funds being spent in an entirely different area. Except as testing for very common predispositions (such as those for coronary artery disease) becomes possible, the number of individuals whose lives will be saved by population-based genetic screening may be too small (politically or even morally) to justify the outlay, even if it is cost saving. A similar investment—for instance, in increasing food supplements to low-income families—might give more children a better chance to develop normally, although it might not mean the difference between life and death for any of them.

Time savings also come into consideration. The time spent counseling a pregnant woman about a test for a 1 in 1,000 risk (e.g., maternal serum AFP testing for neural tube defects) could be spent instead advising her on the avoidance of other risks to her fetus (alcohol, smoking, drugs) whose prevalence—together with the chance of adverse outcomes—is much higher. If it became possible to test for many different genetic disorders without commensurate increases in cost, the discrepancy might be reduced.

The costs to the health care system of not screening for severe disorders are likely to be much higher than the costs of not offering food supplements or counseling on substance abuse. On the other hand, the total costs to parents and to other governmental agencies (welfare, schools) may be greater if the funds are used for genetic testing. Those who determine the allocation of health care dollars—either for testing or for chronic care without testing—are likely to neglect these other social costs.

The compassion argument

Those who argue for testing and abortion from compassion maintain that no person should suffer needlessly. When apparently healthy individuals do not appreciate how much they will suffer because of a genetic susceptibility, their short-sightedness should be overcome by requiring them to be tested. (Logic dictates that they then also be required to take remedial action if their test results are positive.) Prospective parents who cannot foresee the suffering of their unborn children with genetic disease, or their own suffering, should, the argument goes, at least be denied the opportunity to inflict harm on their offspring. In support of this position, Linus Pauling, twice a Nobel Prize winner, wrote of parents who knew they were at risk of having a child with cystic fibrosis: "A father and a mother who, with this knowledge, continue to produce defective children and in this way add to the amount of human suffering should feel guilt for their actions."[102]

Citing the decision of the New Jersey Supreme Court that "the child has a legal right to begin life with a sound mind and body," lawyer-geneticist Margery Shaw points out that a certain number of wanted children "will be physically or mentally defective or diseased and some will have physical pain and suffering that is no less acute than the pain of child abuse. . . . The real tragedy of these tragedies is that the conception or birth of many of these unfortunate children could have been prevented because of advances in our . . . ability to predict many of these adverse conditions. . . . The burden has shifted from the physicians to the parents to act in reasonable ways to prevent the birth of a child who would certainly or likely suffer postnatally."[103]

Proponents of the compassion argument project their views of suffering onto others. There may not always be a consensus, however. As science philosopher Robert Morison asked, "Who is to say that a child with Down's syndrome is more or less happy than the child with an IQ of 150 who spends the first 16 years of his life competing with his peers for admission to an ivy league college?"[104] People without handicaps may assume that those who have them inevitably suffer. Marsha Sexton, a woman with spina bifida and an activist for the rights of the disabled, comments: "Most disabled people have told me with no uncertainty that the disability, the pain, the need for compensatory devices and assistance can produce considerable inconvenience, but that very often these become minimal or are forgotten once individuals make the transition to living their everyday lives."[105] Geneticists Arno Motulsky and Jeffrey Murray contrast the perceptions of handicap based on whether it is congenital or acquired: "A person born blind or deaf who grows to adulthood with that condition may not view himself as particularly 'disabled.' But a person who grew up relying on sight or hearing who loses or imagines losing one of these senses may perceive such a loss as an extreme disability."[106]

Coercion

Once cost savings are demonstrated, the utilitarians will join the "compassionates" in urging widespread use of genetic tests. Data presented in chapter 7 indicate low rates of acceptance of carrier screening, which had been organized primarily by community groups with assistance from dedicated health care professionals. Opposition to abortion does not appear to be widespread enough to provide a complete explanation. Whether it is simply a matter of education, of increasing people's awareness of what the risks are, or of incorporating screening into regular medical care remains to be seen.

If acceptance rates stay low, might there be efforts to promote screening by coercive methods? By "coercion" I mean an effort to gain compliance which goes beyond providing information on the intrinsic merits of the test. A degree of coercion may be present even when informed consent is obtained; people may be persuaded more by authority figures or peers than by their understanding of the test and its implications.

Screening in high schools. When Tay-Sachs carrier screening programs in Montreal failed to reach more than 11 percent of the young adults in the Jewish community, screening was introduced into the high schools. The chief medical officer of the school system recommended testing "in an official letter to all Jewish students . . . and a school assembly was held to discuss the benefits of testing." Specimens were collected in the schools. Information on human genetics was also introduced into the school system's biology curriculum, and awareness of the nature of Tay-Sachs disease and the availability of carrier screening was quite high afterward.[107] A similar strategy was followed for screening for thalassemia carriers.[108] For each disorder, the proportion of high-school students who consented to screening (parental consent was not needed) was over seven times the proportion observed in the adult community!

I suggest that this marked increase was due to external pressure and the ease of being tested in school (especially when one's peers also were being tested) rather than to a better grasp of the problem than young adults had. As I described in chapter 7, after thalassemia screening, only one-third of the carriers and 18 percent of the noncarriers had a correct understanding of the Mendelian probabilities of having an affected child.[109] A survey of a larger segment of the target population, which was conducted before screening but after the distribution of information on thalassemia, determined that fetal diagnosis followed by abortion of affected fetuses was acceptable to only 31 percent.[110] Thus, not all of the students who were screened thought that prenatal diagnosis—the primary reason for screening—was an acceptable option.

Eight years after they were screened in high school, those identified as Tay-Sachs carriers in the Montreal program were surveyed again.[111] Although 95 percent of the carriers who responded said they would want their partner to be screened, nine of the twelve carriers who were married or engaged had a partner who had not been screened. The report does not indicate whether the carriers who were married had told their spouse of their carrier status. This leaves open the question of whether this type of coercion accomplishes very much. As mentioned in chapter 7, young women identified as sickle cell carriers in Greece sometimes failed to tell their spouse of their status.[112]

Compelling health care providers to offer screening. In Maryland, parents must consent before their newborns are screened, but health care providers are required to offer screening. In California, the same holds for maternal serum AFP screening; providers caring for pregnant women are required to offer it. If offering could be done in a way that guaranteed parental autonomy, this would be a fine way of ensuring broad access to genetic tests. As I have already mentioned, physicians may exert some coercion in offering tests out of fear they will be sued should disease eventually become manifest in those who refuse testing (or in their offspring).

Penalties and incentives. The withdrawal or reduction of services (many of which receive governmental support) for long-term care of a disabled child whose condition could have been avoided by prenatal diagnosis and abortion could pressure families to accept carrier screening and prenatal testing. In a 1970 case, the United States Supreme Court upheld setting an absolute maximum of payments to families with dependent children.[113] For poor families, this could serve as an incentive not only for aborting unwanted children but also for using the prenatal diagnosis and abortion of affected but wanted children to keep family expenses down.

Diminished support for research directed at finding treatments for prenatally diagnosable diseases would end the hope of prospective parents that a "cure" might be found, driving them to prenatal diagnosis. For instance, there is less interest today in research to find an effective treatment for Tay-Sachs disease than there was twenty years ago, before the days of carrier screening and prenatal diagnosis.

Mandatory newborn screening. Of the 48 states (plus the District of Columbia) that have statutes governing newborn screening, 45 have made it mandatory.[114] The principal lobbyist for PKU screening was the National Association for Retarded Children (NARC), an organization in which parents of retarded children figured prominently.[115] NARC originally rejected seeking mandatory legislation and instead sought laws that required state health departments to make recommendations for screening. Many departments made such recommendations, but the slow adoption of these recommendations—primarily because of the intransigence of practicing physicians and not because parents were refusing to have their infants tested—led NARC to change its position and advocate mandatory laws. At that point, the American Academy of Pediatrics and the American Medical Association opposed the laws. It is by no means clear that organized medicine will move with greater alacrity to adopt screening or will be any less resistant to governmental intrusions in medical practice in the future than it has been in the past.

As I have indicated, in Maryland, the vast majority of parents accept newborn screening.[116] Nevertheless, ethicists and lawyers persist in talking about a duty of the state to act on behalf of the child and compel testing "if some proportion of parents consistently withheld their consent, even though they have been given appropriate information about the purpose, benefits, and extremely small risks of a test that yields information of great importance to the well-being of children."[117]

Sickle cell screening laws. Seventeen states passed sickle cell screening laws in the early 1970s.[118] In seven of them the screening was mandatory, and in at least five, marriage licenses and school attendance were denied to those who were not willing to be tested or to have their children tested. Because there is no definitive treatment for sickle cell anemia and because the greatest threat to life occurs in infancy (before the tests available in the early 1970s could be applied), the compelling public-health interest served by these laws is difficult to discern. A few states have repealed their original screening laws, others have amended them to make screening voluntary, and others no longer enforce the laws.[119] As Philip Reilly commented on the sickle cell statutes passed in the early 1970s:

> The statutes contained glaring errors, including egregious drafting mistakes that hopelessly muddled the scientific facts about sickle cell anemia. They are a sad commentary on the abyss that separates lawmakers from technical experts. The most consistent error was conferring disease status on sickle cell trait. . . . The Massachusetts law . . . authorized tests on every child "susceptible to the disease known as sickle cell trait or sickle cell anemia." . . . But unquestionably the most egregious provision is found in the opening paragraph of the National Sickle Cell Anemia Control

Act. It states that "sickle cell anemia is a debilitating, inheritable disease that affects approximately two million American citizens and has largely been neglected." About 2,000,000 people in America . . . carry the sickle cell gene, but fewer that 50,000 have sickle cell disease.[120]

Legal support for coercive testing. Demonstrated cost savings of genetic testing might be accepted by some state courts as a justification for mandatory genetic testing. Although a few state courts have demurred, most have used economic arguments to justify the mandatory wearing of helmets by motorcyclists and seat belts by automobile occupants. For example, in upholding a helmet law, a Massachusetts court found: "From the moment of injury, society picks the person up off the road; delivers him to a municipal hospital and municipal doctors; provides him with unemployment compensation if, after recovery, he cannot replace his lost job, and if the injury causes permanent disability, may assume the responsibility for his and his family's continuous subsistence."[121] Society applies this doctrine unevenly; neither cigarettes nor alcohol are prohibited because of the costs they add to health care.

The argument of social costs is more likely to be applied to mandatory testing for genetic susceptibilities to illness in oneself than to testing of one's offspring. But a duty of women to determine the risks to their offspring and to act to minimize them has also been justified legally. I have already mentioned Margery Shaw's views on the responsibilities of prospective parents to avoid the birth of infants who will suffer avoidably. She goes on to argue that "parents might incur a legal duty to obtain an abortion" if a fetus with a birth defect is predicted. Shaw acknowledges that this "violates the concept of parental autonomy held dear by civil libertarians," but continues: "From the viewpoint of the child, a rational argument can be made that non-existence is preferable to existence filled with incapacities and suffering."

Shaw was echoing the words of the California Supreme Court: "We do not think that it is accurate to suggest that this state's public policy establishes—as a mater of law—that under all circumstances 'impaired life' is 'preferable' to 'nonlife.'"[122] In this case, a child with hereditary deafness brought suit against the specialist who failed to warn her parents that they were at risk (the specialist had diagnosed the disorder in their previous child). Had they been warned, her parents maintained, they would never have had another child.

But what if doctors do warn the parents that they are at risk because both are carriers of a recessive disorder, or the mother has an elevated maternal serum AFP level, or prenatal diagnosis indicates a fetus with Down syndrome? In the first two instances, if the parents refuse to determine if the fetus is affected, or in the third, if they refuse to abort, are they then liable to be sued for "wrongful life"? California and five other states have adopted statutes that ban suits for wrongful life by children against their parents.[123] The courts in two other states, Washington and New Jersey, have accepted the concept that a child with an avoidable congenital impairment has a right to bring suit because his or her parents were not warned, but they have side-stepped whether these children would have been better off never being born at all.[124] Neither of these states has statutes prohibiting suits by children against their parents in such an event.

Several other states permit action by parents, but not by affected children, against physicians who fail to warn them; these are known as "wrongful birth" suits. In 1985 a West Virginia court refused to support a "wrongful life" action because the state does not have a statute covering the matter.[125] If a trend toward "wrongful life" develops, statutes establishing the concept may well materialize.

The effect of both wrongful-birth and wrongful-life suits has been to increase physicians' concerns that they might eventually be sued. To protect themselves against malpractice litigation, some may choose to undertake predictive tests without informing or fully discussing them with a pregnant woman, even though she would reject them if given the opportunity.

Legal limits on coercion

Some state courts have specifically rejected the concept of wrongful life, though not that of wrongful birth. In 1967 the Supreme Court of New Jersey wrote: "The right to life is inalienable in our society. . . . Examples of famous persons who have had great achievement despite physical defects come readily to mind, and many of us can think of examples close to home. A child need not be perfect to have a worthwhile life."[126] The rejection of actions for "wrongful life" would make it unlikely that parents could be sued for failing to avoid the birth of children with detectable conditions, as would statutes specifically prohibiting suits against parents. However, that would still not prevent state legislatures or health departments from requiring genetic testing, including carrier and prenatal testing.

The right to privacy. Whether statutes mandating genetic testing would be constitutional is still an unsettled question. Compelling testing early in pregnancy is at odds with the right to privacy accorded the pregnant woman. In *Roe v. Wade*, the United States Supreme Court held that a pregnant woman's reproductive intentions were a private matter in which the state could not interfere up to the point of viability of the fetus.[127] Beyond the point of viability, protection of the health and life of the mother takes precedence over protection of the fetus. Some courts, however, have ordered mothers to undergo Caesarean sections—despite their potential danger to the mother—because physicians have alleged they are required to save the life of the child.[128] (The physicians have not always been right.) Although it is unlikely in the current climate that a mother could be compelled to undergo an abortion to avoid the birth of an infant with a severe defect, giving legal status to wrongful life could lead to such an action. It seems somewhat more likely that mothers could be compelled to undergo prenatal testing, particularly if nonintrusive tests that do not of themselves constitute a threat to the health of either the mother or the fetus are developed.

The unsettled nature of how far the state can go to prevent a fetus at risk of suffering severe disease is suggested by the debate on mandatory premarital or prenatal testing for HIV antibodies to reduce the spread of acquired immune deficiency syndrome (AIDS). Although such screening may have socially desirable consequences, it conflicts with individual autonomy and privacy. In *Eisenstadt v. Baird*, the United States Supreme Court wrote: "If the right to privacy means anything, it is the right of the individual, married or single, to be free from unwarranted governmental intrusions into matters so fundamentally affecting a person as the decision whether to bear or beget a child."[129] This decision struck down a statute that made it illegal for anyone to prescribe, sell, or give an unmarried person a contraceptive except for the prevention of disease.

Would the Supreme Court now uphold the constitutionality of the forced use of contraceptives by married or unmarried sex partners if one or both of them were found to be HIV-positive in order to prevent the conception of a fetus with AIDS? (Enforcing the law might be difficult, but that did not deter the Court from upholding the illegality of consensual sodomy.[130]) Or would the Court uphold the partners' right to privacy in reproductive matters even if they were jeopardizing the health of potential children. If the Court took the former course, it would lay the groundwork for mandating genetic testing and avoidance strategies for couples at risk.

One difference between AIDS and genetic diseases is that the sex partner and the fetus are at risk for contracting AIDS, while only the fetus is at risk for developing a genetic disease. It may well turn out that the probability that a couple at risk will transmit a genetic Mendelian disorder to a fetus is greater than the risk that an HIV-antibody-positive parent will transmit the AIDS virus. Moreover, the diagnosis of genetic disorders can be made prenatally. This is not true of AIDS, so among couples in which at least one partner is HIV-antibody positive, the decision to abort (either mandated by the state or agreed to voluntarily by the parents) would result in the abortion of unaffected fetuses more often than is the case with abortions involving genetic diseases.

Voluntary testing. The National Sickle Cell Anemia Control Act (Public Law 92-294), as well as the National Cooley's Anemia Control Act (Public Law 92-414), both of which were passed in 1972, required that federally supported testing programs for the disorders mentioned in the respective acts were to be entirely voluntary. The concept was then extended to all federally supported genetic testing programs in 1976 with the passage of the National Sickle Cell Anemia, Cooley's Anemia, Tay-Sachs and Genetic Diseases Act (Public Law 94-278). As stated in section 1103 of that act, "The participation by any individual in any program or portion thereof under this part shall be wholly voluntary and shall not be a prerequisite to eligibility for or receipt of any other service or assistance from, or to participation in, any other program." The authorization sections of the Genetic Diseases Act were repealed by the Maternal and Child Health Services Block Grant in 1981 (Public Law 97-35). Nevertheless, section 1103 of the original Act remains the law, even though it is not being enforced. The number of states using federal funds under the block grant to support mandatory newborn screening programs exceeds the number of states offering screening on a voluntary basis.[131]

Maryland requires that genetic screening be wholly voluntary and has promulgated regulations toward that end for newborn screening and sickle cell screening. These decisions have emanated from a statutory Commission on Hereditary Disorders, the majority of whose members are consumers. The Commission has the authority to promulgate regulations for the detection and management of hereditary disorders.[132] Most other states could adopt mandatory genetic testing laws.

A new eugenics?

There's even something somewhat gratifying, one has to admit, about seeing Hitler in a newsreel, with his silly mustache and silly haircut, screaming hysterically and shaking his fist. And one of the reasons we like to see such films or such newsreels is that they give us the reassuring feeling, as we watch them, that we're the sort of people who can recognize evil when it presents itself—the sort of people who will recognize it if it ever should approach us.[133]

I define *eugenics* as any effort to interfere with individuals' procreative choices in order to attain a societal goal. Clearly that is what the early eugenicists did by encouraging the breeding of those with "favorable" attributes and the sterilization of those with "unfavorable" ones.[134] Of course, it was the eugenicists who decided what was favorable and what was unfavorable.

At first glance, it would seem that the early eugenicists had little in common with those who today would impose genetic testing on people to save money or reduce pain and suffering. They attributed the perpetuation of complex traits to genetics rather than to social and cultural transmission. Whether intentional or not, their policies maintained the dominance of the upper classes. The English biometrician R. A. Fisher proposed giving state allowances to high-income families for each child they had.[135] Sterilization was reserved for the inmates of state institutions, among whom few upper-class citizens were likely to be found.[136] Lancelot Hogben pointed out in 1938 that "no eugenicist has publicly proposed sterilization as a remedy for defective kingship" brought on by the presence of hemophilia in the royal houses of Europe.[137]

Those who propose genetic testing for insurance or employment purposes or to avoid the conception or birth of affected offspring may not be aware of the class bias in their proposal. But in the absence of a national health system or guaranteed employment, the poor will suffer from genetic discrimination more than those who have cash reserves to fall back on. The wealthy may be able to afford alternative reproductive strategies to avoid the conception of offspring with severe diseases; the poor will have to settle for abortion. And if the pressure for the abortion of "defective" fetuses comes not from mandatory laws but from the high costs of caring for such infants, the poor will be less able to withstand it than the wealthy.

Some of the early eugenicists were driven by the same forces that today encourage people to advocate coercive testing. In 1926, the American Eugenics Society published what must have been one of the earliest cost-benefit analyses. Sterilization of the original pair of Jukes, who allegedly bred many generations of "social misfits," the Society said, would have cost $150, while the failure to do so had resulted in spending over $2,000,000 on their descendants.[138] The Eugenic Sterilization Law of 1934 in Nazi Germany, which compelled the sterilization of people who suffered from diseases that were alleged to be inherited (including schizophrenia, epilepsy, blindness, and some physical deformities), followed in 1939 by the euthanasia of institutionalized patients with mental and physical disabilities, was justified on the grounds that the public could not assume the expense entailed in maintaining "lives not worth living."[139] Extermination of the Jews came later.[140] In England, H. G. Wells proclaimed: "The children people bring into the world can be no more their private concern entirely, than the disease germs they disseminate or the noises a man makes in a thin-floored flat."[141]

Motivation, therefore, does not provide the principal distinction between the early eugenicists and those who would impose genetic testing on people today. The principal difference is the accuracy of the methods. Regardless of whether their diseases are monogenic or multifactorial, sterilizing *symptomatic* individuals will have little effect on the gene pool and, consequently, on the occurrence of affected offspring in future generations.[142] Although the frequency of late-onset dominant disorders could have been reduced by sterilizing affected individuals before they had children, such individuals were asymptomatic, and hence undiagnosable, until after they had already reproduced. In the case of recessive disorders, disease-causing alleles are maintained primarily by passage from couples in which only one partner is a carrier, not by affected individuals or by couples in which both partners are carriers.[143] In essence, the early eugenicists were unable to identify those who were at risk for passing on "undesirable" traits.

Today, however, predictions of who will, and who will not, have offspring with disease-causing genotypes are amazingly accurate. Moreover, the techniques of carrier detection, alternative reproductive strategies, and abortion of affected fetuses still permit people to have children. (Current prices and reimbursement policies, however, indicate that only the wealthy will be able to afford in vitro fertilization or embryo transfer, each of which literally enables a woman to bear children when they do not contain her own genes.) Unquestionably, many women will undertake pregnancies that would not have been possible without the new techniques. But that still leaves open the question of whether a woman can be denied the opportunity to give birth to an affected child.

The new techniques do, in fact, have the power to reduce deleterious genes in the gene pool. This can be accomplished by avoiding the birth of carriers as well as affected offspring. As outlandish as this may seem, it was suggested by Linus Pauling. Writing in 1963, before prenatal diagnosis was possible, Pauling said that once it has been determined that a disease-causing allele "is not advantageous, even in single dose, then steps should be taken to eliminate it from the pool of human germplasm with the minimum amount of human suffering."[144]

Some genetic counselors share this view. In the extensive survey of genetic counselors mentioned in chapter 7, "a reduction in the number of carriers of genetic disorders in the population" was held to be an "important or somewhat important" goal of counseling by 48 percent of the 202 counselors surveyed.[145] A similar finding was obtained in a survey of American medical geneticists in 1985.[146]

Margery Shaw, who believes that it is a parental duty to avoid fetal abuse, also allows "gene control" to enter her argument: "It should be incumbent upon the law to control the spread of genes causing severe deleterious effects just as disabling pathogenic bacteria and viruses are controlled. . . . Parents should be held accountable to their children if they knowingly and willfully choose to transmit deleterious genes or if the mother waives her right to an abortion if, after prenatal testing, a fetus is discovered to be seriously deformed or mentally defective."[147]

Differences in the targets of the early eugenicists and those who would abrogate individual autonomy today may be more quantitative than qualitative. In the absence of accurate methods to predict who would be "defective," the early American eugenicists attacked on a broad front; the "feeble-minded," the insane, convicted rapists and other criminals, drug fiends, and drunkards all were targets of various state sterilization laws. More sweepingly still, the American eugenicists succeeded in their attack on foreigners by securing passage of the Immigration Restriction Act of 1924.[148] Clearly, the use of recombinant DNA technology will never lead to such an indiscriminate selection of targets. But genes have already been located that play a role in mental retardation, mental illness, cancer, heart disease, deforming conditions such as neurofibromatosis, and even reading disability. The genes responsible for hereditary forms of blindness and deafness will soon be discovered. Other techniques already permit the prenatal detection and abortion of fetuses with common deformities such as spina bifida and conditions with stigmatizing features such as Down syndrome. It is consistent with the notions that the world is "overpopulated" (see the quotation from Bentley Glass above), that resources are scarce, and that family size should be limited, to use all of the accurate techniques at our disposal to ensure that only the healthiest babies are born, that those who are likely to drain society are culled out earlier.

It is interesting to note that in a recent survey of biotechnology companies (table 8.1), eight predicted that genetic testing will be mandatory by the year 2000, and three projected that eugenic applications of these tests will be developed.

> It would be flattering to believe that we are superior in some way to the audiences who cheered for Hitler—more insightful and perceptive, let's say less blood thirsty—but I think it would be more prudent to make the assumption that perhaps we're not. At least we should allow ourselves to imagine that possibility for just a moment. . . . [I]f it should turn out that we're *not* superior, our self-examination might save a lot of people—possibly all people—from being harmed by us.[149]

Attitudes toward the disabled

Laws in the last twenty years have given handicapped individuals greater access to mainstream American society than they have had for some time. "In rural societies disabled people had far more of a social role than they have had in the more urban and industrialized world . . . As work became more structured and formalized, people who 'fit' into the standardized factories were needed. Industrializing America not only forbade the immigration of disabled people from abroad, it shut the ones already here away in institutions."[150] As late as the 1950s, some states continued to prohibit the public presence of persons "diseased, maimed, mutilated or in any way deformed so as to be an unsightly or disgusting object."[151]

Efforts to integrate the handicapped into the mainstream of life have generated annoyance, if not hostility. A professor in the biological sciences who professes liberal leanings lamented to me recently on the inconvenience of having people with hearing impairments in her class; no longer could she talk while she wrote at the blackboard. Marsha Saxton, the woman with spina bifida whom I quoted earlier, maintains that "discriminatory attitudes and thoughtless behaviors" make life difficult for those with handicaps. "The 'suffering' we may experience is primarily a result of not enough human caring, acceptance, and respect," not physical pain.[152]

Physicians might be expected to be more tolerant, but oftentimes they are not. As Saxton points out, "Physicians, by the very nature of their work, often have a distorted picture of disability. Working in hospitals, doctors generally see only those cases of disability where there are complications, poor management, terminal stages, situations where they the physicians, are expected to help."[153] Physicians will often be the instruments of social policy in using predictive tests and recommending actions when the tests are positive. Their distorted perspective may encourage them to do so.

Abortion following prenatal diagnosis may well prove a more economical solution than institutionalization or providing for the needs of the handicapped by mainstreaming. As the opportunity for identifying those at risk and diagnosing affected fetuses increases, I am not sure that our new-found tolerance for the handicapped will endure.

Writing at a time when the possibility of testing every pregnant woman for Down syndrome or a variety of inherited disorders by direct, DNA-based tests seemed remote, Motulsky and Murray did not think the volume of prenatal diagnosis and "selective" abortion testing was likely to change societal attitudes. They cautioned: "If prenatal diagnosis and selective abortion would lead to a sharp decline in a given disease category, and if it were generally known that the disease in question could be avoided by prenatal diagnosis, the public's attitudes toward patients with that disease and their parents might be more critical and could lead to undesirable social consequences."[154] These consequences could range from "social disapproval to selective removal of health care benefits by private insurance companies."[155] In 1973 Leon Kass, physician and philosopher, wrote: "A child with Down's syndrome or with hemophilia or with muscular dystrophy born at a time when most of his (potential) fellow sufferers were destroyed prenatally is liable to be looked upon by the community as one unfit to be alive, as a second class (or even lower) human type. He may be seen as a person who need not have been, and who would not have been, if only someone had gotten to him in time."[156] Only the constant reinforcement of tolerance for differences, which will lead to a truly compassionate society willing to ensure adequate care for those who reject abortion, can prevent this from happening.

Who has the right to decide?

A woman bears children, and her mate joins in nurturing them. It is primarily the parents who bear the emotional costs and most of the economic burden of childrearing, not the state, except in the direst of circumstances and then demeaningly. If the state were to assume all the costs in a "brave new world" scenario, it might then have the right to decide who would be born. Until that dismal time, however, this choice should rest with the parents. Moreover, to fail to heed the desires of a mother-to-be either to have or not to have her baby demeans the status of women. Lawyer George Annas writes: "After birth, the fetus becomes a child and can thereafter be treated in its own right. Before birth, we can obtain access to the fetus only through its mother, and in the absence of her informed consent, can do so only by treating her as a fetal container, a nonperson without rights to bodily integrity."[157]

John Fletcher briefly reviews the views of ethicists, which range from "neither abortion nor infanticide (for genetic reasons) is morally wrong" to the view that both are. Fletcher's position is that "until the fetus is separate, the pregnant woman's interests ought to be morally overriding, because greater harm could be done (in the name of doing good) to the moral and legal traditions of choice in human reproduction by following a policy of coercion than by a policy of persuasion limited by the woman's consent."[158] Although I agree with Fletcher's position, his use of the word *persuasion* runs counter to the concept of nondirective counseling, which, I believe, should be paramount.[159]

Who but the parents would have the wisdom to decide whether they can cope or not? As I have pointed out repeatedly, the list of conditions for which genetic testing—including prenatal testing—exists is growing steadily. Who will determine which tests have a sufficiently high predictive value, and which diseases are severe enough or of early enough onset or of sufficient cost to warrant prenatal diagnosis and abortion? The slope is slippery. Speaking of policies to decide which genetic traits should be exorcised, geneticist James Neel wrote: "We do not possess the wisdom or knowledge to make them."[160]

In contrast to other species, humans have used their brains and hands to overcome the loss of genes (e.g., the gene for hairiness) that afforded protection from hostile environments.[161] Humans have also used their ingenuity to overcome genetic predispositions, with the result that some traits are no longer incapacitating. The wearing of eyeglasses to overcome genetically conditioned myopia and other refractive errors not only corrects vision defects but provides employment for "an industry of ophthalmologists, opticians, and spectacle frame makers. Analogously, in the distant future human beings might require injections and pills for a variety of genetic infirmities—a development that we currently view as unhealthy. However, our descendants might consider this state of affairs to be as 'normal' as we consider the wearing of clothing or eyeglasses today."[162] As the great geneticist Theodosius Dobzhansky pointed out, "Usefulness and harmfulness are not the intrinsic properties of a variant gene; genes are useful, neutral, or harmful only in a certain environment. . . . What is good in the Arctic is not necessarily good on the equator; what was good in man in the ice age is not necessarily good now; what is good in a democracy is not necessarily good in a dictatorship."[163]

When fully educated and informed, most people will probably accept carrier testing, prenatal diagnosis, and the abortion of fetuses who are destined to develop severe disease in infancy or childhood. Regardless of how many refuse testing, society's imposing its will on them may exact a greater price in tearing our social fabric than would caring for their affected offspring.

Summary and Conclusions

It is possible to override the autonomy of individuals in deciding whether they want to have genetic tests. Those who do this sometimes justify their actions (paternalistically) as being in the best interests of the individual. That is the case when physicians perform tests without obtaining their patients' informed consent or when they exert pressure on patients to accept testing. (Once they obtain positive genetic test results that may be important to fiancé(e)s or relatives, physicians can also override the autonomy of patients who do not want the results revealed, by informing others of their findings.) An overzealous promotion of community programs also can override personal autonomy.

Concern for preventing the pain and suffering of those who refuse tests or of their unborn but potentially affected offspring may partially account for state-mandated programs. It is difficult, however, to tease apart the motive of benevolence from the motive of saving society money by avoiding the birth of infants who are destined to require long-term, expensive care. Thus far, most genetic testing programs that have been analyzed econometrically have proved to be cost saving, but such analyses overlook the fact that in time people born free of detectable disease will develop other diseases and incur other costs.

In some cases, testing is undertaken explicitly to serve the best interests of third parties. Adoptive parents may want to know the genetic status of an infant or of its biological parents before accepting the child. This could result in the rejection of some children for adoption. A justified use of testing is to determine that the donor of an egg or sperm to a couple seeking to use an alternative reproductive strategy to avoid the birth of an infant with a genetic disease is not a carrier of the disease to be avoided. When sperm, eggs, or wombs (in the case of surrogate mothers) are being sold, there is justification for performing genetic tests on the "vendor" regardless of the reason for using a particular reproductive strategy.

Once predictive genetic tests are used in medical practice, and patients are informed of the results and their implications, insurance companies will be at a disadvantage in selling individual insurance if they do not know the results. Individuals or couples at risk for future disease are likely to want to purchase additional life and health insurance to protect them. This will ultimately result in an increase in the standard premium. As the ability to distinguish the risks of one individual from another increases, the concept of private insurance (which was attractive to large numbers of people precisely because their risks could not be distinguished), will come into question. To protect themselves, insurance companies may require genetic testing. For people with negative results, genetic testing by insurers may result in a lowering of premiums or, in the case of those who would not be insured on the basis of family history alone, the opportunity to purchase insurance. For those with positive test results, genetic testing may lead to a diminished quality of life or increased suffering as the disease develops and they are inadequately insured and have no means of support.

Genetic testing may be included in preemployment examinations to screen out job seekers who have genetic susceptibilities to harmful reactions from workplace exposures as well as applicants who are at increased risk of developing diseases that have little to do with workplace exposures. In the first case, employers can claim increased safety and productivity as a justification for not hiring such people. However, genetic testing will not protect job applicants who have unidentifiable susceptibilities to workplace exposures. (Employers often reject the alternative policy of making the workplace safe for all employees as too costly.) In both cases, employers will save money by having to pay fewer health and disability claims under employee benefits programs and workers' compensation. If preemployment testing becomes widespread, people with positive genetic test results may be unemployable. The burden of caring for them is already beginning to shift from the private to the public sector, which thus far has not succeeded in providing either jobs or adequate health care for everyone.

The legal barriers to overriding individual autonomy in genetic testing vary between states and are not particularly strong. Federal statutes apply only to those employed by the federal government or to those contracting with it. The U.S. Civil Rights Act protects minority groups and women from discrimination based on genetic tests, but genetic disorders that do not occur with greater prevalence in a group protected by the Act are not covered. Broader protection against harm from workplace exposures is afforded by the Occupational Safety and Health Act. Both it and the Civil Rights Act provide protection only to the extent feasible, however; there is no absolute right of all workers to be protected regardless of susceptibility. The Rehabilitation Act may provide some protection to federal workers who are at risk for a future handicap, even if they are asymptomatic at the time of hiring. State rehabilitation laws vary in the extent of protection they afford. In some states, the laws have been so narrowly interpreted as to give no protection to those who are at risk for future disability.

Federal law requires that federally supported screening programs be wholly voluntary, but it is not clear that this has been strictly enforced. Only a few states have provisions for voluntary genetic testing. The courts might uphold the refusal of persons to have genetic tests for reproductive purposes under the right to privacy in reproductive matters as defined explicitly in a number of Supreme Court decisions—most notably *Roe v. Wade*—but this right is not absolute.

Recent efforts to impose genetic tests, which may be neither in the best interests nor consonant with the values of those being tested—especially those with positive results—constitute a new eugenics. The motives in some cases may not be different from those of the early eugenicists, but the techniques are far more accurate. Still, no group possesses the wisdom to mandate genetic testing or to dictate reproductive choices to pregnant women without doing grave harm to the principles of tolerance and individual freedom.

Chapter 9

What Is (Going) to Be Done?

In the previous three chapters, I have traced the development of genetic tests from basic research in university laboratories to the commercial sector and finally to the public. I have drawn heavily on experiences with a limited number of neoclassical genetic tests to suggest the ways in which DNA-based tests will be used for a much larger number of disorders. I have emphasized the possibilities for misuse of these tests. The reasons for misuse are numerous: inadequate procedures for ensuring validity and reliability; an insufficient number of adequately trained health care providers; a lack of public understanding of genetics and genetic testing; and, finally, efforts to override individual autonomy. In this final chapter, I offer some predictions of what is going to be done in the way of test proliferation (without regard to potential misuse), and conclude with some suggestions about what can be done to ensure that genetic tests will be used with a minimum of harm.

The Future of Genetic Testing

In this section, I examine how tests are likely to be used to predict disorders for which genes have already been located or for which there is a high probability that such genes will be located. Existing tests and screening programs (e.g., for PKU or hemoglobinopathies) are not considered. I assume that direct tests for the disease-causing or susceptibility-conferring allele(s) will be available, and that they will be no more expensive than currently available tests for screening. I separate tests into those for disorders that are always or almost always expressed and in which the manifestations are fairly consistent and severe, and those that have variable expressivity. After considering tests categorically, I turn to a consideration of who will provide them.

The effect of expressivity and interventions on the use of genetic tests

When it is certain that disease-causing genotypes will be expressed, both health care providers and consumers will be interested in testing for them; the predictive value of positive results—measured in terms of the future occurrence of disease—will be high. Most highly expressed disorders will be single gene in origin. For disorders whose frequency is greater than 1 in 10,000 live births, carrier screening is likely to occur when avoidance is deemed to be the principal means of reducing the burden of the disorder. Direct tests for cystic fibrosis will probably be the first to fit into this category. The purpose of these tests will be to identify couples at risk of having affected offspring. It is unlikely that efforts to curtail the procreation of carriers (regardless of the carrier status of their mate) will be undertaken in the near future. The extent of acceptance of carrier screening for cystic fibrosis will indicate the future of genetic testing for reproductive purposes.

DNA-based screening for carriers of severe X-linked diseases like hemophilia A and Duchenne muscular dystrophy may be undertaken despite the fact that new mutations will not be detected. A lack of sensitivity (which results from the failure to detect new mutations) will not detract from the proliferation of carrier screening as much as low predictive value. Low maternal serum AFP concentrations are capable of detecting fewer than one-third of fetuses with Down syndrome in women under the age of 35, but they are increasingly being used for that purpose because they are much less expensive and much safer than collecting fetal cells to karyotype every woman.

When it becomes possible to obtain fetal cells from the maternal circulation at no risk to the fetus, chromosome-specific DNA probes will be widely used. They will be much more sensitive predictors of Down syndrome and other trisomies than AFP tests, and less expensive than karyotyping, even though they will not detect as many conditions.

I doubt that carrier or chromosome screening will become mandatory, but it is likely that physicians will be required to offer them. As they become part of standard procedure, it may be more difficult for women to refuse them.

Limiting direct tests for disease-causing alleles for disorders like cystic fibrosis or Duchenne muscular dystrophy to families in which the disease has occurred will not have much impact on the occurrence of new cases in the long run. Members of cystic fibrosis families constitute a small fraction of all those at risk of having offspring with this disorder. (The same holds true for members of families in which other autosomal recessive disorders have occurred. They will account for only a small proportion of all new cases.) The fraction is larger for X-linked or autosomal dominant disorders. If testing is used by families with any type of Mendelian disorder to avoid the birth of affected offspring, then within a couple of generations few family members will recollect that they might carry the disease-causing allele. Population-wide carrier screening in each successive generation would rectify this problem.

Carrier screening is less likely to be undertaken for disorders with incidences of less than 1 in 10,000. When, however, effective treatments for highly expressed rare disorders are developed, screening for presymptomatic individuals will become more likely. DNA-based tests for urea-cycle abnormalities can be performed on the blood spot collected on newborns and would fit into this category. Even when early treatment does not prevent disease manifestations but alleviates them, screening will be undertaken. This is already the case for newborn screening for sickle cell anemia and cystic fibrosis.

For rare, late-onset dominant disorders like Huntington disease and adult polycystic kidney disease, testing will continue to be limited to families in which the disease has occurred, even after direct tests for disease-causing alleles are developed. Only when the technology evolves to the point that many different diseases can be tested on the same specimen at minimal expense (which it will) might population screening be undertaken for these rare disorders. Even then, however, concerns about knowing one has an untreatable disorder or about avoiding the birth of offspring with late-onset disorders will limit the extent of this screening.

As tests for disorders of high expressivity become standard practice, insurance companies will not only reimburse for them but will also want to know the results, and may even require testing if these conditions are potentially costly in terms of future health and disability insurance claims. They are also unlikely to provide life insurance to individuals whose test results predict an increased risk of early death.

The extent of testing for disorders of variable expressivity is more uncertain. One might expect wide use of testing for genotypes that will always or almost always cause disability in the face of exposures to common but avoidable environmental agents. The few attempts to screen high-risk populations for glucose-6-phosphate dehydrogenase (G6PD) deficiency have not been very successful. Tests that identify workers who will *consistently* develop disease in the presence of substances used in the workplace, at the concentrations used in the workplace, will find a place in preemployment examinations.

At the present time, we do not know how frequently those who have genotypes capable of causing common diseases like bipolar affective disorder, Alzheimer disease, or coronary artery disease will actually manifest the disease if they live long enough. Regardless of the expressivity of the genotype, I doubt that population-wide screening will be adopted for bipolar affective disorder or Alzheimer disease; there is no evidence that presymptomatic intervention would improve the outcomes. If randomized controlled trials were to prove otherwise, screening might be undertaken. In the absence of effective interventions, I doubt that many people in the general population would want to know they are at risk or would want to take action to avoid the birth of affected offspring (unless, in the latter case, the expressivity of the disease-causing genotype was very high). On the other hand, members of families with a high rate of these disorders might want to use tests for either or both purposes. If tests for these disorders were highly predictive, even if their sensitivity was low, insurance companies might be eager to use them.

Tests for genetic predispositions to heart disease might be used for screening if the predictive value of positive results proved to be considerably better than that of current tests for high- and low-density lipoprotein cholesterol, if they accounted for at least the same proportion of early heart attack victims as cholesterol screening (or supplemented those identified by cholesterol screening), and if early dietary therapy proved to be effective in preventing or delaying the occurrence of myocardial infarction in those with genetic predispositions. If drugs were needed to improve the outcome, it is more likely that testing would be limited to families at risk.

Employers will use tests that predict the future occurrence of conditions that will raise their outlays for health and disability claims. As long as there is a plentiful supply of labor, they will not be deterred by tests of low predictive value.

Tests for identifying young people with genetic predispositions to lung cancer from smoking might be used to discourage them from taking up the habit. From what is known so far, it is doubtful that positive test results will have high predictive values. I am not sure how popular such screening would be among adolescents or how much it would add to current efforts to reduce smoking. It could have the harmful effect of encouraging people to smoke who might be at lower risk for lung cancer but at greater risk for other diseases for which genetic predispositions have not yet been discovered or do not exist.

Genetic screening is likely to be used to identify individuals at greater-than-average risk for diseases whose outcome can be improved by early, but expensive, presymptomatic monitoring. For instance, screening young women for a susceptibility-conferring genotype for breast cancer could reduce the burden of disease if those with positive tests received annual mammograms, a procedure that is recommended on an annual basis only in women over the age of 50. Monitoring those with genetic predispositions to insulin-dependent diabetes mellitus, colorectal cancer, neurofibromatosis, retinoblastoma, or Wilms tumor for the purpose of detecting early manifestations of the disease might prove beneficial. Discovering those with genetic predispositions could be accomplished either by population-wide screening or, less completely, by testing families in which disease has already occurred.

Who will provide genetic testing?

The field of medical genetics will grow, and those with specialized training will begin to compete with established university-based genetic centers to counsel clients and perform additional tests. The major source of their clients will be referrals from primary-care physicians, nongeneticist specialists, and health department clinics. These clients tend to fall into two categories: (1) members of families in which a genetic disease has already occurred who are concerned about the risks to future offspring; and (2) individuals or couples found by screening to be at risk of having affected offspring. Associations between medical geneticists and obstetricians who will perform prenatal diagnosis are likely to increase.

The number of medical geneticists will be insufficient to provide carrier screening to young couples, or chromosome screening to all pregnant women regardless of age. This task will increasingly be performed by family physicians and obstetricians. These physicians, particularly when they practice in groups, may hire their own genetic counselors rather than refer their patients to separate geneticists. Screening will also be conducted in health department clinics and at the worksite (although employers will not necessarily be given access to the results.)

The testing of newborns for presymptomatic, treatable disease will be added to current newborn screening programs, which are largely regulated by state health departments. The screening of older individuals for genetic susceptibilities will be performed by primary-care physicians and nongenetic specialists who are caring for families in which disease in their area of expertise has already occurred. These specialists—including internists and psychiatrists—will manage persons who have had positive test results themselves, although if concerns about risks to offspring arise, they may refer them to geneticists.

The types of laboratories performing DNA-based genetic tests will change as the technology evolves and becomes more automated and simplified. While the testing remains complex, a few highly specialized commercial laboratories as well as some laboratories in universities and free-standing groups of medical specialists will perform most of the analyses. When complex tests are performed primarily for reproductive purposes, laboratories affiliated with medical geneticists (in and outside universities) will have the edge over commercial laboratories because they will be able to provide counseling. They may also be geographically closer to the clients.

As the technology becomes simpler, multipurpose medical laboratories will offer genetic tests. Eventually, tests to screen for carriers and presymptomatic individuals at risk will be easy enough for physicians to perform in their offices.

How to Stop Worrying and Learn to Live with Genetic Tests

The preceding summary suggests that predictive genetic tests for a wide variety of diseases will soon be upon us and will be offered by physicians whose ability to use them may not be optimal. Yet genetic testing will not be held back by a lack of adequately trained health care providers. Commercial efforts to market tests as the technologies become available will prevail. Physicians will be more frightened of not using genetic tests at all (for fear of litigation) than of using them incorrectly.

Professional education

As a physician and teacher, I must speak out first about current inadequacies of medical education. These extend far beyond genetics, as the inverse relation between problem solving and amount of medical education (see chapter 7) indicates. The current emphasis on memorizing a forever-expanding body of knowledge detracts from the ability of physicians to reason and help people choose between different options. The emphasis given to disease in its advanced stages, as evidenced by the central role of hospitals providing highly specialized care in medical education, ill prepares health care providers to deal with the prevention and avoidance of disease. Moreover, as cost ceilings shorten hospital stays, less time is available for students to spend with patients. A new paradigm for medical education is needed, one that stresses methods of finding information rather than memorizing, that improves reasoning ability and communication skills, and that downplays paternalism and prepares physicians to accept the role of patients in making decisions relevant to their own health.

Medical genetics should be a required course in the curriculum of every medical school, with emphasis on common, gene-influenced diseases. The concepts of heterogeneity and variable expressivity should be stressed. They will help move medical students away from typological thinking "in which patients are perceived as representatives of the class rather than of themselves—so that variation and individuality, while certainly not ignored, are too often accorded only a back seat."[1] Genetics lends itself to teaching probability. Teaching the proper use of genetic tests introduces the idea (which should be self-evident, but often is not) that rates of disease (incidence and prevalence) provide probabilistic information that is useful in solving a wide array of clinical and diagnostic problems, including the predictive value of laboratory tests.

As genetic tests increase in volume and importance, other health professionals, including nurses and medical social workers, will be called upon to contribute to patient understanding. Much greater attention should be paid to genetics in schools of nursing and social work. The training of master's-level genetic counselors should be modified to permit them to function independently of medical geneticists—for instance, in primary-care facilities and with the nongeneticist specialists who will increasingly offer genetic tests. They could also assume, with medical geneticists, a teaching role for nurses and social workers. According to the director of one counseling program, the absence of trained minority and Spanish-speaking genetic counselors is a pressing issue that is not being adequately addressed.[2]

How people make decisions when confronted with probabilities rather than certainties is poorly understood. It will be impossible for physicians to communicate appropriately with clients—a process that requires an understanding of the clients' concerns, values, and other factors that influence their decisions regarding genetic risks—until more knowledge is gained in this area.

Educating the public

Pregnancy is not the best time to begin educating women, or their partners, about the chances of disease in the fetus or about the purposes of genetic tests. Because many people do not go to college, high school presents the last opportunity to reach most of the young, prereproductive population with information on probability and genetics. (Many who go on to college will never have a genetics course either.) Neither subject is adequately taught in secondary schools. If probability was taught, people might include probabilistic considerations in reaching value-loaded decisions in uncertain circumstances. Probability is sometimes introduced into the teaching of genetics, but seldom is the question of risk put in terms of choice—of what the student would do, given a 25 percent chance or a 50 percent chance of having an affected offspring. Such discussions—in math as well as biology classes—might bring home the subjective as well as the objective components of decision making. As students begin to realize that they differ from each other in the risks they are willing to take and to understand the reasons behind these differences, they might—given sufficient skill on the part of the teacher—develop a greater tolerance for those with different personal preferences. Some secondary school systems are incorporating sections on human genetics, but as a result of bureaucratic intransigence and the opposition of creationists and antiabortion groups, many graduates will be ill prepared to appreciate the implications of the genetic tests with which they will be confronted.

Another obstacle is the lack of teachers with sufficient knowledge of genetics and awareness of the ethical dilemmas posed by testing. The applications of modern science are too numerous for educators to permit high-school courses to dwell only on theory and not on the effects of science on students' lives and their environment. Until a new cadre of teachers is trained that is comfortable dealing with the social as well as the theoretical aspects of science, the danger will be greater (some danger will always be present) that teachers will transmit their own biases to students.

How to improve the quality of high-school teaching is beyond the scope of my expertise, but I would argue that—genetics aside—the task is important enough to warrant paying higher salaries and providing benefits competitive with other jobs requiring similar educational attainments.

Demonstrating the validity of genetic tests

In chapter 7, I described the Food and Drug Administration's (FDA's) procedures for approving medical devices, the category in which genetic tests fits. There are a number of loopholes that manufacturers could use to avoid having to provide evidence on the safety and effectiveness of genetic tests. Manufacturers could, for instance, claim "substantial equivalence" to existing devices, provided that the intended use of the new test is the same as that of the previous one. The number of uses to which new DNA-based genetic tests can be put, however, will almost always be greater than those to which existing tests are applied, even if the manufacturer claims that a new test is being marketed only for the same purposes as an existing test. Manufacturers could also present evidence of a test's ability to predict correctly the presence or absence of a disease-causing allele (or alleles)—something that is quite easy to do—but they might not be required to present evidence of how often a positive test correctly predicts the occurrence of a disease (the problem of variable expressivity) or how often a negative result is associated with the subsequent appearance of a disease (the problem of genetic heterogeneity). These loopholes can be closed by denying the use of "substantial equivalence" in categorizing new DNA-based genetic tests and treating them instead as class III devices, which require a premarketing demonstration of their safety and effectiveness.

The collection of this information may take considerable time, however, and it may be inappropriate to deny health care providers the use of the device until final estimates of its safety and effectiveness can be made. Under existing FDA procedures (Investigational Device Exemptions) the information can be collected. During this stage, health care providers could be permitted to offer the test, provided they informed their patients that the test was still under investigation and that its validity was not yet known.

An alternative to this premarket-approval approach would be to permit marketing of the test (on the basis of limited evidence of its validity), but to have the FDA continue to collect data on its sensitivity, specificity, and predictive values through postmarket surveillance. As noted in chapter 7, current procedures for postmarket surveillance are inadequate. Such surveillance might be facilitated by restricting the use of the test to a relatively small number of laboratories. These laboratories could be required to keep records of test results, and health care providers using the laboratories could be required to report all subsequent occurrences of the disease. These laboratories could then determine the sensitivity, specificity, and predictive value of the disease. This approach would be useful for disorders whose manifestations appear shortly after the test is given, but not for those that do not become manifest until long after the test is performed. In the latter case, other methods are needed (see chapter 5). One of them involves making comparisons between the laboratories' rate of positive test results and the observed rate of disease occurrence in a population comparable to the one screened. This provides a crude estimate of how often the disease is expressed (assuming reliable performance of the test).

Ensuring the reliability of genetic tests

Like many other commercial ventures in the United States, the proliferation of screening laboratories is based more on the opportunity to make money than on population needs. Until California limited the number of laboratories it licensed to perform newborn screening, 200 laboratories provided the test,[3] undoubtedly more per capita than in most other states. At that time, California accounted for a disproportionate number of the PKU infants missed by screening.[4] The picture improved after the number of laboratories was reduced to 7 and strict quality-control requirements were instituted.[5] Similar restrictions for laboratories performing DNA-based tests seem appropriate, at least until the technology becomes much less complex than it is at present. Depending on how the technology evolves, it may prove efficient to have tests for certain disorders performed in one or a few labs, and to have tests for other disorders done in a few other laboratories.

The interpretation of genetic test results often requires knowledge of the expressivity of the disorder and an awareness of the many issues that arise in providing information on reproductive risks. One arrangement that might ensure adequate interpretation and counseling is the requirement that laboratories have a working relationship with medical geneticists. (This is now the case for MSAFP testing in California.) Centralizing the entire screening process by providing a state coordinating agency would probably improve the quality of testing, particularly when it operated in conjunction with a state (or in the case of small states, a regional) laboratory. This agency could track specimens for the completeness and adequacy of collection, timely transmission to the laboratory, and correct reporting of results and follow-up.[6]

A centralized proficiency-testing program for DNA-based tests should be established. The Centers for Disease Control, the American Society of Human Genetics, one of the country's regional genetics groups, or the College of American Pathologists could sponsor such a program. States should require not merely participation in the program but adequate performance before licensing. Federal regulation of laboratories is limited to those receiving specimens across state lines or to those receiving federal reimbursement (e.g., Medicare) for services rendered. Satisfactory performance in a proficiency-testing program should be required of these labs.

It will be much harder to ensure the quality of laboratory performance or the interpretation of test results when genetic tests can be performed in physicians' office laboratories. At the very least, states will need to regulate these laboratories in some meaningful way. For instance, it might be helpful if states required physicians to demonstrate an understanding of genetic tests (and how to interpret them) before entitling them to use them in their offices. I hope that the technology will not improve faster than the physicians' understanding of genetics, but it might.

Even when genetic tests are approved for marketing by the FDA, states can regulate their use. California has done this for MSAFP testing, and Maryland's Commission on Hereditary Disorders has the authority to do it.

Limiting genetic testing by insurers and employers

The use of valid genetic tests to deny individual insurance to people with positive results represents victim blaming of the most blatant sort, for people have no control over the genes they inherit. Such a policy may be advantageous to insurance companies and those with negative test results, but it places a heavy burden on those with positive results and, perhaps, their beneficiaries. Except when surviving beneficiaries are highly dependent on income from the affected person, the effects of denying life insurance will generally be less serious than those of denying health insurance. The establishment of high-risk pools—already done by some states—provides insufficient relief. People at greater-than-average risk will have to pay more. Denial of insurance and employment based on test results has already occurred with AIDS.

One way of solving the problem is to prohibit insurance companies from using genetic tests or from obtaining their results from applicants' personal physicians. I do not think this is a good solution. If only a few (mostly small) states ban testing, companies will stop offering insurance in those states. If the bans are more widespread, the insurance companies will find themselves losing money as those persons who are tested confidentially and learn they are at increased risk purchase more insurance. The companies will have to raise premiums, thereby excluding people with negative test results who can no longer afford coverage. A better solution would be to recognize that health care is a right—regardless of differences in risk—and to establish a national health system in which everyone is guaranteed adequate health care coverage, genetic and other predictive tests are used entirely on a voluntary basis, and individuals with positive test results are not penalized.

It does make sense to prohibit the use of genetic tests as a condition of employment when the results have no direct bearing on ability to perform the job but affect only employee health-benefit costs. To this end, current federal law prohibiting the firing of covered employees for reasons related to employee benefits should be extended to prohibiting discrimination in hiring for the same reasons. States should adopt such laws as well. The only justification for genetic testing in hiring should be that it provides important information about the ability of applicants to perform the specific jobs for which they are being considered. (Maryland places such restrictions on the information gathered in preemployment examinations.)[7] Even then, employment should be denied only when an industry can demonstrate conclusively that it cannot accommodate at-risk persons in other ways.

Access to genetic tests

Charges for some genetic tests (and some options that follow a positive test result) place them out of the financial reach of many people. Sometimes third-party reimbursement for counseling (which should be an inherent part of testing for reproductive purposes) is not provided, and at other times it is inadequate. Although insurance companies will increasingly reimburse for genetic tests (as they realize the savings in doing so), the potential for discrimination (e.g., failing to renew individual health insurance policies after a test result is known) makes a national health system that covers voluntary testing, confirmatory studies, counseling, and the abortion of affected fetuses a better way to eliminate inequities. A somewhat problematic question is whether such a system would reimburse for expensive procedures such as in vitro fertilization to avoid the conception of affected children, since the alternative of avoiding their birth by prenatal diagnosis and abortion could be used. If there are people who would use avoidance-of-conception but not avoidance-of-birth options, their reproductive freedom would be impaired by the lack of reimbursement for the former. I doubt that there are many such people.

At the present time, geographical differences in the availability of genetic testing services exist. This is, of course, true of other elements of health care as well. Through a national health system, the federal government could redress geographical inequities. It did so partially with allocations under the Genetic Diseases Act, but on a per capita basis, state allocations for genetic services still varied markedly after federal assistance.[8]

Many young adults, who could benefit from genetic testing for reproductive purposes, do not have a regular source of care or seek care only when they are ill. Performing genetic tests for the first time when a woman comes for prenatal care deprives her of some avoidance options and may not give her adequate time to make a reasoned decision. Testing could be provided in childhood, but there is no guarantee that the child or his or her parents will remember the results or comprehend them later in life. Recording the results of genetic tests on a medical record, which the subject retains and makes available to physicians who provide care subsequently, is one solution, provided confidentiality is maintained. Mass screening—in communities or schools—is another, but the dangers of coercion are too great for me to commend this approach. Perhaps when the barriers to medical care are removed through the provision of comprehensive care as part of a national health system, people of all ages will more readily seek and obtain care.

Protecting individual autonomy

Competent adolescents and adults should always have the right to decide whether to have a genetic test. Parents should have that right regarding the testing of their infant or child: "It is more important for society to follow a conscious policy of protecting individual autonomy in assessing the social implications of one's individual genotype than to mobilize social resources behind a coercive model of genetic 'normality.'"[9]

How is autonomy to be ensured? Certainly the knowledge people bring to a situation in which testing is offered is important, as I have already discussed, but informed consent is the touchstone of any genetic testing program. To be fully informed, people need to know the following:

(1) the purposes of the test (e.g., to determine whether they are carriers of a specific allele for a recessive disease or are at risk for the disease themselves);

(2) the risk of the test itself;

(3) the chance that the test results will be incorrect;

(4) the implications of a positive result (e.g., the need for further testing to confirm the result, or the likelihood of disease);

(5) the nature of the condition the test is intended to detect, including its range of severity and age of onset (particularly important when the person being tested is unfamiliar with the disease);

(6) the options available to reduce the burden of disease in the event of a confirmed positive result;

(7) the alternatives if the individual decides not to have the test.

In families in which disease has already struck, individuals coming for testing will have some idea of the severity of the condition. Often, they will not appreciate the risks to their own offspring or the options for avoiding the conception or birth of affected offspring. In population-wide screening, the vast majority of those coming for testing will have no personal experience with the condition, and may have distorted notions of its severity, little idea of how its expression can vary, and a poor understanding of the risks to their offspring.

In situations where sex partners differ on whether the woman should undergo prenatal diagnosis, the woman's views should prevail. She has the greater stake, since she will carry the child and, in this society, do more of the nurturing.

Requiring informed consent is consonant with individual autonomy, but does not guarantee it. People are not really free to choose if they know that penalties will be exacted for refusing to be tested or for refusing to take certain actions, such as abortion, if the test results are positive. The withdrawal or curtailment of support for the care of infants born with avoidable handicapping conditions is one such penalty. Because many people will elect to terminate such pregnancies regardless of the level of support offered, the money saved can be used to assure optimal care for the affected offspring of parents who refuse abortion.

Women and men who wish to donate or sell their ova or sperm, respectively, to other couples, or women who are willing to serve as surrogates (to be inseminated by another woman's husband), should not be permitted to do so unless they consent to genetic tests to determine that they are not at risk of transmitting genetic disease to the offspring. For the genetic testing of biological parents who wish to place their children for adoption, or of the children themselves, the consent of the biological parents should be required. The effect of that information on the adoption process needs to be studied. Ensuring that adoptive parents will receive full compensation for the added costs of caring for children with genetic disorders that could have been detected, makes less likely the chance that infants whose parents refuse testing will not be adopted. The biological parents should be told in advance of testing that the results may provide them with information about the risks of genetic disease to future offspring of their own or to themselves. They should have the option to decide whether they want to be given this information or not.

Preserving confidentiality

Consent to be tested is not perfectly autonomous if the results are made known to others without the permission of the person being tested, or, in the case of a child, of his or her parents. Some people who know that the results are likely to be released to insurance companies or employers will refuse testing on that ground alone. For this reason, results should be released only after permission is granted by the person being tested or by his or her parents. Permission to release results, stipulating to whom they are to be released, could be included in the consent solicited prior to testing, or could be obtained at any time after testing when the question of releasing results comes up. Some people who consent to testing and to the release of the results may not be aware of how the results can be used by third parties to the disadvantage of those with positive results. For this reason, physicians or others who are asked to release results should discuss the possible consequences of disclosure with patients before obtaining their permission to release test information.

A thorny question is whether test results should be provided to one's spouse. The argument for doing so is less strong in the case of genetic testing than in those cases (HIV-antibody testing, for instance) in which both the spouse and the prospective offspring are endangered. Nonetheless, a woman who is not given her partner's test results might choose never to become pregnant; or if she had the information, she might choose prenatal diagnosis to determine whether the fetus was at risk for disease. Consequently, in obtaining a patient's consent to undergo tests that will determine if he or she is a carrier for a recessive or X-linked condition, or for a late-onset dominant condition, in which the results carry information about the risks to prospective offspring, I would indicate that I plan to release positive results to the spouse, provided the couple intends to have additional children. If the individual then refuses the screening, I personally would not test. I do not think such situations would arise very often. Except in the case of tests for late-onset dominant disorders, the principal reason that people want to be tested is either to avoid, or to prepare for, the birth of an affected offspring. I believe that one's spouse should be included in either case. One might also argue that a commitment to communicate with one's spouse carries with it an obligation to inform future spouses, if the test is performed prior to marriage, or to inform living offspring or siblings, if they have a chance of transmitting the disease-causing allele or of being affected. Although I believe that physicians should encourage their patients to communicate test results to relatives at risk, I also believe that requiring physicians to communicate to relatives other than the spouse places too much burden on the physician, who may not be caring for these relatives. Moreover, as testing becomes well established, it is likely that these people will be offered testing independently. (Of course, they might refuse, not knowing they are at increased risk.)

Disclosure of the test results for people wishing to donate or sell their gametes or to serve as surrogates should not include the person's name (although in embryo donation or surrogacy the identity may be known to the receiving parents).

Summary and Conclusions

Genetic testing based on recombinant DNA technology will not transform medical practice overnight. The first tests offered may nevertheless affect large numbers of people. The opportunities provided by the first tests will be primarily the avoidance of the conception or birth of affected children, the long-term use of drugs or life-style changes whose effectiveness has not always been demonstrated, or an increased monitoring for signs of illness that still may not result in cure. For some disorders (primarily those that are single gene in origin) the tests will prove to be highly accurate predictors. When genetic heterogeneity and variable expressivity characterize a disease, positive test results will increase the chances that the disorder will occur but will not predict it with certainty.

Genetic tests could soon be used by insurance companies to exclude or limit coverage for people found to be at risk for diseases whose management costs are high; they could be used by employers for the same reason and also to exclude from employment workers with genetic predispositions to diseases caused by workplace exposures.

With such limited and controversial benefits, the question can be asked, Why proceed at all? The most primitive answer is that we have no choice. As I have shown in earlier chapters, biotechnology companies are already developing and marketing genetic tests. It would go against the grain of our economic system to prohibit such tests. Even if commercial development were sharply curtailed, academic institutions would provide tests on a quasi-investigational basis, and such tests would be exempt from quality assurance and regulation. Moreover, test laboratories in universities might not be able or willing to satisfy the demand for testing; unequal access would result.

The prospect of prohibiting the performance of genetic tests in research-oriented university laboratories brings me to a second reason why such testing should not be curtailed: curtailment would decelerate the rate at which we come to understand genetic diseases and thus the rate at which we develop the means to prevent—not simply avoid—or effectively manage them. The interventions that are currently used following the finding of positive test results are halfway technologies. The interim solutions they provide should not be accepted as "final solutions." If we do not continue research into the basic mechanisms of detectable diseases—and genetic testing to identify those at risk—people will be forced to rely on the halfway technologies.

To prohibit testing when only halfway technologies (under which I include avoidance strategies) are available would deny people the opportunity to use such technologies. Just as I deplore the imposition of testing on anyone—or the imposition of any action pursuant to a positive test result—so I deplore withholding these technologies from those who would freely and knowledgeably choose to use them. The major dangers of genetic testing in the recombinant DNA era are its unbridled development without assurance of test validity and reliability; inadequate knowledge on the part of providers and potential recipients; inequities in test use and ensuing care; and, finally, restrictions on individual autonomy and confidentiality. I have suggested a number of policies to minimize these dangers.

There is no retreating from the use of genetic tests. Their widespread adoption using public funds, however, requires close scrutiny. Public funding would reduce barriers to access and availability, but widespread testing might be accomplished at the expense of other programs that would improve health. So long as military expenditures consume an inordinate percentage of the federal budget (in relation to the threat of war or to the use of negotiation to reduce the threat), I will not be willing to say that we have reached the limit of public spending to improve health care. In the foreseeable future, however, choices will continue to be made on expenditures within the health sector. The nation's policy makers must decide whether publicly supported genetic testing deserves high priority in the provision of adequate health care to all people.

Notes

Introduction: The Shape of Things to Come

1. Ludmerer KM. Genetics and American society. Baltimore: Johns Hopkins University Press, 1972. See also Kevles DJ. In the name of eugenics. New York: Alfred A. Knopf, 1985.

2. Committee for the Study of Inborn Errors of Metabolism (CSIEM). Genetic screening: programs, principles, and research. Washington, D.C.: National Academy of Sciences, 1975.

3. Ibid.:27–29. See also Holtzman NA. Anatomy of a trial. Pediatrics 1977;60:932–34; and Berwick DM, Cretin S, Keeler E. Cholesterol, children, and heart disease: an analysis of alternatives. New York: Oxford University Press, 1980:12–14.

4. Tourian A, Sidbury JB. Phenylketonuria and hyperphenylaninemia. In: Stanbury JB, Wyngaarden JB, Fredrickson DS, Goldstein JL, Brown MS, eds. The metabolic basis of inherited disease. New York: McGraw-Hill, 1983:270–286.

5. Holtzman NA, Mellits ED, Meek AG. Neonatal screening for phenylketonuria. I. Effectiveness. JAMA 1974;229:667–670.

6. Reilly P. Genetics, law, and social policy. Cambridge, Mass.: Harvard University Press, 1977.

7. Stamatoyannopoulos G. Problems of screening and counseling in the hemoglobinopathies. In: Motulsky AG, Lenz W, eds. Birth defects. Amsterdam: Excerpta Medica, 1974:268–276.

8. U.S. Congress, Office of Technology Assessment (OTA). The role of genetic testing in the prevention of occupational disease. Washington, D.C.: U.S. Government Printing Office, 1983. See also Calabrese EJ. Ecogenetics: genetic variation in susceptibility to environmental agents. New York: John Wiley, 1984; and Omenn GS, Gelboin HV, eds. Genetic variability in responses to chemical exposure. Cold Spring Harbor Laboratory, 1984; Banbury Report 16.

9. Holtzman NA. Dietary treatment of inborn errors of metabolism. Ann Rev Med 1970;21:335–356.

10. Murray RF, Jr. Problems behind the promise: ethical issues in mass genetic screening. Hastings Center Report 1972;2 (April):10–13.

11. Holtzman NA. The impact of the federal cutback on genetic services. Amer J Med Genet 1983;15:353–365.

12. As most infants with neural tube defects are born into families without any previous history, the greatest reduction of neural tube defects would result from testing every pregnant woman. The low cost of the test makes this feasible. However, given the incidence of neural tube defects in the United States, approximately thirty to fifty false positive test results would be obtained for every true positive. Unless those receiving the results recognized the importance of obtaining more specific follow up tests, unnecessary abortions might result.

13. U.S. Department of Health and Human Sevices. Alpha-fetoprotein test kits: proposed restrictions and proposed additional quality control and testing requirements. 45 Fed. Reg. 74158–74176 (1980).

14. U.S. Department of Health and Human Sevices. Alpha-fetoprotein test kits: withdrawal of proposed rule. 48 Fed. Reg. 27780–27782 (1983).

15. Thomas L. The future place of science in the art of healing. J Med Educ 1976;51:23–29.

Chapter 1: The Structural Basis of Genetic Differences

1. Mayr E. The growth of biological thought. Cambridge, Mass.: Harvard University Press, 1982:710–722.

2. Garrod AE. Inborn errors of metabolism. 1909. Reprint. New York: Oxford University Press, 1963.

3. Garrod AE. Inborn factors of disease. New York: Oxford University Press, 1931.

Chapter 2: The Complexity of Diseases: No More Magic Bullets

1. Galston I. The meaning of social medicine. Cambridge, Mass.: Harvard University Press, 1954:38.

2. McKeown T. The role of medicine: dream, mirage, or nemesis? Princeton: Princeton University Press, 1979. See also McKinlay J, McKinlay S. The questionable contribution of medical measures to the decline of mortality in the United States in the twentieth century. Milbank Mem Fund Q/Hlth & Soc 1977;55:405–428. Because rates were quite low by the time vaccines and antibiotics appeared, their effect is much more evident when log mortality rates rather than the rates themselves are plotted.

3. National Center for Health Statistics (NCHS). Advance report of final mortality statistics, 1985. Hyattsville, Md.: Public Health Service, 1987; DHHS publication no (PHS) 87-1120. (Mo Vit Stat Rep 36 [5 suppl]).

4. U.S. Department of Commerce, Bureau of the Census. Mortality statistics, 1910. Washington, D.C.: U.S. Government Printing Office; 1913:533.

5. NCHS, Advance report.

6. Kalter H, Warkany J. Congenital malformations: etiologic factors and their role in prevention. New Engl J Med 1983;308:424–431, 491–497. Single-gene and chromosomal disorders account for at least 8 percent of these abnormalities, a more significant component than those caused by maternally acquired infection.

7. Doll R, Hill AB. Lung cancer and other causes of death in relation to smoking. Brit Med J 1956;2:1071–1081.

8. Kannel WB, Gordon T, eds. The Framingham study. Washington, D.C.: U.S. Government Printing Office, 1976; DHEW publication no (NIH) 76-1083, sec. 31: The results of the Framingham study applied to four other U.S.-based epidemiologic studies of cardiovascular disease. Data calculated from tables 6 and 25.

9. Sorensen TIA, Orholm M, Bentsen K, Hoybye G, Eghoje K, Christoffersen P. Prospective evaluation of alcohol abuse and alcoholic liver injury in men as predictors of development of cirrhosis. Lancet 1985;2:241–244.

10. Tsuji S, Choudary PV, Martim BM, et al. A mutation in the human glucocerebroside gene in neuronopathic Gaucher's disease. N Engl J Med 1987; 316:570–575.

11. Friend SH, Bernards R, Rogelj S, et al. A human DNA segment with properties of the gene that predisposes to retinoblastoma and osteosarcoma. Nature 1986;323:643–646.

12. Bodmer WF, Bailey CJ, Bodmer J, et al. Localization of the gene for familial polyposis on chromosome 5. Nature 1987;328:614–616.

13. Solomon E, Voss R, Hall V, et al. Chromsome 5 allele loss in human colorectal carcinomas. Nature 1987;328:616–619.

14. Goldstein JL, Brown MS. Familial hypercholesterolemia. In: Stanbury JB, Wyngaarden JB, Fredrickson DS, Goldstein JL, Brown MS, eds. The metabolic basis of inherited disease. New York: McGraw-Hill, 1983:672–712. See also Goldstein JL, Brown MS. Familial hypercholesterolemia: a genetic receptor disease. Hosp Prac 15 November 1985:35–46.

15. Kueppers F. The effect of smoking on the development of emphysema in alpha-1-antitrypsin deficiency. In: Omenn GS, Gelboin HV, eds. Genetic variability in responses to chemical exposure. Cold Spring Harbor Laboratory, 1984; Banbury Report 16:345–356.

16. Cited by Martin JB. Molecular genetics: applications to the clinical neurosciences. Science 1987;238:765–772.

17. Comings DE, Comings BG. A controlled study of Tourette syndrome. I. Attention-deficit disorder, learning disorders, and school problems. Am J Hum Genet 1987;41:701–741.

18. Marmot MG, Shipley MJ, Rose G. Inequalities in death—specific explanations of a general pattern? Lancet 1984;1:1003–1006.

19. Tokuhata GK. Familial factors in human long cancer and smoking. Am J Pub Hlth 1964;54:24–32.

20. Nora JJ, Lortscher RH, Spangler RD, Nora AH, Kimberling WJ. Genetic-epidemiologic study of early-onset ischemic heart disease. Circulation 1980;61: 503–508.

21. Berg K. Genetics of coronary heart disease. Prog Med Genet 1983;5:35–90. See also Breslow, JL. Apolipoprotein defects. Hosp Prac 15 December 1985:43–49; and Motulsky AG. Genetic research in coronary heart disease. In: Rao DC, Elston RC, Kuller LH, Feinleib M, Carter C, Havlik R, eds. Genetic epidemiology of coronary heart disease. New York: Alan R. Liss, 1984:541–548.

22. Udall JN, Dixon M, Newman AP, Wright JA, James B, Bloch KJ. Liver disease in alpha-1-antitrypsin deficiency. JAMA 1985;253:2679–2682. It is possible that human milk is protective.

23. Kueppers, The effect of smoking.

24. Thacker SB, Veech RL, Vernon AA, Rutstein DD. Genetic and biochemical factors relevant to alcoholism. Alcoholism: Clin Exp Res 1984;8:375–383. For a

list of disorders in which both genetic and environmental factors have been implicated see Williams R. Understanding genetic and environmental risk factors in susceptible persons. Western J Med 1984;141:799–806.

25. Dubos R. Mirage of health. New York: Harper & Row, 1959:278,281.

26. A very high dose of a toxic substance might cause disease by itself. A mutation that caused extreme alterations in the gene product (e.g., none synthesized), particularly when it is present in double dose, is likely to result in a different clinical entity than mutations causing less extreme defects (e.g., diminished enzyme activity).

27. Individuals with early age of clinical manifestations of several common disorders are more likely to have the disease on a genetic basis than those with later onsets. See Childs B, Scriver CR. Age at onset and causes of disease. Perspect Biol Med 1986;29:437–460.

28. Holtzman NA, Khoury MJ. Monitoring for congenital malformations. Ann Rev Pub Hlth 1986;7:237–266.

29. Because humans cannot be bred at will, segregation analysis is not always straightforward even when only a single locus is involved, but corrections can be made. See Emery AEW. Methodology in medical genetics. London: Churchill, 1976:38–50.

30. King M-C, Lee GM, Spinner NB, et al. Genetic epidemiology. Ann Rev Pub Hlth 1984;5:1–52. See also Susser M. Separating heredity and environment. Am J Prev Med 1985;1(2):5–23.

31. St. George–Hyslop PH, Tanzi RE, Polinsky RJ. The genetic defect causing familial Alzheimer's disease maps on chromosome 21. Science 1987;235:885–890.

32. Mendlewicz J, Simon P, Sevy S, et al. Polymorphic DNA marker on X chromosome and manic depression. Lancet 1987;1:1230–1232.

33. Egeland JA, Gerhard DS, Pauls DL, et al. Bipolar affective disorders linked to DNA markers on chromosome 11. Nature 1987:325:783–787.

34. Goldstein JL, Schrott HG, Hazzard WR, et al. Hyperlipidemia in coronary heart disease. II. Genetic analysis of lipid levels in 176 families and delineation of a new inherited disorder, combined hyperlipidemia. J Clin Invest 1973;52:1544–68. See also Brown MS, Goldstein JL. A receptor-mediated pathway for cholesterol homeostasis. Science 1986;34–47.

35. Vessell ES, Penno MB. Impact of multiple dynamically interacting genetic and environmental factors on methods to detect new polymorphisms of hepatic drug oxidation. In: Omenn and Gelboin, eds. Genetic variability:117–123.

36. Holtzman, Khoury. Monitoring for congenital malformations.

37. Ibid. A recent exception is isotretinoin (Accutane®), a potent teratogen used to treat a severe form of acne.

38. Ibid. See also Khoury MJ, Holtzman NA. On the ability of birth defects monitoring to detect new teratogens. Am J Epidemiol 1987;126:136–143.

39. Piper JM, Tonascia J, Matanoski GM. Heavy phenacetin use and bladder cancer in women aged 20 to 49 years. N Engl J Med 1985;313:292–295.

40. Ritchie JC, Sloan TP, Idle JR, Smith RL. Toxicological implications of polymorphic drug metabolism. In: Evered D, Lawrenson G, eds. Environmental chemicals, enzyme function, and human disease. Ciba Foundation Symposium 76. Amsterdam: Excerpta Medica, 1980:219–244.

41. Payami H, Khan MA, Grennan DM, Sanders PA, Dyer A, Thomson G.

Analysis of genetic interrelationship among HLA-associated diseases. Am J Hum Genet 1987;41:331–349.

42. Nagel RL, Fabry ME, Pagnier J, et al. Hematologically and genetically distinct forms of sickle cell anemia in Africa: the Senegal type and the Benin type. N Engl J Med 1985;312:880–884.

43. Holtzman NA. The goal of preventing early death. In: Blendon R, Duval MK, Hiscock W McC et al., eds. Conditions for change in the health care system. Washington, D.C.: U.S. Department of Health, Education, and Welfare, Public Health Service, Health Resources Administration, 1977; DHEW publication no (HRA) 78-642:107–132. See also Farquhar JW, Fortmann SP, Maccoby N, et al. The Stanford five-city project: design and methods. Am J Epidemiol 1985;122:323–334; and Puska P, Nissinen A, Tuomilehto J, et al. The community-based strategy to prevent coronary heart disease: conclusions from the ten years of the North Karelia project. Ann Rev Pub Hlth 1985;6:147–193.

Chapter 3: The Role of Genes in Disease

1. Harris H. The principles of human biochemical genetics. 3rd ed. Amsterdam: Elsevier, 1980. See also Neel JV. A revised estimate of the amount of genetic variation in human proteins: implications for the distribution of DNA polymorphisms. Am J Hum Genet 1984;36:1135–1148; and Goldman D, Goldin LR, Pathnagiri P, et al. Twenty-seven protein polymorphisms by two-dimensional electrophoresis of serum, erythrocytes, and fibroblasts in two pedigrees. Am J Hum Genet 1985:37:898–911. Enzymes are more likely to be polymorphic than proteins involved in cell structure, and serum proteins are more likely to be polymorphic than cellular proteins. These differences are not as pronounced as originally believed. See ibid.

2. The frequency of a specific allele is the proportion of that allele to all alleles at that locus present in the population. Since individuals have two alleles at the locus, then for uncommon alleles, for which the frequency of homozygotes can be neglected, the allele frequency is one half the frequency of heterozygotes for the allele in the population.

3. If there are two alleles in the population, with frequencies of p and q respectively $(p + q = 1)$, the heterozygote frequency $= 2pq$, and the frequency of q homozygotes $= q^2$. Thus, if the allele frequency, q, for a disease that manifests in heterozygotes is .001, the frequency of heterozygotes, $2pq$, is 2(.999)(.001), or .002. The homozygous (disease) frequency, q^2, is .0001. This is 20 times less than the frequency of heterozygotes.

4. Harris. Principles of human biochemical genetics.

5. Tonegawa S. Somatic generation of antibody diversity. Nature 1983;302:575–581.

6. Weitkamp LR, Schacter BZ. Transferrin and HLA: spontaneous abortion, neural tube defects, and natural selection. N Engl J Med 1985;313:925–932. See also Jones JS, Partridge L. Tissue rejection: the price of sexual acceptance. Nature 1983;304:484–485. These authors hypothesize that when the parents share too many MHC proteins, the fetus cannnot elicit an immune response strong enough to prevent a later attack by maternal cells.

7. Nebert DW. P450 genes and evolutionary genetics. Hosp Prac 15 March 1987:63–74.

8. Miller LH, Mason SJ, Clyde DF, et al. The resistance factor to plasmodium vivax in blacks. N Engl J Med 1976;296:302–304.

9. Childs B, Moxon R, Winkelstein J. Genetics and infectious diseases. In: King RA, Rotter JI, Motulsky A, eds. The genetic basis of common disease. New York: McGraw-Hill. [In press].

10. Rotter JL, Rimoin DL. The genetics of diabetes mellitus. Hosp Prac 15 May 1987:79–88. See also Erlich H, Stetler D. HLA Class II DNA polymorphisms: markers for genetic predisposition to insulin-dependent diabetes. In: Omenn GS, Gelboin HV, eds. Genetic variability in responses to chemical exposure. Cold Spring Harbor Laboratory, 1984; Banbury Report 16:321–331.

11. McDevitt HO. The HLA system and its relation to disease. Hosp Prac 15 July 1985:57–72.

12. Rotter, Rimoin. Genetics of diabetes.

13. McDevitt. The HLA system. See also Arnett FC. HLA genes and predisposition to rheumatic diseases. Hosp Prac 15 December 1986:89–100; Childs, Moxon, Winkelstein. Genetics and infectious diseases; Kostyu DD, Amos DB. The histocompatibility complex: genetic polymorphism and disease susceptibility. In: Stanbury JB, Wyngaarden JB, Fredrickson DS, Goldstein JL, Brown MS, eds. The metabolic basis of inherited disease. New York: McGraw-Hill, 1983:77–98; and King M-C, Lee GM, Spinner NB, et al. Genetic epidemiology. Ann Rev Pub Hlth 1984;5:1–52. It is likely that susceptibility to the three diseases mentioned is due to the product of specific HLA alleles. In addition, several other disorders have been associated with the region because disease-causing alleles reside at gene loci that are tightly linked to HLA genes; these include hemochromatosis and congenital adrenal hyperplasia.

14. William RC, Raizada V, Prakash K, et al. Studies of streptococcal membrane antigen-binding cells in acute rheumatic fever. J Lab Clin Med 1985;105:531–536. The allele responsible for this product, which has been detected by monoclonal antibody, may reside at the HLA DR locus.

15. Petersen GM, Silimperi DR, Scott EM, Hall DB, Rotter JI, Ward HI. Uridine monophosphate kinase 3: a genetic marker for susceptibility to haemophilus influenzae type B disease. Lancet 1985;2:417–418.

16. Ritchie JC, Sloan TP, Idle JR, Smith RL. Toxicological implications of polymorphic drug metabolism. In: Evered D, Lawrenson G, eds. Environmental chemicals, enzyme function, and human disease. Ciba Foundation Symposium 76. Amsterdam: Excerpta Medica, 1980:219–244.

17. Price Evans DA. Survey of the human acetylator polymorphism in spontaneous disorders. J Med Genet 1984;21:243–253.

18. Batchelor JR, Welsh KI, Tinoco RM, et al. Hydralazine-induced systemic lupus erythematosus: influence of HLA-DR and sex on susceptibility. Lancet 1980;1:1107–1109.

19. Nebert DW. P450 genes. See also Gonzalez FJ, Jaiswal AK, Nebert DW. P450 genes: evolution, regulation, and relationship to human cancer and pharmacogenetics. Cold Spring Harbor Symp Quant Biol 1986;51(pt 2):879–890.

20. Ayesh R, Idle JR, Ritchie JC, Crothers MJ, Hetzel MR. Metabolic oxidation phenotypes as markers for susceptibility to lung cancer. Nature 1984;312:169–170.

21. Evans DAP, Harmer D, Downham DY, et al. The genetic control of sparteine and debrisoquine metabolism in man with new methods of analysing bimodal distributions. J Med Genet 1983;20:321–329.

22. Lennard MS, Silas JH, Freestone S, Ramsay LE, Tucker GT, Woods HF. Oxidation phenotype—a major determinant of metoprolol metabolism and response. N Engl J Med 1982;307:1558–1560.

23. Ritchie et al. Toxicologic implications. Toxic effects (agranulocytosis) of metiamide were observed in some extensive metabolizers; they rapidly converted the thiourea side-chain of the drug to a toxic compound. The side-chain was not essential for pharmacological activity (histamine H_2-receptor antagonist) and was replaced by cyanoguanidine in cimetidine, thereby removing toxicity. Poor metabolizers are more likely to develop toxic reactions from phenacetin because the drug itself, not the oxidation product, is readily converted to a toxic metabolite by an enzyme under independent genetic control.

24. Galloway SM, Perry PE, Meneses J, et al. Cultured mouse embryos metabolize benzo(a)pyrene during early gestation: genetic difference detectable by sister chromatid exchange. Proc Natl Acad Sci USA 1980;77:3524–3528.

25. Shum S, Jensen NM, Nebert DW. The murine Ah locus: in utero toxicity and teratogenesis associated with genetic differences in benzo(a)pyrene metabolism. Teratology 1979;20:365–376.

26. Manchester D, Jacoby E. Decreased placental monooxygenase activities associated with birth defects. Teratology 1984;30:31–37. See also Manchester DK, Parker NB, Bowman CM. Maternal smoking increases xenobiotic metabolism in placenta but not umbilical vein endothelium. Pediatr Res 1984;18:1071–1075. Induction of at least one P450 enzyme depends on receptor sites that are separate from the structural gene for the enzyme, and others that are contiguous with it. See Jones PBC, Galeazzi DR, Fisher JM, Whitlock JP, Jr. Control of cytochrome P-450 gene expression by dioxin. Science 1985;227:1499–1502.

27. Strickler SM, Dansky LV, Miller MA, Seni M-H, Andermann E, Spielberg SP. Genetic predisposition to phenytoin-induced birth defects. Lancet 1985;2:746–749.

28. Harris. Principles of human biochemical genetics:173–190.

29. Beutler E. Sensitivity to drug-induced hemolytic anemia in glucose-6-phosphate dehydrogenase deficiency. In: Omenn, Gelboin, eds. Genetic variability:205–211.

30. Jackson-Cook CK, Flannery DB, Corey LA, Nance WE, Brown JA. Nucleolar organizer region variants as a risk factor for Down syndrome. Am J Hum Genet 1985;37:1059–1061.

31. Hassold TJ, Jacobs PA. Trisomy in man. Ann Rev Genet 1984;18:69–98.

32. Antonarakis SE, Kittur SD, Metaxotou C, Watkins PC, Patel AS. Analysis of DNA haplotypes suggests a genetic predisposition to trisomy 21 associated with DNA sequences on chromosome 21. Proc Natl Acad Sci USA 1985;82:3360–3364.

33. See note 3.

34. On the basis of findings in a number of recessive diseases, Vogel concluded that "the present evidence, fragmentary as it looks, suggests the possibility that slight phenotypic manifestations in humans heterozygous for autosomal recessive diseases might be the rule rather than the exception." The manifestations usually could not be classified as diseases, but were deviations from normal labo-

ratory findings. Given stressful environmental situations, or the presence of certain alleles at other loci, heterozygotes with such findings might be more prone to certain diseases. See Vogel F. Clinical consequences of heterozygosity for autosomal-recessive diseases. Clin Genet 1984;25:381–415.

35. Goldstein JL, Brown MS. Familial hypercholesterolemia: a genetic receptor disease. Hosp Prac 15 November 1985:35–46.

36. Boers GHJ, Smals AGH, Trijbels FJM, et al. Heterozygosity for homocystinuria in premature peripheral and cerebral occlusive arterial disease. N Engl J Med 1985;313:709–715.

37. Swift M, Reitnauer PJ, Morrell D, Chase CL. Breast and other cancers in families with ataxias-telangiectasia. N Engl J Med 1987;316:1289–1294. Female heterozygotes may account for 1–8 percent of all women with breast cancer in the United States.

38. Frorath B, Schmidt-Preuss U, Siemers U, Zollner M, Rudiger HW. Heterozygous carriers for Bloom syndrome exhibit a spontaneously increased micronucleus formation in cultured fibroblasts. Hum Genet 1984;67:52–55. Epidemiological studies on the risk of cancer in parents of children with Bloom syndrome have not yet been reported.

39. Gadek JE, Crystal RG. Alpha-1-antitrypsin deficiency. In: Stanbury et al. Metabolic basis of inherited disease:1450–1467. See also Cohen BH, Ball WC, Jr., Brashears S, et al. Risk factors in chronic obstructive pulmonary disease (COPD), Am J Epidemiol 1977;105:223–232.

40. Prokop DJ. Mutations in collagen genes. J Clin Invest 1985;75:783–787.

41. Antonarakis SE. Hemophilia A persistence and gene mutational variability. Hosp Prac 15 December 1987:73–82.

42. Harris. Principles of human biochemical genetics:348.

43. The gene for G6PD is on the X-chromosome. Female carriers of the G6PD deficiency allele who ingest fava beans may have a reproductive advantage over female noncarriers. In addition, carriers may have more female offspring—half of whom would be carriers—than noncarriers, in order to compensate for the increased loss of sons with G6PD deficiency. Their carrier daughters would also be at an advantage. For the effect of fava bean components on malarial parasitization in G6PD deficiency, see Golenser J, Miller J, Spira DT, et al. Inhibitory effect of a fava bean component on the in vitro development of Plasmodium falciparum in normal and glucose-6-phosphate dehydrogenase deficient erythrocytes. Blood 1983;61:507–510. See also Friedman MJ. Expression of inherited resistance to malaria in culture. In: Evered D, Whelan J, eds. Malaria and the red cell. Ciba Foundation Symposium 94. London: Pitman, 1983:196–205.

44. Childs, Moxon, Winkelstein. Genetics and infectious diseases.

45. Cavalli-Sforza LL, Bodmer WF. The genetics of human populations. San Francisco: W. H. Freeman, 1971:45–62.

46. Costa T, Scriver CR, Childs B. The effect of Mendelian disease on human health: a measurement. Am J Med Genet 1985;21:231–242.

47. Neel JV. Diabetes mellitus: a thrifty genotype rendered detrimental by "progress"? Am J Hum Genet 1962;14:356–362. See also Neel JV. The thrifty genotype revisited. In: Kobberling J, Tattersall R, eds. The genetics of diabetes mellitus. London: Academic Press, 1982:283–293. One might also speculate that the synthesis of new chemicals, to which humans had not been exposed through most of their evolution, might leave the majority with inadequate genetic mecha-

nisms. On the other hand, it is possible that the use of fire exposed primitive man to most chemical moieties and that modern chemistry has added very little that is fundamentally different from a metabolic viewpoint. This argument is less applicable to modern man's ability to concentrate other forms of energy, such as ionizing radiation. It is possible that alleles for the most efficient enzymes for coping with larger doses of radiation—for example, those that trigger DNA repair—have not yet reached their maximum frequency. Alleles for enzyme variants that impair DNA repair are known; whether heterozygotes for them are at a disadvantage, so that allele frequency would decline as ambient levels of radiation increased, is difficult to prove.

48. Stanbury et al. Metabolic basis of inherited disease:22. See also Lander E, Botstein D. Mapping complex genetic traits in humans: new methods using a complete linkage map. Cold Spring Harbor Symp Quant Biol 1986;51(pt 1):49–62.

49. Antonarakis. Hemophilia A.

50. Antonarakis SE, Kazazian HH, Jr., Orkin SH. DNA polymorphism and molecular pathology of the human globin gene clusters. Hum Genet 1985;69:1–14.

51. Harris. Principles of human biochemical genetics.

52. Goldstein, Brown. Familial hypercholesterolemia.

53. Guttler F, Ledley FD, Lidsky AS, DiLella, Sullivan SE, Woo SL. Correlation between polymorphic DNA haplotypes at phenylalanine hydroxylase locus and clinical phenotypes of phenylketonuria. J Pediatr 1987;110:68–71.

54. Kalter H, Warkany J. Congenital malformations: etiologic factors and their role in prevention. N Engl J Med 1983;308:424–431, 491–497.

55. Comings DE, Comings BG. A controlled study of Tourette syndrome. I. Attention-deficit disorder, learning disorders, and school problems. Am J Hum Genet 41:701–741.

56. Czeizel A, Sankaranarayanan K. The load of genetic and partially genetic disorders in man. I. Congenital anomalies: estimates of detriment in terms of years of life lost and years of impaired life. Mutat Res 1984;128:73–103.

57. Childs, Moxon, Winkelstein. Genetics and infectious diseases.

58. Baird PA, Anderson TW, Newcombe HB, Lowry RB. Genetic disorders in children and young adults: a population study. Am J Hum Genet 1988;677–693. The rate of Mendelian disorders was 3.6 per 1,000 live births; chromosomal disorders, 1.8 per 1,000; genetic etiology unknown, 1.2 per 1,000; multifactorial disorders, 46.4 per 1,000. Although the estimates of multifactorial disorders are conservative (and do not count conditions that would appear after age 25), the authors assume that *all* cases of disorders like diabetes mellitus, schizophrenia, and mental retardation reported before age 25 are genetic in origin. This remains to be proved.

59. King M-C, et al. Genetic epidemiology. See also Childs B, Scriver CR. Age at onset and causes of disease. Perspect Biol Med 1986;29:437–460; and Childs B. Causes of essential hypertension. Prog Med Genet 1983;5:1–34.

60. Goldstein JL, Schrott HG, Hazzard WR, et al. Hyperlipidemia in coronary heart disease. II. Genetic analysis of lipid levels in 176 families and delineation of a new inherited disorder, combined hyperlipidemia. J Clin Inv 1973;52:1544–1568.

61. Brown MS, Goldstein JL. A receptor-mediated pathway for cholesterol homeostasis. Science 1986;34–47.

62. The nature of the clinical abnormality or the altered concentration of a par-

ticular amino acid or sugar may suggest which enzyme, or which metabolic pathway (involving enzymes that act consecutively on the product of the previous enzymatic reaction in the pathway), should be assayed.

63. Pauling L, Itano HA, Singer SJ, Wells IC. Sickle cell anemia: a molecular disease. Science 1949;110:543–548.

64. Beet EA. The genetics of the sickle-cell trait in a Bantu tribe. Eugenics 1949;14:274–284. See also Neel JV. The inheritance of sickle cell anemia. Science 1949;110:64–66. Beet and Neel independently reported that in every family they studied, both parents of the patients with sickle cell anemia demonstrated the sickling phenomenon.

65. Taliaferro WH, Huck JG. The inheritance of sickle-cell anemia in man. Genetics 1923;8:594–598.

66. Ingram VM. A specific chemical difference between the globins of normal human and sickle-cell anaemia haemoglobin. Nature 1956;178:792–794.

67. The medium on which electrophoresis has been conducted (paper or some type of gel) is exposed to a solution containing the substrate of the enzyme of interest, any necessary cofactors of the enzyme, and a dye whose color changes only when the reaction occurs. After rinsing, only those electrophoretic bands containing the enzyme for the reaction show the expected color of the dye.

68. Harris. Principles of human biochemical genetics.

69. In the two-dimensional technique, proteins obtained from preparations of the organ or tissue of interest are dissociated into their respective polypeptide chains. They are then separated according to their charge characteristics (isoelectric points) in the first dimension. Polypeptides with the same charge characteristics are separated from each other in the second dimension if they differ in size (molecular weight). Because the proteins are denatured into polypeptides, enzyme-specific stains cannot be applied. Recently, radioactively labeled peptides and very sensitive stains have been developed, but these still do not permit determination of the function of the polypeptide.

70. Calin A. HLA-B27: to type or not to type? Ann Intern Med 1980;92:208–211.

71. Stanbury et al. Metabolic basis of inherited disease.

72. Pyeritz R. Heritable disorders of connective tissue. Hosp Prac 15 February 1987:153–168.

73. In animals that can be bred selectively it often does not take many generations to develop separate lines that have marked differences in disease susceptibility—for example, hypertension or sensitivity to specific infectious agents (see Childs, Moxon, Winkelstein. Genetics and infectious diseases; and Childs. Causes of essential hypertension). The fewer the generations that accomplish this difference, the fewer the number of gene loci involved. Given the results of animal studies, and some work with humans, it seems likely that for each of a few common diseases a few gene loci exert major effects.

Chapter 4: Finding Gene Loci and Alleles Implicated in Disease

1. A detailed source of information on recombinant DNA technology, which provides many of the basic references, is Watson JD, Tooze J, Kurtz DT, eds. Recombinant DNA: a short course. New York: W. H. Freeman, 1983. Applications to

medicine can be found in a series in Lancet entitled "DNA in Medicine" (Nov–Dec 1984). See also Weatherall DJ. Genetics and clinical practice. New York: Oxford University Press, 1985; and Childs B, Holtzman NA, Kazazian HH, Jr., Valle DL, eds. Molecular genetics in medicine [Prog Med Genet, new series, 1987;7]. New York: Elsevier, 1988.

2. The sequences recognized by many restriction enzymes are palindromes; when read from the 5' end, each strand has the same sequence as the other when read from the 3' end. Although offset from the other, the cut made by one of these restriction enzymes in each strand is between the same two nucleotides.

3. A nonspecific polydeoxythymidine primer, which is complementary to the string of adenine nucleotides that most mRNAs have at their 3' end, can be used, in which case all mRNAs present will be reverse transcribed. Or a primer consisting of the correct complementary anti-codons for a short sequence on the mRNA can be constructed (see figure 4.1, top), in which case reverse transcriptase will initiate the synthesis of the "correct" cDNA much more efficiently than it will trigger the synthesis of other cDNAs. The construction of such a specific primer requires knowledge of the amino acid sequence of at least part of the candidate protein. The cDNA made by using a specific primer will not contain the sequence of nucleotides 3' to the primer's complementary sequence on the mRNA.

A number of other techniques can be used to obtain at least partially purified mRNA from which cDNA can be derived. Antibodies against the protein of interest can be used to isolate the nascent mRNA-polypeptide complex. The mRNA from this complex can then be reverse transcribed into cDNA using a polydeoxythymidine primer for the reverse transcriptase. mRNAs can also be separated by their size differences, and cDNAs can be made for each size. Clones of bacteria containing only the cDNAs of one size of mRNA can be assayed to determine which are synthesizing the candidate protein. Cloning is discussed further below.

4. Woo et al. used this method to obtain a probe for human phenylalanine hydroxylase, the enzyme defective in PKU. See Woo SLC, Lidsky AS, Guttler F, Chandra T, Robson KJH. Cloned human phenylalanine hydroxylase gene allows prenatal diagnosis and carrier detection of classical phenylketonuria. Nature 1983;306:6451–6455.

5. Kazazian HH, Jr. The nature of mutation. Hosp Prac 15 February 1985:55–69. See also Antonarakis SE, Kazazian HH, Jr., Orkin SH. DNA polymorphism and molecular pathology of the human globin gene clusters. Human Genetics 1985;69:1–14.

6. The safety of cloning was a major issue in the 1970s. The use of "disabled" bacteria has reduced the likelihood that potentially harmful organisms will escape from the laboratory, but as the types of DNA inserted and the number of different vectors employed increases, the danger cannot be eliminated. See Alexander M. Ecological consequences: reducing the uncertainties. Issues Sci Tech 1985;1:57–68; and Ozonoff D. Just when you thought it was safe: an update on the risks of recombinant DNA technology. In: Milunsky A, Annas GJ, eds. Genetics and the law. III. New York: Plenum, 1985:467–474. Studies involving tumor viruses may entail somewhat greater risks. As important as this safety issue is, I will not deal with it further here, because it is not unique to, or even particularly likely in, the identification of genes involved in human genetic diseases.

7. When a radioactive 32P-labeled probe is used, the bands to which the probe has hybridized are made visible by placing unexposed X-ray film over the mem-

brane. Several days later, developing the film reveals dark bands wherever the probe has bound to the membrane. When a biotinylated probe is used, the hybridized bands bind avidin or strepavidin conjugated to an enzyme capable of converting a colorless substrate to a colored product. Addition of the conjugated enzyme and its colorless substrate colors the band within a few hours. The biotin method is less sensitive than the use of ^{32}P labeled probes, requiring more DNA on the bands.

8. Chang JC, Kan YW. A sensitive new prenatal test for sickle-cell anemia. N Engl J Med 1982;307:30–32.

9. Lehrman MA, Schneider WJ, Sudhof TC, Brown MS, Goldstein JL, Russell DW. Mutation in LDL receptor: alu-alu recombination deletes exons encoding transmembrane and cytoplasmic domains. Science 1985;227:140–146.

10. Kan YW, Dozy AM. Antenatal diagnosis of sickle-cell anemia by DNA analysis of amniotic-fluid cells. Lancet 1978;2:910–912.

11. Chakraborty R, Lidsky AS, Daiger SP, et al. Polymorphic DNA haplotypes at the human phenylalanine hydroxylase locus and their relationship with phenylketonuria. Human Genet 1987;76:40–46. More recently, the disease-causing mutations that account for 60 percent of PKU among northern Europeans have been identified. See DiLella AG, Huang W-M, Woo SLC. Screening for phenylketonuria mutations by DNA amplification with the polymerase chain reaction. Lancet 1988;1:497–499.

12. Kidd VJ, Wallace RB, Itakura K, Woo SLC. Alpha-1-antitrypsin deficiency detection by direct analysis of the mutation in the gene. Nature 1983;306:230–234.

13. Saiki RK, Scahrf S, Faloona F, et al. Enzymatic amplification of beta-globin genomic sequences and restriction site analysis for diagnosis of sickle cell anemia. Science 1985;230:1350–1354.

14. Erlich H. Personal communication, November 1987.

15. Kogan SC, Doherty M, Gitschier J. An improved method for prenatal diagnosis of genetic diseases by analysis of amplified DNA sequences: application to Hemophilia A. N Engl J Med 1987;317:985–990.

16. Embury S, Scharf SJ, Saiki RK, et al. Rapid prenatal diagnosis of sickle cell anemia by a new method of DNA analysis. N Engl J Med 1987;316:656–660.

17. Kogan SC, Doherty M, Gitschier J. An improved method for prenatal diagnosis of genetic diseases by analysis of amplified DNA sequences: application to Hemophilia A. N Engl J Med 1987;317:985–990.

18. DiLella, Huang, Woo. Screening for phenylketonuria mutations.

19. Myers RM, Larin Z, Maniatis T. Detection of single base substitutions by ribonuclease cleavage at mismatches in RNA;DNA duplexes. Science 1985;230:1242–1246. Not all mismatches will be detected. The proportion can be increased by preparing RNAs for both the coding and noncoding strands of DNA.

20. Ibid.

21. Caskey CT. Disease diagnosis by recombinant DNA methods. Science 1987;236:1223–1228.

22. Myers RM, Maniatis T. Recent advances in the development of methods for detecting single base substitutions associated with human genetic diseases. Cold Spring Harbor Symp Quant Biol 1986;51(pt 1):275–284.

23. Wong C, Dowling CE, Saiki RK, Miguchi RG, Erlich HA, Kazazian HH, Jr.

Characterization of beta thalassemia mutations using direct genomic sequencing of amplified single copy DNA. Nature 1987;330:384–386.

24. In the case of Alzheimer, a "candidate chromosome" was suggested by the frequent occurrence of neuropathologic findings of Alzheimer disease in older patients with Down syndrome, sometimes accompanied by clinical symptoms of Alzheimer disease. Because patients with Down syndrome have an extra dosage of at least some genes on chromosome 21, this chromosome was singled out for linkage studies. A locus for Alzheimer has been found on chromosome 21, but it is not in the region that is always present in Down syndrome. See St. George–Hyslop PH, Tanzi RE, Polinsky RJ, et al. The genetic defect causing familial Alzheimer's disease maps on chromosome 21. Science 1987;235:885–890.

25. Botstein D, White RL, Skolnick M, Davis RW. Construction of a genetic linkage map in man using restriction fragment length polymorphisms. Am J Hum Genet 1980;32:314–331. See also Cooper DN, Schmidke J. DNA restriction fragment length polymorphisms and heterozygosity in the human genome. Hum Genet 1984;66:1–16; and Antonarakis SE. DNA diagnosis of genetic disorders. N Engl J Med. [In press].

26. Cooper, Schmidke. DNA restriction fragment length polymorphisms. See also Neel JV. Genetic variation in human proteins. Am J Hum Genet 1984;36: 1135–1148.

27. Nakamura Y, Leppert M, O'Connell P, et al. Variable number of tandem repeat (VNTR) markers for human gene mapping. Science 1987;235:1616–1622.

28. White R, Leppert M, Bishop DT, et al. Construction of linkage maps with DNA markers for human chromosomes. Nature 1985;313:101–105. See also Marx JL. Putting the human genome on the map. Science 1985;229:150–151; and Saltus R. Biotech firms compete in genetic diagnosis. Science 1986;234:1318–1320.

29. Felix J, Badman WS. Human DNA repository. Science 1986;231:203.

30. U.S. Congress, Office of Technology Assessment (OTA). Mapping our genes. Washington, D.C.: U.S. Government Printing Office, 1988; OTA-BA-373.

31. Several methods of obtaining isolated human chromosomes are available. The older ones depend on the retention of one or a few human chromosomes by mouse-human somatic cell hybrids as the others are randomly lost in successive cell divisions. In a more recently developed method—chromosome-mediated gene transfer—single human chromosomes are endocytosed by mouse cells, broken into smaller fragments, and replicated with the mouse cell. One can then identify the human chromosomes present using cytogenetic techniques, or by determining the presence of human proteins or of RFLPs that have already been assigned to a specific chromosome. Chromosomes in human somatic cells can be stained with fluorochromes, and the fluorescence-activated cell sorter used to separate them on the basis of their different patterns of fluorescence. See Ruddle F, Bentley K, Ferguson-Smith A. Physical mapping review. Contractor report prepared for the U.S. Congress, Office of Technology Assessment. [Unpublished, 1987].

32. Harper ME, Saunders GF. Localization of single copy DNA sequences on G-banded human chromosomes by in situ hybridization. Chromosoma 1981;83: 431–439. See also Jones C, Morse HG, Kao FT. Human T-cell receptor alpha-chain genes: location on chromosome 14. Science 1985;228:83–85.

33. White et al. Construction of linkage maps.

34. Even when the disease can be traced to the same mutation many generations earlier (founder effect), the distance between the polymorphism and the disease locus is likely to be great enough that crossing over between the two in earlier generations (not observed in the study at hand) results in linkages to different forms of the polymorphism in different families. The disease could also arise from independent mutations at the same locus in different families.

35. Gusella JF, Tanzi RE, Manderson MA, et al. DNA markers for nervous system diseases. Science 1984;225:1320–1326. The LOD score (see note 40) for the haplotype locus was 12.1 with a recombination fraction of 0.02. This is equivalent to odds of slightly over one trillion to one.

36. Folstein SE, Phillips JA, III, Meyers DA, et al. Huntington's disease: two families with differing clinical features show linkage to the G8 probe. Science 1985;229:779–779. See also Youngman S, Sarfarazi M, Harper PS, Quarrell OW, Shaw D, Gusella JF. G8 typing of Huntington's disease families in South Wales. Am J Hum Genet 1985;37(suppl):A185.

37. Wang HS, Greenberg CR, Hayden M. Subregional assignment of a DNA marker (G8) linked to Huntington disease by *in situ* hybridization. Am J Hum Genet 1985;37(suppl):A121. See also Gusella J, Tanzi R, Gibbons K, et al. Mapping of the Huntington's disease–linked G8 (D4S10) DNA marker to 4p16. Am J Hum Genet 1985;37(suppl):A155. In the latter study, individuals with another disorder in which the terminal portion of the short arm of chromosome 4 was missing on one of their chromosomes were found to have only one G8 haplotype, which is consistent with its location on the part of their chromosome 4 that was missing.

38. Beaudet A, Bowcock A, Buchwald M, et al. Linkage of cystic fibrosis to two tightly linked DNA markers: joint report from a collaborative study. Am J Hum Genet 1986;39:681–693.

39. Since recombination is directly proportional to the distance between two loci, this distance can be expressed as the frequency of recombinations between the two loci. The unit for this measurement is the centiMorgan (cM); one cM is defined as that distance between two loci which results in crossing over in 1 percent of meioses. In terms of physical distance, it is equivalent to about one million nucleotide pairs. The average distance between markers over the entire human genome at the present time is about ten million nucleotide pairs. (In some regions, the distances are considerably shorter.) Crossing over between two markers this distance apart would be expected in 10 percent of meioses. Crossing over between one of these markers and a disease-related locus midway between it and the other would occur 5 percent of the time.

40. The probability that the observed associations are caused by linkage is calculated, using the recombination fraction that gives the maximum likelihood of linkage. Then the probability that the observations arose by chance (no linkage) is calculated. The ratio of these two probabilities is the odds ratio for linkage. The overall odds ratio is obtained by multiplying the odds ratios in independent families. Usually, however, the logarithm (base 10) of the odds ratio (LOD) in each family is calculated and the LOD "scores" are added together. With a combined LOD score of 3 (log of base 10), the odds are 1,000 to 1 in favor of linkage. See Cavalli-Sforza LL, Bodmer W. The genetics of human populations. San Francisco: W. H. Freeman, 1971:873–878; and Lander ES, Botstein D. Mapping complex genetic traits in humans: new methods using a complete RFLP map. Cold Spring Harbor Symp Quant Biol 1986;51(pt 1):49–62.

41. Lander, Botstein. Mapping complex genetic traits.

42. Verellen-Dumoulin CH, Freund M, De Meyer R, et al. Expression of an X-linked muscular dystrophy in a female due to translocation involving Xp21 and non-random inactivation of the normal X chromosome. Hum Genet 1984;67:115–119. See also Kunkel LM, Monaco AP, Middlesworth W, Ochs HD, Latts, SA. Specific cloning of DNA fragments absent from the DNA of a male patient with an X chromosome deletion. Proc Natl Acad Sci USA 1985;82:4778–4782; and Kunkel LM, Hejtmancik JF, Caskey CT, et al. Nature 1986;322:73–77.

43. See ref. 3 in Lee W-H, Bookstein R, Hong F, Young L-J, Shew J-Y, Lee EY-HP. Human retinoblastoma susceptibility gene: cloning, identification, and sequence. Science 1987;235:1394–1399.

44. Francke U, Ochs HD, de Martinville B, et al. Minor Xp21 chromosome deletion in a male associated with expression of Duchenne muscular dystrophy, chronic granulomatous disease, retinitis pigmentosa, and McLeod syndrome. Am J Hum Genet 1985;37:250–267.

45. Kunkel et al. Specific cloning.

46. Friend SH, Bernards R, Rogelj S, et al. A human DNA segment with properties of the gene that predisposes to retinoblastoma and osteosarcoma. Nature 1986;323:643–646.

47. Monaco AP, Neve R, Colletti-Fenner C, Bertelson CJ, Kurnit DM, Kunkel LM. Isolation of candidate cDNA for portions of the Duchenne muscular dystrophy gene. Nature 1986;323:646–650.

48. Friend et al. A human DNA segment.

49. Monaco et al. Isolation of candidate cDNA. Hoffman EP, Monaco AP, Feener CC, Kunkel LM. The DMD gene transcription and predicted protein sequence in human and mouse muscle. Am J Hum Genet 1987;41:A219.

50. Royer-Pokora B, Kunkel LM, Monaco AP, et al. Cloning the gene for an inherited human disorder—chronic granulomatous disease—on the basis of its chromosomal location. Nature 1986;322:32–38.

51. Friend et al. A human DNA segment. See also Lee W-H et al. Human retinoblastoma susceptibility gene.

52. Royer-Pokora et al. Cloning of the gene for an inherited human disorder.

53. Koenig M, Hoffman EP, Bartelson CJ, Monaco AP, Feener A, Kunkel LM. Complete cloning of the Duchenne muscular dystrophy (DMD) cDNA and preliminary genomic organization of the DMD gene in normal and affected individuals. Cell 1987;50:509–517. Use of the cDNA probe indicated that about half of the cases of DMD studied were attributable to deletions.

54. Kunkel. Personal communication, December 1987.

55. Hoffman EP, Knudson CM, Campbell KP, Kunkel LM. Subcellular fractionation of dystrophin to the triads of skeletal muscle. Nature 1987;330:754–758.

56. Lee W-H, Shew JY, Hong FD, et al. The retinoblastoma susceptibility gene encodes a nuclear phosphoprotein associated with DNA binding activity. Nature 1987;329:642–645.

57. Dinauer MC, Orkin SH, Brown R, Jesaitis AJ, Parkos CA. The glycoprotein encoded by the X-linked chronic granulomatous disease locus is a component of the neutrophil cytochrome B complex. Nature 1987;327:717–720.

58. Yeast vectors are capable of incorporating fragments up to 500 kb long. See Burke DT, Carle GF, Olson MV. Cloning of large segments of exogenous DNA into

yeast by means of artificial chromosome vectors. Science 1987;236:801–812.

59. Schwartz DC, Cantor CR. Separation of yeast chromosome–sized DNAs by pulsed field gradient gel electrophoresis. Cell 1984;37:67–75.

60. Estivill X, Farrall M, Scambler PJ, et al. A candidate for the cystic fibrosis locus isolated by selection for methylation-free islands. Nature 1987;326:840–845.

61. The long fragment was obtained by digesting human DNA with a "rarely cutting" restriction enzyme, Notl. This enzyme recognizes a sequence of eight nucleotides in which guanine–unmethylated cytosine (GC) dinucleotides predominate. The occurrence of an eight-nucleotide sequence is less frequent than that of a four-nucleotide sequence. Consequently, the number of nucleotides between eight-nucleotide sequences will be larger than that between four-nucleotide sequences recognized by "frequently cutting" restriction enzymes. Moreover, GC dimers occur less frequently than expected by chance in mammalian DNA. Notl fragments over 1,000 kb in length have been obtained. The presence of the Notl site in the fragments was determined by using an oligonucleotide probe for the sequence of the Notl site.

62. Often, the neighboring sequences are also rich in GC sequences four nucleotides long, in which the cytosine is unmethylated. These sequences are digested by frequently cutting enzymes, such as HpaII, which recognizes CCGG when the cytosine is unmethylated. Such a region is known as an "HpaII tiny fragment" (HTF). HTFs are not found around all structural genes, however.

63. Roberts L. Race for cystic fibrosis gene nears end. Science 1988;240:282–285.

64. Another approach to determining the relationship of distant sites to each other involves bringing the two sites closer together by circularizing a segment of DNA that contains them both. Digestion with restriction enzymes at sites other than the one at which the original two ends were joined, and Southern blotting with appropriate probes, brings the sites closer together than they were in the natural DNA. See Little P. Restriction fragment length polymorphisms: finding the defective gene. Nature 1986;321:558–559.

65. The observation of linkage disequilibrium suggests that a sufficient number of generations have not elapsed since the CF mutation occurred on a chromosome with one haplotype to permit the number of crossovers that will eventually lead to equilibrium. This will be reached when the proportion of CF cases with the haplotype in question is equal to the frequency of the haplotype in the population. Linkage disequilibrium also occurs when an allele causing a recessive disease confers an advantage to the heterozygote, as has been documented for sickle cell anemia. In such instances, a neutral variation linked to the disease-related mutation would benefit from the heterozygote advantage and would also increase in frequency.

66. Childs B, Scriver CR. Age at onset and causes of disease. Perspect Biol Med 1986;29:437–460.

67. Egeland JA, Gerhard DS, Pauls DL, et al. Bipolar affective disorders linked to DNA markers on chromosome 11. Nature 1987;325:783–787.

68. St. George–Hyslop PH, Tanzi XE, Polinsky RJ. The genetic defect causing familial Alzheimer's. Science 1987;235:885–890.

69. Bodmer WF, Bailey CJ, Bodmer J, et al. Localisation of the gene for familial adenomatous polyposis on chromosome 5. Nature 1987;328:614–616.

70. Brown MS, Goldstein JL. A receptor-mediated pathway for cholesterol homeostasis. Science 1986;232:34–47.

71. Lander, Botstein. Mapping complex genetic traits.

72. Ibid. A high frequency of a susceptibility-conferring allele at one locus will increase the chances for homozygosity, making linkage to it in succeeding generations impossible to find. Not all of the people with either a single or a double dosage of the allele will have the disease, however, because they lack the susceptibility-conferring alleles at the other loci. Lander and Botstein estimate that linkage should be possible with allele frequencies of less than 10 percent.

73. Childs B, Moxon R, Winkelstein J. Genetics and infectious diseases. In: King RA, Rotter JI, Motulsky A, eds. The genetic basis of common disease. New York: McGraw-Hill. [In press]. See also Childs B. Causes of essential hypertension. Prog Med Genet 1983;5:1–34.

74. Owerbach D, Nerup J. Restriction fragment length polymorphism of the insulin gene in diabetes mellitus. Diabetes 1982;31:275–277.

75. Mandrup-Poulsen T, Owerbach D, Mortensen SA, et al. DNA sequences flanking the insulin gene on chromosome 11 confer risk of atherosclerosis. Lancet 1984;1:250–252. The authors' original findings of an association can be attributed largely to poorly matched groups of controls. Although they used better matching in their later studies, they did not make intrafamily comparisons. In the later studies, the authors did find a weak, but statistically significant, association between an insertion polymorphism near the insulin gene and angiographically proven coronary artery disease in nondiabetics. This association was not confirmed in another population. See Jowett NI, Rees A, Caplin J, Williams LG, Galton DJ. DNA polymorphisms flanking insulin gene and atherosclerosis. Lancet 1984;2:348.

76. Ordovas JM, Schaefer EJ, Salem D, et al. Apolipoprotein A-I gene polymorphism associated with premature coronary artery disease and familial hypoalphalipoproteinemia. N Engl J Med 1986;314:671–677. Other risk factors (hypertension, cigarette smoking, and diabetes) were present less often in coronary artery disease patients with the form of the RFLP linked to coronary artery disease than in patients with the other form of the RFLP, which suggests that the disease is associated with an independent risk factor. Some people who have the form associated with disease have normal levels of Apo A-I.

77. Hegele RA, Huang L-S, Herbert PN, et al. Apolipoprotein B-gene DNA polymorphisms associated with myocardial infarction. N Engl J Med 1986;315:1509–1515.

78. Childs B, Motulsky AG. Recombinant DNA analysis of multifactorial disease. Prog Med Genet 1987;7:180–194. See also Breslow JL. Apolipoprotein defects. Hosp Prac 15 December 1985:43–49.

79. Brown, Goldstein. A receptor-mediated pathway for cholesterol homeostasis.

80. Todd JA, Acha-Orbea H, Bell JI, et al. A molecular basis for MHC class II–associated autoimmunity. Science 1988;240:1003–1009.

81. Ibid. See also Todd JA, Bell JI, McDevitt HO. HLA-DQ$_\beta$ gene contributes to susceptibility and resistance to insulin-dependent diabetes mellitus. Nature 1987;329:599–604. The specific DR alleles that confer susceptibility may do so because they are in linkage disequilibrium with the DQ susceptibility-conferring

allele, but they may also contribute independently to the risk of IDDM; other alleles may contribute to resistance.

82. So far, alanine, valine, and serine have been found in diabetics. It is interesting to note that in the mouse analog to human IDDM an allele containing a serine at position fifty-seven of the mouse equivalent of the DQ_β beta chain is present. This allele is not found in mice that are resistant to diabetes. Ibid.

83. Gusella et al. DNA markers for nervous system diseases.

84. Egeland et al. Bipolar affective disorders.

85. Lander, Botstein. Mapping complex genetic traits.

86. Egeland et al. Bipolar affective disorders.

87. Barker D, Wright E, Nbguyen K, et al. Gene for von Recklinghausen neurofibromatosis is in the periconetromeric region of chromosome 17. Science 1987;236:1100–1102. There is another locus for a neurofibromatosis-like disorder in which bilateral acoustic neurofibromas and other central nervous system tumors figure more prominently. It has been linked to chromosome 22. See Rouleau GA, Wertelecki W, Superneau DW, Conneally PM, Gusella JF. Genetic linkage of bilateral acoustic neurofibromatosis to DNA markers on chromosome 22. Am J Hum Genet 1987;41:A236.

88. Riccardi V. Personal communication, October 1987.

89. Lander, Botstein. Mapping complex genetic traits.

Chapter 5: Genetic Testing in Health Care

1. It is also possible to use linkage studies in families in which disease has not yet occurred but in which couples at risk have been identified by neoclassical tests. Some of these tests—for instance for thalassemia or alpha-1-antitrypsin deficiency—cannot be used safely for prenatal diagnosis, but DNA-based testing can. In some families at risk for these disorders, linkage studies will be needed.

2. For instance, prenatal diagnosis of an X-linked disorder for which only a linked RFLP marker is available does not always require testing of previously affected males in the family. In the case of previously affected sons, the mother is an obligate carrier of the disease-causing allele. If she is heterozygous at the marker locus with RFLP alleles A and B, and a healthy living son has allele A (remember that males have only one X chromosome [axiom 2]), then a male fetus would have to have allele B in order to be affected, barring the occurrence of recombination.

To take another example, a young, apparently healthy woman is at risk for Huntington disease (HD), a late-onset autosomal dominant disorder, because her father died from it. She wants to have a child, but not if it will be at risk for HD. Since no treatment is available for HD, she is not eager to learn whether she has the disease. Assuming that HD has not occurred on the husband's side, the chance that any of their offspring will be affected is 25 percent. (If the mother is affected, there is a 50 percent chance that each of her offspring will be affected; but the mother has only a 50 percent chance of being affected.) If the young woman had a hypothetical allele, C, at the linked marker locus that was not present in either her mother or her husband, the presence of this allele in the fetus would increase its risk from 25 percent to 50 percent. The absence of this allele would reduce the risk to 0. We know that allele C had to come from the woman's affected father, but we do not know whether it was on the chromosome that contained the

HD allele. We can now say that the fetus inherited one chromosome from its maternal grandfather; this raises its risk to 50 percent, the same as in its mother. Both of these examples indicate that diagnosis is possible in these families only when informative genotypes are present at the marker loci.

3. The new mutation may have occurred in the mother's germ cell (or its precursor), in which case only the offspring of her affected child are at risk. Or it may have occurred in a grandparent's germ cell (or further back, but without the birth of affected male children), so that the mother has the mutation in all of her germ cell precursors. In that case, each of her male children has a 50 percent risk of being affected. The only way these possibilities can be distinguished is if unaffected male siblings of the affected child have the same RFLPs as he does. Barring the occurrence of crossing over, this distinction indicates that the mutation arose in the mother's germ cell.

4. Antonarakis SE. DNA diagnosis of genetic disorders. N Engl J Med. [In press].

5. In recessive diseases two different alleles can cause the disease (see chapter 4), but the same two will be present in all affected siblings.

6. Antonarakis. DNA diagnosis of genetic disorders.

7. Darras BT, Harper JF, Francke U. Prenatal diagnosis and detection of carriers with DNA probes in Duchenne's muscular dystrophy. N Engl J Med 1987; 316:985–992.

8. Kan YW, Dozy AM. Antenatal diagnosis of sickle-cell anemia by DNA analysis of amniotic-fluid cells. Lancet 1978;2:910–912.

9. Estivill X, Farrall M, Scambler PJ, et al. A candidate for the cystic fibrosis locus isolated by selection for methylation-free islands. Nature 1987;326:840–845.

10. At the present time, carriers would be determined by linkage studies that show that they carry one of the chromosomes on which the disease-causing allele resides in their affected sibling(s).

11. Antonarakis. DNA diagnosis of genetic disorders.

12. Arnheim N, Erlich HA. Commercial uses of recombinant DNA technology in human genetic disease. Prog Med Genet 1987;7:195–219.

13. Relative risk is determined by case-control methods, in which the presence of the marker allele is sought in patients with the disease in question and in suitable controls. In studies of this type, unaffected, approximately age-matched family members might be more appropriate than unrelated controls matched on other factors as well as age. A significant odds ratio would establish the associated marker allele as a risk factor. If the probability of developing the disease (incidence) is known, if the controls are representative of the general population, and if the disease is relatively uncommon (affecting less than 10 percent of the general population), the probability that the disease will develop—as well as the relative risk, given the presence of the marker—can be determined.

14. For instance, two different hemoglobins can migrate to the same position during electrophoresis; one causes the disease that is being screened for, but the other does not. Errors also result when a particular diet or drug interferes with an enzyme assay or the measurement of a metabolite.

15. Committee for the Study of Inborn Errors of Metabolism (CSIEM). Genetic screening: programs, principles, and research. Washington, D.C.: National Academy of Sciences, 1975.

16. Holtzman NA, Meek AG, Mellits ED, Kallman C. Neonatal screening for phenylketonuria. III. Altered sex ratio: extent and possible causes. J Pediatr 1974;85:174–181. See also McCabe ERB, McCabe L, Mosher GA, Allen RJ, Berman JL. Newborn screening for phenylketonuria: predictive validity as a function of age. Pediatrics 1983;72:390–398; and Committee on Genetics. New issues in newborn screening for phenylketonuria and congenital hypothyroidism. Pediatrics 1982;69:104–106.

17. For most such tests, the range of concentrations of the substance being measured will overlap between affected and unaffected persons. When persons with the disease have increased concentrations, lowering the cutpoint will show more affected people with abnormal results (increased sensitivity), but it will also show more unaffected people with abnormal results (decreased specificity).

18. This method has serious drawbacks for genetic tests at the gene product level; the alteration observed in people with clinically overt disease may not be present in presymptomatic individuals. Testing for disease-causing genotypes, which do not change during the course of the disease, overcomes this problem.

19. Farrell P. Personal communication, January 1988. For a preliminary report on the early findings for the screened group and a discussion of "false positives," see Farrell P, Rock M, Mischler E, et al. Infant screening test for cystic fibrosis (CF) [abstract]. Pediatr Res. 1988;23 (pt 2):563A.

20. Hayes A, Costa T, Scriver CR, Child B. The effect of Mendelian disease on human health. II. Response to treatment. Am J Med Genet 1985;21:243–255.

21. This possibility was suggested to me by John Fletcher and Leroy Walters, two prominent bioethicists. Their scenario is based on the assumption that other forms of treatment for recessive disorders will be so successful that the frequency of recessives in the population will increase to the point that matings between them become probable. I find this highly improbable, for reasons that will be discussed later in this chapter.

22. Verlinsky Y, Pergament E. Preimplantation genetic diagnosis by embryonic biopsy. Am J Hum Genet 1984;36:199S.

23. Stanbury JB, Wyngaarden JB, Fredrickson DS, Goldstein JL, Brown MS, eds. The metabolic basis of inherited disease. New York: McGraw-Hill, 1983. See also Holtzman NA. Dietary treatment of inborn errors of metabolism. Ann Rev Med 1970;21:335–356.

24. Caskey CT. Genetic therapy: somatic gene transplants. Hosp Prac 15 August 1987:115–132.

25. Holtzman NA, Kronmal RA, van Doorninck W, Azen C, Koch R. Effect of age at loss of dietary control on intellectual performance and behavior of children with phenylketonuria. N Engl J Med 1986;314:593–598.

26. Holtzman. Dietary treatment of inborn errors of metabolism.

27. Andrews LB. State laws and regulations governing newborn screening. Chicago: American Bar Foundation, 1985. See also U.S. Congress, Office of Technology Assessment (OTA). Healthy children: investing in the future. Washington, D.C.: U.S. Government Printing Office, 1988; OTA-H-345.

28. Consensus Conference. Newborn screening for sickle cell disease and other hemoglobinopathies. JAMA 1987;258:1205–1209.

29. Rosenstein B. Newborn screening for cystic fibrosis. Contemp Pediatr. 1987;4:71–91. See also Farrell P, Rock M, Mischler E, et al. Infant screening test for cystic fibrosis. Pediatr Res 1988;23(4 pt 2):563A.

30. Brusilow SW. Disorders of the urea cycle. Hosp Prac 15 October 1985:65–72.

31. McCabe ERB, Huang S-Z, Seltzer WK, Law ML. DNA microextraction from dried blood spots on filter paper blotters: potential applications to newborn screening. Hum Genet 1987;75:213–216.

32. See note 16.

33. Holtzman NA, Leonard CO, Farfel MR. Issues in antenatal and neonatal screening and surveillance for hereditary and congenital disorders. Ann Rev Med 1981;2:219–251.

34. Erlich H. Personal communication, April 1987.

35. Keown PA, Stiller CR. Cyclosporine: a double-edged sword. Hosp Prac 15 May 1987:147–160. See also Bougneres PF, Carel JC, Castano L, et al. Factors associated with early remission of type I diabetes in children treated with cyclosporine. N Engl J Med 1988;318:663–670.

36. Bodansky HJ, Grant PJ, Dean BM, et al. Islet-cell antibodies and insulin autoantibodies in association with common viral infections. Lancet 1986;2:1351–1353.

37. Olson RE. Mass intervention vs screening and selective intervention for the prevention of coronary heart disease. JAMA 1986;255:2204–2207.

38. American Academy of Pediatrics, Committee on Nutrition. Toward a prudent diet for children. Pediatrics 1983;71:78–80.

39. Multiple Risk Factor Intervention Trial Research Group. Multiple risk factor intervention trial: risk factor changes and mortality results. JAMA 1982;248:1465–1477. The failure to observe a significant change in the subjects of this study was attributed to the health consciousness of men in the control group, who lowered their dietary fat intake. If the use of low-fat diets is already widespread, little is to be gained by identifying men with genetic risk factors and admonishing them to change their diets.

40. Lipid Research Clinics Program. The lipid research clinics coronary primary prevention trial results. I. Reduction in incidence of coronary heart disease. JAMA 1984;251:351–364.

41. Vega GL, Grundy SM. Treatment of primary moderate hypercholesterolemia with lovastatin (mevinolin) and colestipol. JAMA 1987;257:33–38.

42. Kraemer KM, DiGiovanna JJ, Moshell AN, Tarone RE, Peck GL. Prevention of skin cancer in xeroderma pigmentosum with the use of oral isotretinoin. N Engl J Med 1988;318:1633–1637.

43. Ritchie JC, Sloan TP, Idle JR, Smith RL. Toxicological implications of polymorphic drug metabolism. In: Evered D, Lawrenson G, eds. Environmental chemicals, enzyme function, and human disease. Ciba Foundation Symposium 76. Amsterdam: Excerpta Medica, 1980:219–244.

44. Strickler SM, Dansky LV, Miller MA, Seni M-H, Andermann E, Spielberg SP. Genetic predisposition to phenytoin-induced birth defects. Lancet 1985;2:746–749.

45. Craik CS, Largman C, Fletcher T, et al. Redesigning trypsin: alteration of substrate specificity. Science 1985;228:291–297.

46. Andrews LB. New reproductive technologies: the genetic indications and the genetic consequences. Paper prepared for U.S. Congress, Office of Technology Assessment. [Unpublished, 1987].

47. Ibid.

48. Ibid. See also Curie-Cohen M, Lutree L, Shapiro S. Current practice of artificial insemination in the United States. N Engl J Med 1979;30:585–590; and Garver KL, Holtzman NA, Snyder DL, Marchese SG. Genetic evaluation of prospective semen donors in sperm banking institutions. [Unpublished, 1985].

49. Bernhardt B, Bannerman RM. The pro-life bonus of amniocentesis. N Engl J Med 1980;302:925. See also Dumars K. Questionnaire to medical genetics units listed in the National Foundation directory, pertinent to pregnancies "saved" by the availability of amniocentesis and prenatal genetic counseling. Am J Hum Genet 1979;31:400.

50. Hook EB, Chambers GM. Estimated rates of Down syndrome in live births by one year, maternal age intervals for mothers aged 20–49 in a New York State study—implications of the risk figures for genetic counseling and cost-benefit analysis of prenatal diagnosis programs. Birth Defects 1977;13(3a):123–141.

51. Covone AE, Johnson PM, Mutton D, Adinolfi M. Trophoblast cells in peripheral blood from pregnant women. Lancet 1984;2:841–843.

52. Ludman MD, Grabowski GA, Goldberg JD, Desnick J. Heterozygote detection and prenatal diagnosis for Tay-Sachs and Type I Gaucher diseases. In: Carter TP, Wiley AM, eds. Genetic disease: screening and management. New York: Alan R. Liss, 1986:19–48.

53. Stamatoyannopoulos G. Problems of screening and counseling in the hemoglobinopathies. In: Motulsky AG, Lenz W, eds. Birth defects. Amsterdam: Excerpta Medica, 1974:268–276.

54. Slamon DJ. Proto-oncogenes and human cancers. N Engl J Med 1987;317:955–957.

55. Solomon E, Voss R, Hall V, et al. Chromosome 5 allele loss in human colorectal carcinomas. Nature 1987;328:616–619.

56. Brauch H, Johns B, Hovis J, et al. Molecular analysis of the short arm of chromosome 3 in small-cell and non–small cell carcinoma of the lung. N Engl J Med 1987;317:1109–1113. See also Ali IU, Lidereau R, Theillet C, Callahon R. Reduction to homozygosity of genes on chromosome 11 in human breast neoplasia. Science 1987;238:185–188.

57. Johnson K. DNA "fingerprinting" tests becoming a factor in courts. New York Times, 7 February 1988:1. See also Marx JL. DNA fingerprinting takes the witness stand. Science 1988;240:1616–1618.

58. Jacobs PA, Brunton M, Melville MM, et al. Aggressive behavior, mental subnormality, and the XYY male. Nature 1965;208:1351–1352.

59. Several controlled, prospective studies, which generally show few significant differences between XYY and normal males, are reported in Ratcliffe SG, Paul N, eds. Prospective studies on children with sex chromosome aneuploidy. Birth Defects: Orig Art Ser 1986;22.

60. Chorever SL, as cited by Gould SJ. The mismeasure of man. New York: W. W. Norton, 1981:144–145.

Chapter 6: Technology Transfer: From Research to the Commercial Development of Genetic Tests

1. Kuhn TS. The structure of scientific revolutions. Chicago: University of Chicago Press, 1970.

2. U.S. Congress, Office of Technology Assessment (OTA). Commercial bio-

technology: an international analysis. Washington, D.C.: U.S. Government Printing Office, 1984; OTA-BA-218:307–312. Extramural research is that done off the NIH campus, primarily at universities. It constitutes about 75 percent of all NIH research support. With the recent federal commitment to mapping the human genome, support will continue to increase.

3. Fredrickson DS. Epochal decisions. Bethesda, Md.: Howard Hughes Medical Institute, 1985.

4. Public Law 97-219. 96 Stat 217–21 (1982).

5. Culliton B. NIH role in biotechnology debated. Science 1985;229:147–148.

6. Quoted by Makulowich J. Biotech's growth depletes academic ranks. Gen Eng News 1987;7(9):1.

7. OTA. Commercial biotechnology:414.

8. Sylvester EJ, Klotz LC, eds. The gene age. New York: Charles Scribner's Sons, 1983:128.

9. Dickson D. The new politics of science. New York: Pantheon, 1984:89.

10. Ibid.:89.

11. Kobbe B. Cohen-Boyer plasmid patent: an analysis of the issues. Gen Eng News 1984;4(8):3. For details of the agreement see Yoxen E. The gene business. New York: Harper & Row, 1983:76–77. The income thus far represents about 2 percent of Stanford's annual research budget of approximately $150,000,000. A second patent on the recombinant plasmids themselves was issued to Stanford after much controversy in 1984.

12. Collaborative Research, Inc. Annual report. Lexington, Mass., 1984. The method, based on gene mapping and described in chapter 4, was originally published in 1980 (Botstein D, White RL, Skolnick M, Davis RW. Construction of a genetic linkage map in man using restriction fragment length polymorphisms. Am J Hum Genet 1980;32:314–331). The four coauthors of the original paper were all affiliated with the company; two of them were on its Scientific Advisory Board.

13. National Institutes of Health. NIH policy relating to reporting and distribution of unique biological materials produced with NIH funding. NIH Guide 1987;16(35):1–2.

14. OTA. Commercial biotechnology:417–18, 574–77. See also Dickson. New politics:65–68.

15. Blumenthal D, Gluck M, Louis KS, Wise D. Industrial support of university research in biotechnology. Science 1986;231:242–246.

16. Blumenthal D, Gluck M, Louis KS, Stoto MA, Wise D. University-industry research relationships in biotechnology: implications for the university. Science 1986;232:1361–1366.

17. See note 14. A number of other universities, including Johns Hopkins and Harvard, have followed suit.

18. Abelson P. Evolving state-university-industry relations. Science 1986;231:317. See also Abelson P. Academic-industrial interactions. Science 1988;240:265; and OTA. Commercial biotechnology:418.

19. Gatz RL, Scantland DA, Minshall CD. The Dallas approach to commercializing university research. Bio/technology 1985;3:695–699.

20. Dibner MD. An analysis of state-sponsored biotech centers in the United States. Gen Eng News 1988(Jan):21. The largest number of new centers, nine, were started in 1987.

21. Pyeritz RE, Tumpson JE, Bernhardt BA. The economics of clinical genetics services. I. Preview. Am J Hum Genet 1987;41:549–558.

22. OTA. Commercial biotechnology:11.

23. Ibid.:332–333, 547–549.

24. Survey of the National Academy of Sciences. Cited by Makulowich. Biotech's growth.

25. Blumenthal et al. Industrial support.

26. My discussions with scientists who were consultants to companies, but who retained their university positions, indicated a broad range of research in their university laboratories. Some are working on basic methodology that eventually will have commercial application. Others are conducting basic research on common diseases for which a commercial role in either diagnosis or treatment is foreseeable. Others have completely separated their two activities; their university research has no apparent commercial application.

27. Berg EN. Small concerns battle cancer. New York Times, 28 December 1985: Business Day, 29.

28. Blumenthal et al. University-industry research relationships.

29. Blumenthal et al. Industrial support.

30. Makulowich. Biotech's growth.

31. Blumenthal et al. University-industry research relationships.

32. The companies were Cetus Corp., Emeryville, Calif.; Collaborative Research, Inc., Lexington, Mass.; Genentech, Inc., South San Francisco, Calif.; Genetics Institute, Cambridge, Mass.; Integrated Genetics, Inc., Framingham, Mass.; Molecular Diagnostics, Inc., West Haven, Ct.

33. The survey was conducted while I was at the Office of Technology Assessment (OTA), with partial support from OTA. Some of the findings appear in an OTA Staff Paper: Hewitt M, Holtzman NA. The commercial development of tests for human genetic disorders. February 1988. The paper is unpublished, but is available from the Health Program, OTA.

34. Rogers EM. Diffusion of innovations. New York: Free Press (Macmillan), 1983:141. According to Rogers, a phase of technological competition will follow in which firms that fail to improve the technology will be eliminated.

35. Klausner A, Wilson T. Gene detection technology opens doors for many industries. Bio/technology 1983;1:471–478.

36. Integrated Genetics, Inc. Prenatal diagnosis and carrier detection of inherited disease. Framingham, Mass., n.d. (ca. 1987).

37. Collaborative Research, Inc. DNA diagnostic services. Waltham, Mass., n.d. (ca. 1987).

38. Donis-Keller H, Green P, Helms C, et al. A genetic linkage map of the human genome. Cell 1987;51:319–337.

39. Collaborative Research, Inc. First genetic map of human genome completed by Collaborative Research. Bedford, Mass., 7 October 1987.

40. Integrated Genetics, Inc. Current concepts in DNA-probe analysis: Alzheimer's disease. Genetic Reference Laboratory at Integrated Genetics. Framingham, Mass., October 1987.

41. Kolata G. Reducing risk: a change of heart? Science 1986;231:669–670.

42. Frossard P. Personal communication, November 1987.

43. Henderson N. Biomark program draws high-tech portraits of employees' health risks. Washington Post, 17 March 1986: Business. According to the article,

the company will attempt to get licenses for DNA probes and other methods, which were developed in university and other companies' laboratories, to use in their tests. "Focus plans to license different markers and pull them together into one package, while financing research to develop new tools."

44. L. McCarthy, president of Focus Technologies. Personal communication, June 1988.

45. Klausner, Wilson. Gene detection technology opens doors.

46. Food and Drug Administration (FDA). Clinical studies of safety and effectiveness of orphan products: availability of grants; request for applications. 206 Fed. Reg. 39996–39999 (1987).

47. Collaborative Research, Inc. DNA diagnostic services.

48. The meeting took place on 17 January 1986. The NIH representatives present were Fred Bergmann, Cheryl Corsaro, Felix de la Cruz, Delbert Dayton, Jeanette Felix, and Robert Katz. They emphasized that the elegance of a proposed study, not the frequency of a given disease, is a major determinant of whether an application for the study of that disease is funded. When scores of applications dealing with rare diseases are of borderline acceptability, special efforts are made to support them.

49. Integrated Genetics, Inc. Report to the Securities and Exchange Commission. Framingham, Mass., 1984.

50. Integrated Genetics, Inc. Prenatal diagnosis.

51. DiMaio MS, Baumgarten A, Greenstein RM, Sasl HM, Mahoney MJ. Screening for fetal Down's syndrome in pregnancy by measuring maternal serum alpha-fetoprotein levels. N Engl J Med 1987;317:342–346.

52. Amniotic fluid AFP and cholinesterase are used to follow up MSAFP elevations. At many genetic centers the policy is also to karyotype the fetal cells, even when there is no indication of increased risk of chromosome abnormality.

53. Genentech has combined with another company to form Travenol-Gentech Diagnostics. Currently, it is concentrating on diagnostics for infectious diseases, including hepatitis and the AIDS virus (HIV).

54. Cetus Corp. Annual report. Emeryville, Calif., 1984.

55. Saiki RK, Scahrf S, Faloona F, et al. Enzymatic amplification of beta-globin genomic sequences and restriction site analysis for diagnosis of sickle cell anemia. Science 1985;230:1350–1354. For a brief description see Marx JL. New sickle cell test. Science 1985;230:1365.

56. Embury S, Scharf SJ, Saiki RK, et al. Rapid prenatal diagnosis of sickle cell anemia by a new method of DNA analysis. N Engl J Med 1987;316:656–660.

57. Erlich H. Personal communication, November 1987.

58. Orkin SH. Genetic diagnosis by DNA analysis: progress through amplification. N Engl J Med 1987;317:1023–1025.

59. Saltus R. Biotech firms compete in genetic diagnosis. Science 1986;234:1318–1320.

60. Although one company gave as its reason for not constructing probes for human DNA its concern about protecting its proprietary position, this area of recombinant DNA technology does not seem to be more prone than any other to having patents rapidly become obsolete. If patents are awarded for methods, such as the use of RFLPs (see above), or for denaturing gradient gels or for RNA-DNA heteroduplexes (see chapter 4), the companies holding them (or exclusive licenses for them) will have a considerable advantage.

61. Saltus. Biotech firms compete.

62. Tsui L-C, Buchwald M, Barker D, et al. Cystic fibrosis locus defined by a genetically linked polymorphic DNA marker. Science 1985;230:1054–1057.

63. White R, Woodward S, Leppert M, et al. A closely linked genetic marker for cystic fibrosis. Nature 1985;318:382–384. This manuscript was received by Nature on November 1. Simultaneously, Collaborative Research, Inc., reported that its markers also were on chromosome 7. Knowlton RG, Cohen-Haguenauer O, Van Cong N, et al. A polymorphic DNA marker linked to cystic fibrosis is located on chromosome 7. Nature 1985;318:380–382. This article was received by Nature on November 11.

64. White R. The search for the cystic fibrosis gene. Science 1986;234:1054–1055. See also Roberts L. The race for the cystic fibrosis gene. Science 1988;240:141–144.

65. Collaborative Research, Inc. First genetic map of human genome.

Chapter 7: Technology Transmittance: From Commercial Development to the Widespread Use of Genetic Tests

1. Gusella JF. Probes in Huntington's chorea. Nature 1986;320:21–22.

2. Watt DG, Lindenbaum RH, Jonasson JA, Edwards JH. Probes in Huntington's chorea. Nature 1986;320:21. After establishing the unlikelihood of a second locus, Gusella announced that the probe would be made available to other institutions for clinical testing as long as the program was approved by a local institutional review board or ethics committee. See Gusella JF. Accuracy of testing for Huntington's disease. Nature 1986;323:118.

3. McDermott W. Evaluating the physician and his technology. Daedalus 1977;106:135–157.

4. Gjestland T. The Oslo study of untreated syphilis: an epidemiologic investigation of the natural course of the syphilitic infection based on a restudy of the Boeck-Bruusgard material. Acta Derm Venereol 1955;35(suppl):11. See also Wooley PD, Anderson AJ. Prevalence of undiagnosed syphilis in the elderly. Lancet 1986;2:1034.

5. Farrant W. Stress after amniocentesis for high serum alpha-fetoprotein concentrations. Brit Med J 1980;3:452.

6. Fearn J, Hibbard BM, Laurence KM, Roberts A, Robinson JO. Screening for neural-tube defects and maternal anxiety. Brit J Obstet Gynaec 1982;89:218–221.

7. Smithells RW. AFP screening and maternal anxiety. Lancet 1980;1:772–773.

8. Sorenson JR, Levy HL, Mangione TW, Sepe SJ. Parental response to repeat testing of infants with "false-positive" results in a newborn screening program. Pediatrics 1984;73:183–187. See also Bodegard G, Fyro F, Larsson A. Psychological reactions in 102 families with a newborn who has a falsely positive screening test for congenital hypothyroidism. Acta Paediatr Scand 1983;304(suppl):3–21.

9. The evidence for this comes from my personal observation of the late age of diagnosis of PKU in cases missed by newborn screening in which the parents bring suit against the screening laboratory and/or the infant's physician. From time to time, I am called upon to provide an opinion in such cases.

10. U.S. Congress, Office of Technology Assessment (OTA). Federal policies

and the medical device industry. Washington, D.C.: U.S. Government Printing Office, 1984; OTA-H-230.

11. 21 C.F.R. 807.81–807.97 (1988).

12. U.S. General Accounting Office (GAO). Medical devices: early warning of problems is hampered by severe underreporting. Washington, D.C.: U.S. General Accounting Office, 1987; GAO/PEMD-87-1.

13. U.S. Department of Health and Human Services (DHHS), Public Health Service, Food and Drug Administration. Regulatory requirements for medical devices: a workshop manual. Washington, D.C.: U.S. Government Printing Office, 1983; DHHS publication no (FDA) 83-4165.

14. 51 Fed. Reg. 140 (1986), Premarket approval of medical devices, pp. 23342–26364.

15. 21 C.F.R. 862, 864, 868 (1988).

16. Those applying for investigational-device exemptions are required to demonstrate that the testing of the device will be initially and continually reviewed by an institutional review board (IRB), that appropriate informed consent will be obtained, and that certain records and reports will be maintained. See DHHS. Regulatory requirements.

17. Hellman K, FDA. Personal communication, October 1987.

18. GAO. Medical devices.

19. Ibid.

20. Young FE. DNA probes: fruits of the new biotechnology. JAMA 1987;258:2404–2406.

21. 21 C.F.R. 809.10 (1987).

22. Young. DNA probes.

23. 48 Fed. Reg. 118 (1983), Alpha-fetoprotein test kits; withdrawal of proposed rule, Food and Drug Administration, pp. 27780–27782.

24. Young. DNA probes.

25. GAO. Medical devices.

26. Thacker SB, Berkelman RL. Surveillance of medical technologies. J Hlth Pol 1986;7:363–377.

27. OTA. Federal policies.

28. 21 C.F.R. § 812.3(m) (1988).

29. Holtzman NA, Hewitt M. How new technology becomes routine procedure: the case of DNA-based tests for genetic disorders. In: Willey AM, ed. Nucleic acid probes in the diagnosis of human genetic diseases. [In press].

30. Bucci VA, Reiss JB. Technology assessment of medical devices under Medicare: who should examine "safety and effectiveness"? Food Drug Cosmet Law J 1985;40:445–455. Although part of the reason for a repeat evaluation may be concern over safety, a more important consideration to HCFA—which decides whether Medicare will reimburse for the procedure—is cost. The FDA does not take cost into consideration in its premarket approval process.

31. Emergency Care Research Institute. The growth of physician office laboratories. J Hlth Care Technol 1986;3:95–115. See also Eisenberg JM, Myers LP, Pauly MV. How will changes in physician payment by Medicare influence laboratory testing? JAMA 1987;258:803–808; and Holtzman, Hewitt. How new technology becomes routine procedure.

32. Bogdanich W. Medical labs, trusted as largely error-free, are far from infallible. Wall Street Journal, 2 February 1987.

33. Cited by Eisenberg et al. How will changes in physician payment by Medicare influence laboratory testing?

34. Bogdanich. Medical labs.

35. Ibid.

36. U.S. Congress, Office of Technology Assessment (OTA). Healthy children: investing in the fetus. Washington, D.C.: U.S. Government Printing Office, 1988; OTA-H-375.

37. Bogdanich. Medical labs.

38. Ibid.

39. Roberts L. Measuring cholesterol is as tricky as lowering it. Science 1987;238:482–483.

40. Bogdanich. Medical labs.

41. Holtzman NA, Meek AG, Mellits Ed. Neonatal screening for phenylketonuria. I. Effectiveness. JAMA 1974;229:667–670.

42. Holtzman C, Slazyk WE, Cordero JF, et al. Descriptive epidemiology of missed cases of phenylketonuria and congenital hypothyroidism. Pediatrics 1986;78:553–558.

43. Sola AM. Legal high risk areas in genetic screening: programs and what to expect when you are sued. In: Andrews LB, ed. Legal liability and quality assurance in newborn screening. Chicago: American Bar Foundation, 1985:119–127.

44. Andrews, ed. Legal liability:2.

45. Kazazian H. Personal communication, October 1987.

46. Holtzman C, et al. Descriptive epidemiology. The reasons for most of the remainder could not be determined or were the result of miscellaneous causes.

47. Ibid. Only data on congenital hypothyroidism were available for this estimate. The authors point out that data on missed cases could well have been more complete from the large programs, thereby making the discrepancy even greater.

48. Tuerck JM, Buist NRM, Skeels MR, Miyahira RS, Beacg PG. Computerized surveillance of errors in newborn screening. Am J Pub Hlth 1987;77:1528–1531.

49. U.S. Bureau of the Census. Statistical Abstract of the United States, 1982–83. Washington, D.C.: U.S. Government Printing Office, 1982. See also National Center for Health Statistics. Advance report of final natality statistics, 1985. Hyattsville, Md.: National Center for Health Statistics; DHHS publication no (PHS) 87-1120. (Mo Vit Stat Rep 1987;36[4 suppl]).

50. DNA markers that have been associated with insulin-dependent diabetes have population frequencies of about 5 percent. The combined frequency of markers for alleles conferring susceptibility to coronary heart disease also is approximately 5 percent. For familial forms of bipolar affective disorder or Alzheimer disease, variable expressivity can be expected, and the combined heterozygote frequency of susceptibility-conferring alleles could also approach 5 percent. Because the point of this analysis is to demonstrate the large volume of positive test results following the marketing of DNA-based tests, it should be noted that even if the markers for the disorders shown in table 7.2 occur on average in only 1 percent of the population, over 160,000 positive results per year will still be obtained.

51. Ottman R, Pike MC, King M-C, Casagrande JT, Henderson BE. Familial breast cancer in a population-based series. Am J Epidemiol 1986;123:15–21.

52. Sorenson JR, Swazey JP, Scotch NA. Reproductive pasts, reproductive futures: genetic counseling and its effectiveness. New York: Alan R. Liss, 1981:84–88.

53. National Center for Education in Maternal and Child Health. State treatment centers for metabolic disorders. Washington, D.C.: NCEMCH, 1986.

54. Kessler S. Genetics associates/counselors in genetic services. Am J Med Genet 1980;7:323–334.

55. American Board of Medical Genetics. Personal communication, October 1987.

56. Finley WH, Finley SC, Dyer RL. Survey of medical genetics personnel. Am J Hum Genet 1987;40:374–377.

57. Forsman I. Non-physician health providers and expanded genetic testing. Paper prepared for the Office of Technology Assessment. [Unpublished, 1987].

58. Bernhardt BA, Weiner J, Foster EC, Tumpson JE, Pyeritz RE. The economics of clinical genetic services. II. A time analysis of a medical genetics clinic. Am J Hum Genet 1987;41:559–565.

59. Finley et al. Survey of medical genetics personnel.

60. American Society of Human Genetics. Guide to human genetics training programs in North America. Rockville, Md.: American Society of Human Genetics, 1986, 1988.

61. Cypress BK. Patients' reasons for visiting physicians: National Ambulatory Medical Care Survey, United States, 1977–78. Washington, D.C.: U.S. Government Printing Office, 1982; DHHS publication no (PHS) 82-1717. (Vit Hlth Stat; series 13; no 56).

62. Committee for the Study of Inborn Errors of Metabolism (CSIEM). Genetic screening: programs, principles, and research. Washington, D.C.: National Academy of Sciences, 1975:161–164. For more detailed information see Rosenstock IM, Childs B, Simopoulos AP. Genetic screening: a study of knowledge and attitudes of physicians. Washington, D.C.: National Academy of Sciences, 1975. It is likely that had physicians more readily adopted newborn screening in the early 1960s, fewer mandatory laws for screening, which ironically were opposed by physician organizations, would have been passed.

63. Chwalow AJ, Faden R, Holtzman NA. Informed consent for newborn genetic-metabolic screening. Am J Hum Genet 1978;30:108A. In this survey, chiefs of obstetric and pediatric services in Maryland hospitals were interviewed.

64. Gordis L, Childs B, Roseman MG. Obstetricians' attitudes toward genetic screening. Am J Pub Hlth 1977;67:469–471.

65. Childs B, Gordis L, Kaback MM, Kazazian HH, Jr. Tay-Sachs screening: motives for participating and knowledge of genetics and probability. Am J Hum Genet 1976;28:537–549. See also Rothschild H, Ivker FB. Advocacy and compliance factors in a voluntary selective screening program. South Med J 1977;70: 184–186; and Beck E, Blaichman S, Scriver C, et al. Advocacy and compliance in genetic screening: behavior of physicians and clients in a voluntary program of testing for the Tay-Sachs gene. N Engl J Med 1974;291:1166–1170. In a survey of Jews of reproductive age who had not been the target of any campaign for screening, 71 percent thought physicians should have the primary responsibility for testing compared to "State Governments—by law" (43 percent) or "Community (potentially affected religious or ethnic groups)" (27 percent). See Massarik F, Kaback

M. Genetic disease control: a social psychological approach. Beverly Hills, Calif.: Sage, 1981:88.

66. Holtzman NA, Faden R, Leonard CO, Chase G, Chwalow AJ, Richmond S. Effect of education on physicians' knowledge of a new technology: the case of alpha-fetoprotein screening for neural tube defects. [Submitted for publication]. California recognized the problem of getting obstetricians to adopt AFP screening when it issued regulations requiring physicians to offer the test to pregnant women.

67. National Center for Health Statistics. Health, United States, 1983. Washington, D.C.: U.S. Government Printing Office, 1983; DHHS publication no (PHS) 84-1232:33–34.

68. Sepe SJ, Markes JS, Oakley GP, Manley AF. Delivery of genetic services in the United States. JAMA 1982;248:1733–1735. See also Bernhardt BA, Bannerman RM. The influence of obstetricians on the utilization of amniocentesis. Prenat Diagn 1984;4:43–49; and Lippman-Hand A, Cohen DI. Influence of obstetricians' attitudes on their use of prenatal diagnosis for the detection of Down's syndrome. Can Med Assoc J 1980;122:1381–1385. Pregnant women in low socioeconomic groups have high utilization rates when amniocentesis services are made available to them. See Marion JP, Kassam GR, Fernhoff PM, et al. Acceptance of amniocentesis by low-income patients in an urban hospital. Am J Obstet Gynecol 1980;138:11–15. See also Ferguson-Smith MA. Prenatal chromosome analysis and its impact on the birth incidence of chromosome disorders. Brit Med Bull 1983;39:355–364; and Hewitt M. Hospital-based analyses of amniocentesis utilization. Am J Hum Genet 1986;39(3 suppl):A177.

69. American Cancer Society. Survey of physicians' attitudes and practices in early cancer detection. CA 1985;35:197–231.

70. Nader PR, Taras HL, Sallis JF, Patterson TL. Adult heart disease prevention in childhood: a national survey of pediatricians' practices and attitudes. Pediatrics 1987;79:843–850.

71. Rogers EM. Diffusion of innovations. New York: Free Press, 1983:241–270.

72. CSIEM. Genetic screening:162.

73. Riccardi VM, Schmickel RD. Human genetics as a component of medical school curricula: a report to the American Society of Human Gentics. Am J Hum Genet 1988;42:639–643.

74. Childs B, Huether CA, Murphy EA. Human genetics teaching in U.S. medical schools. Am J Hum Genet 1981;33:1–10.

75. Ibid.

76. Bertram DA, Brooks-Bertram PA. The evaluation of continuing medical education: a literature review. Hlth Educ Monog 1977;5:330–362. See also Sibley JC, Sackett DL, Neogeld V, Gerrard B, Rudnick KV, Frase W. A randomized trial of continuing medical education. N Engl J Med 1982;306:511–515; Lloyd JS, Abramson S. Effectiveness of continuing medical education; a review of the evidence. Eval Hlth Prof 1979;2:251–280; Berg AO. Does continuing medical education improve the quality of medical care? A look at the evidence. J Fam Prac 1979;8:1171–1174; and Stein LS. The effectiveness of continuing medical education: eight research reports. J Med Educ 1981;56:103–110.

77. Holtzman et al. Effect of education on physician knowledge.

78. Casscells W, Schoenberger A, Graboys TB. Interpretation by physicians of clinical laboratory results. N Engl J Med 1978;299:999–1001. See also Berwick

DM, Fineberg HV, Weinstein MC. When doctors meet numbers. Am J Med 1981;71:991–998; and Billings PR, Bernstein MS. Physicians poor at prevalence and positive predictive value. JAMA 1985;254:1173–1174.

79. Holtzman NA. Rare diseases, common problems: recognition and management. Pediatrics 1978;62:1056–1060.

80. Holtzman et al. Effect of education on physician knowledge.

81. If test results were positive for 5 percent of the unaffected population, 50 healthy people out of 1,000 would have a positive result. Since only one person in 1,000 has the disease, the probability that a person with a positive result actually has the disease is 1/51, or 2 percent. The proportion of incoming students who had taken undergraduate courses in statistics or computers was about the same in the classes studied. Statistics had not been taught to the students at the Hopkins medical school before they were asked the question. I obtained approximately the same high score in two subsequent classes of first-year medical students.

82. Tversky A, Kahneman D. Judgment under uncertainty: heuristics and biases. Science 1974;185:1124–1131.

83. Collins DL. Results of the NSGC professional status survey. Perspect Genet Counsel 1987;9(2):1–4.

84. Cohen FL. Clinical genetics in nursing practice. Philadelphia, Pa.: J. B. Lippincott, 1984. See also Jensen MD. Maternity care. 2nd ed. St. Louis: C. V. Mosby, 1981. Waechter EN, Philips J, Holoday B. Nursing care of children. 10th ed. Philadelphia, Pa.: J. B. Lippincott, 1985; and Whaley LF. Nursing care of infants and children. St. Louis: C. V. Mosby, 1979.

85. American Nurses' Association. Facts about nurses, 1984–85. Kansas City, Kans., 1985.

86. Cohen F. Genetic knowledge possessed by American nurses and nursing students. J Adv Nurs 1979;4:493–501.

87. Williams JK. Pediatric nurse practitioners' knowledge of genetic disease. Pediatr Nursing 1983;9:119–121.

88. Rauch J. Genetic content for graduate social work education practice course. Council on Social Work Education publication no 86-71596. Washington, D.C.: CSWE, 1986.

89. Forsman. Non-physician health providers.

90. Marks J. Personal communication, August 1987.

91. Avorn J, Soumerai SB. Improving drug therapy decisions through educational outreach: a randomized controlled trial of academically based "detailing." N Engl J Med 1983;308:1457–1463.

92. Gibbs JO, Henes C, Kaplan GN. Health Services Foundation, Blue Cross and Blue Shield Association. Final report: genetic services benefit study. Chicago, Ill., 1987.

93. Ibid.

94. Holtzman N, personal observation. For evidence that physicians have been sued in conjunction with the screening of newborns, see Holtzman et al. Descriptive epidemiology of missed cases of phenylketonuria.

95. Andrews LB. Medical genetics: a legal frontier. Chicago: American Bar Foundation, 1987:138–147. See also Coplan J. Wrongful life and wrongful birth: new concepts for the pediatrician. Pediatrics 1985;75:65–72; and Shaw MW. To be or not to be? That is the question. Am J Hum Genet 1984;36:1–9. Court decisions have been based on two doctrines, wrongful birth and wrongful life. In wrongful-

birth rulings, damages are awarded for the special care involved in bringing up a child with a disability and for the emotional distress caused the parents. More recently, courts have begun to accept wrongful-life suits that permit the child to recover damages for being born with a disability. California, Colorado, Illinois, New Jersey, and Washington recognize a cause of action for wrongful life.

96. Quoted by Annas GJ, Elias S. Maternal serum AFP: educating physicians and the public. Am J Pub Hlth 1985;75:1374–1375.

97. Holtzman et al. Effect of education on physician knowledge.

98. U.S. Congress, Office of Technology Assessment (OTA). New developments in biotechnology—background paper: public perceptions of biotechnology. Washington, D.C.: U.S. Government Printing Office, 1987; OTA-BP-BA-45.

99. McInerney J. DNA in medicine: school-based education. Am J Hum Genet 1988;42:635–636.

100. Kan YW, Dozy AM. Polymorphism of DNA sequence adjacent to human β-globin structural gene: relationship to sickle mutation. Proc Natl Acad Sci 1978; 75:5631–5635.

101. Association of American Publishers, American Library Association, and Association for Supervision and Curriculum Development. Limiting what students shall read: books and other learning materials in our public schools: how they are selected and how they are removed. Washington, D.C., 1981.

102. McInerney J. Personal communication, March 1987.

103. There are a few model programs. The Human Genetics and Bioethics Education Laboratory at Ball State University, for instance, provides an intensive summer session for high-school teachers on addressing ethical and public policy issues in genetics in the classroom. The North Carolina Biotechnology Center in Research Triangle Park is developing instructional materials and conducting workshops for teachers. A Cold Spring Harbor program, with support from the National Science Foundation, introduces teachers to the laboratory techniques of genetic engineering in school districts throughout the Northeast with the help of a mobile van. The demand for continuing education may increase as teachers are required to prove subject competence and remain conversant with developments in their respective fields. See McInerney J. Testing for human genetic disorders using recombinant DNA technology: the role of the schools in developing public understanding. Paper prepared for the Office of Technology Assessment. [Unpublished, 1987].

104. Rothschild, Ivker. Advocacy and compliance factors in a voluntary selective screening program. This estimate may not be representative, as only 32 percent of randomly selected nonparticipants from Jewish community census lists responded to the survey.

105. Volodkevich H, Huether CA. Causes of low utilization of amniocentesis by women of advanced maternal age. Soc Biol 1981;28:176–186.

106. Kodanaz A, Ziegler D. Genetic counseling in Huntington's disease. [Unpublished manuscript]. Cited by Wexler N. Genetic jeopardy and the new clairvoyance. In: Bearn A, Motulsky A, Childs B, eds. Prog Med Genet, new series, 1985;6:277–304. It could be argued that the staff assumed that families knew about the genetic implications of the disorder. Nevertheless, they made no effort to provide information or to check the accuracy of the family's knowledge. When they made referrals for additional help, they often did not follow them up.

107. Gibbs et al. Final report: genetic service benefit study:47.

108. Sorenson et al. Reproductive pasts. See also Wertz DC, Sorenson JR. Client reactions to genetic counseling: self-reports of influence. Clin Genet 1986; 30:494–502.

109. Golbus MS, Loughman WD, Epstein CJ, Halbasch G, Stephens JD, Hall BD. Prenatal genetic diagnosis in 3000 amniocenteses. N Engl J Med 1979;300: 157–163. See also Bannerman DM, Gillick D, Coevering RV, Knobloch NL, Ingall GB. Amniocentesis and educational attainment. N Engl J Med 1977;297:449–450.

110. OTA. New developments in biotechnology.

111. Persons who said that religion was very important in their daily life were less likely to favor testing (63 percent in both cases compared to 73 and 72 percent, respectively, of people who said religion was not too important or was unimportant). Differences in education did not have a significant effect.

112. Faden RR, Chwalow AJ, Holtzman NA, Horn SD. A survey to evaluate parental consent as public policy for neonatal screening. Am J Pub Hlth 1982;72: 1347–1352.

113. Chase G, Kwiterovich PO, Bachorik P. The Columbia population study. III. Volunteer status, educational background, and plasma total cholesterol level in a prepaid health care program. Johns Hopkins Med J 1981;148:191–195. The volunteers had lower plasma cholesterol levels than plan participants who did not volunteer but were sampled on a random basis. The differences were observed for both men and women at all educational strata, so socioeconomic factors do not account for the effect. A "healthy volunteer effect" may explain the lower-than-expected coronary heart disease death rate in a number of clinical trials in both treated and untreated (control) subjects. See, for instance, Lipid Research Clinic Program. The lipid research clinics coronary primary prevention trial results. I. Reduction in incidence of coronary heart disease. JAMA 1984;251:351–363.

114. Jaffe FS, Lindheim BL, Lee PR. Abortion politics: private morality and public policy. New York: McGraw-Hill, 1981:99–111.

115. Faden RR, Chwalow AJ, Quaid K, et al. Prenatal screening and pregnant women's attitudes toward the abortion of defective fetuses. Am J Pub Hlth 1987; 77:288–290. When the question was put in terms of whether abortion was justified for other women, 84 percent of the respondents favored it for serious mental handicap, and 73 percent supported it for serious physical handicap.

116. Cao A, Furbetta, M, Galanello R, et al. Prevention of homozygous beta-thalassemia by carrier screening and prenatal diagnosis in Sardinia. Am J Hum Genet 1981;33:592–605.

117. Stamatoyannopoulos G. Problems of screening and counseling in the hemoglobinopathies. In: Motulsky AG, Lenz W, eds. Birth defects. Amsterdam: Excerpta Medica, 1974:268–276.

118. McCormack MK, Leiblum S, Lazzarini A. Attitudes regarding utilization of artificial insemination by donor in Huntington disease. Am J Med Genet 1983;14:5–13. Only 44 and 25 percent of these two groups, respectively, thought AID was the "best" alternative, while 81 and 58 percent of the corresponding groups of women thought it was.

119. Goldstein MS, Greenwald S, Nathan T, Massarik F, Kaback MM. Health behavior and genetic screening for carriers of Tay-Sachs disease: a prospective study. Soc Sci Med 1977;11:515–520. See also Rothschild, Ivker. Advocacy and compliance factors in a voluntary selective screening program; Beck et al. Ad-

vocacy and compliance; and Kaback MM, Zeiger RS, Reynolds LW, Sonneborn M. Tay-Sachs disease: a model for the control of recessive genetic disorders. In: Motulsky AG, Lenz W, eds. Birth defects. Amsterdam: Excerpta Medica, 1974: 248–262.

120. Even among Hassidic Jews who oppose abortion, Tay-Sachs screening is used. Marriage brokers in the Hassidic community in Brooklyn, N.Y., take Tay-Sachs carrier status into consideration when arranging marriages. This may also occur in Israel, which has a national Tay-Sachs screening program. I surveyed Tay-Sachs screening results and the number of cases of Tay-Sachs detected by prenatal diagnosis or by diagnosis after birth in Israel in 1981. Even adjusting for outbreeding, the expected number of cases is greater than the number observed, suggesting fewer matings between carriers than expected from the frequency of carriers.

121. Goldstein et al. Health behavior and genetic screening.

122. Massarik, Kaback. Genetic disease control:53.

123. For a succinct summary see CSIEM. Genetic screening: 164–174.

124. For the extent of sickle cell screening in Maryland in 1980 by primary-care providers, hospitals, and other organizations, see Farfel M, Holtzman NA. Education, consent, and counseling in sickle cell screening programs: report of a survey. Am J Pub Hlth 1984;74:373–375.

125. Scriver CR, Bardanis M, Cartier L, Clow CL, Lancaster GA, Ostrowsky JT. Beta-thalassemia disease prevention: genetic medicine applied. Am J Hum Genet 1984;36:1024–1038.

126. Modell B, Ward RHT, Fairweather DVI. Effect of introducing antenatal diagnosis on reproductive behaviour of families at risk for thalassemia major. Brit Med J 1980;280:1347–1350.

127. Cao et al. Prevention of homozygous beta-thalassemia.

128. Quaid KA, Brandt J, Folstein SE. The decision to be tested for Huntington's disease [letter]. JAMA 1987;257:3362.

129. Mastromauro C, Myers RH, Berkman B. Attitudes toward presymptomatic testing in Huntington disease. Am J Med Genet 1987;26:271–282.

130. Zerres K, Stephan M. Attitudes to early diagnosis of polycystic kidney disease. Lancet 1986;2:1395. The outcome of the disease can be improved by kidney transplantation.

131. Faden et al. Prenatal screening and pregnant women's attitudes.

132. Marion et al. Acceptance of amniocentesis. See also Ferguson-Smith. Prenatal chromosome analysis. Hewitt. Hospital-based analyses of amniocentesis utilization.

133. Holtzman, NA. Screening for congenital abnormalities. Intl J Tech Assess Hlth Care 1985;1:805–819. See also Rowley PT. Response of pregnant women to hemoglobinopathy carrier identification. In: Carter TP, Willey AM. Genetic disease: screening and management. New York: Alan R. Liss, 1986:151–172; and Boehm CD, Antonarakis SE, Phillips JA, Stetten G, Kazazian HH, Jr. Prenatal diagnosis using DNA polymorphisms: report on 95 pregnancies at risk for sickle-cell disease or alpha-thalassemia. N Engl J Med 1983;308:1054–1058.

134. Baltimore Sun, from New York Times News Service, 12 February 1985. Demands, lawsuits reduce appeal of obstetrics, p. 3a.

135. Kaback M, Zippin D, Boyd P, et al. Attitudes toward prenatal diagnosis of cystic fibrosis among parents of affected children. In: Lawson D, ed. Cystic fibrosis: horizons. New York: John Wiley, 1985:15–28. For 65 percent of the fam-

ilies the child with cystic fibrosis was the last child born; no adjustment was made for parity, however.

136. Ibid.

137. Ibid. Leonard CO, Chase GA, Childs B. Genetic counseling: a consumers'[sic] view. N Engl J Med 1972;287:433–439. See also Ad Hoc Committee Task Force on Neonatal Screening, Cystic Fibrosis Foundation. Neonatal screening for cystic fibrosis: position paper. Pediatrics 1983;73:741–745.

138. Saxton M. Born and unborn: the implications of reproductive technologies for people with disabilities. In: Arditti R, Duelli Klein R, Minden S, eds.. Test tube women: what future for motherhood? London: Pandora Press, 1984:298–312.

139. Andrews LB. State laws and regulations governing newborn screening. Chicago: American Bar Foundation, 1985.

140. Farfel, Holtzman. Education, consent, and counseling.

141. Cassileth BR, Zupkis RV, Sutton-Smith K, et al. Informed consent—why are its goals imperfectly realized? N Engl J Med 1980;302:896–900. See also Meisel A, Roth LH. What we do and do not know about informed consent. JAMA 1981;246:2473–2477; Morrow G, Gootnick J, Schmale A. A simple technique for increasing cancer patients' knowledge of informed consent to treatment. Cancer 1978;42:793–799; and Andrews. Medical genetics:108–110.

142. Lorenz RP, Botti JJ, Schmidt CM, Ladda RL. Encouraging patients to undergo prenatal genetic counseling before the day of amniocentesis: its effect on the use of amniocentesis. J Reprod Med 1985;30:933–935.

143. Finley SC, Varner PD, Vinson PC, Finley WH. Participants' reaction to amniocentesis and prenatal genetic studies. JAMA 1977;238:2377–2379.

144. Rothman BK. The tentative pregnancy. New York: Viking, 1986:39. Rothman interviewed 25 genetic counselors, but her book does not indicate what criteria she used in selecting them.

145. Rothman BK. Personal communication, August 1987.

146. Fearn J, Hibbard BM, Laurence KM, Roberts A, Robinson JO. Screening for neural-tube defects and maternal anxiety. Brit J Obstet Gynaec 1982;89:218–221.

147. Sorenson et al. Parental response to repeat testing of infants with "false-positive" results. The parents who had not been told the truth had no greater anxiety or depression than those who had.

148. Hampton ML, Anderson J, Lavizzo BS, Bergman AB. Sickle cell "non-disease." Am J Dis Child 1974;128:58–61.

149. Goldstein et al. Health behavior and genetic screening.

150. McQueen D. Social aspects of genetic screening for Tay-Sachs disease: the pilot community screening program in Baltimore and Washington. Soc Biol 1975; 22:125–133. In this survey, 60 percent of the respondents said they would change their plans if both mates were found to be carriers.

151. Scriver CR, Bardanis M, Cartier L, Clow CL, Lancaster GA, Ostrowsky JT. Beta-thalassemia disease prevention: genetic medicine applied. Am J Hum Genet 1984;36:1024–1038.

152. Chase G, Faden RR, Holtzman NA, et al. The assessment of risk by pregnant women: implications for genetic counseling. Soc Biol 1986;33:57–64. Ninety percent of college graduates and 66 percent of women who were not college graduates answered correctly.

153. Evers-Kiebooms G, van den Berghe H. Impact of genetic counseling: a review of published follow-up studies. Clin Genet 1979;15:465–474.

154. Sorenson et al. Reproductive pasts.

155. Wertz DC, Sorenson JR, Heeren TC. Clients' interpretation of risks provided in genetic counseling. Am J Hum Genet 1986;39:253–264.

156. Rothman. The tentative pregnancy:43. This change coincides with increased use of prenatal diagnosis for risks of one in one hundred or fewer cases (for trisomies in older pregnant women). Thus women might be encouraged not to take risks that a decade ago were considered negligible.

157. Wertz DC, Sorenson JR, Heeren TC. Genetic counseling and reproductive uncertainty. Am J Med Genet 1984;18:79–88. Having a living affected child was another factor causing "pessimistic" interpretations of risk. Because genetic tests will increasingly be used by people without a family history, this factor has less bearing on genetic testing than how risks are communicated.

158. McNeil BJ, Pauker SG, Sox HC, Tversky A. On the elicitation of preferences for alternative therapies. N Engl J Med 1982;306:1259–1262.

159. McKormick JS, Skrabanek P. Holy dread. Lancet 1984;2:1155–1156.

160. Schoenbach VJ, Wagner EH, Beery WL. Health risk appraisal: review of evidence for effectiveness. Hlth Serv Res 1987;22:553–580.

161. Lippman-Hand A, Fraser FC. Genetic counseling—the postcounseling period. I. Parents' perceptions of uncertainty. Am J Med Genet 1979;4:51–71. For some people, a risk of occurrence of a disorder of 10 percent may be perceived no differently than a 50 percent risk if they believe they cannot cope with the situation.

162. Wertz et al. Genetic counseling and reproductive uncertainty. In the multicenter study, factors that were not often discussed included the effects of an affected child on family life, costs, and caring for the affected child at home.

163. Wertz DC, Sorenson JR, Heeren TC. Communication in health professional–lay encounters: how often does each party know what the other wants to discuss? In: Rubin BR, ed. Information and behavior. II. New Brunswick, N.J.: Transaction Books, Rutgers University Press, 1987.

164. Clow CL, Scriver CR. Knowledge about and attitudes toward genetic screening among high-school students: the Tay-Sachs experience. Pediatrics 1977;59:86–91. See also Childs B, Gordis L, Kaback MM, Kazazian HH, Jr. Tay-Sachs screening: social and psychological impact. Am J Hum Genet 1976;28:550–558.

165. Zeesman S, Clow CL, Cartier L, Scriver CR. A private view of heterozygosity: eight-year follow-up study on carriers of the Tay-Sachs gene detected by high-school screening in Montreal. Am J Med Genet 1984;18:769–778. Fewer than one third of those involved in the screening replied to the follow-up questionnaire mailed to them.

166. Clow, Scriver. Knowledge about and attitudes toward genetic screening.

167. See Fletcher J. Moral problems and ethical guidance in prenatal diagnosis: past, present, and future. In: Milunsky A, ed. Genetic disorders and the fetus. New York: Plenum, 1986:819–859.

168. Froese AP, Rose V, Allen DM. Emotional implications of primary familial hyperlipoproteinemia in childhood and adolescence. Pediatrics 1980;65:469–472.

169. Bergman AB, Stamm SJ. The morbidity of cardiac nondisease in school children. N Engl J Med 1967;276:1008–1013.

170. American Academy of Pediatrics, Committee on Nutrition. Toward a prudent diet for children. Pediatrics 1983;71:78–80.

171. Nader. Adult heart disease prevention in childhood.

172. Cadman D, Chambers LW, Walter SD, Ferguson R, Johnston N, McNamee J. Evaluation of public health preschool child developmental screening: the process and outcomes of a community program. Am J Pub Hlth 1987;77:45–51.

173. Mastromauro. Attitudes toward presymptomatic testing. Fourteen other people who thought they might be suicidal said they would not want to be tested.

174. Fraser FC. Genetic counseling. Am J Hum Genet 1974;26:636–659.

Chapter 8: Testing: In Whose Best Interest?

1. Hawthorne N. The scarlet letter. New York: Harper & Row, 1968:106.

2. Holtzman NA, Leonard CO. Maryland's MSAFP pilot program. II. Physicians' attitudes and knowledge. In: Haddow JE, Wald NJ, eds. Proceedings of the Third Annual Scarborough Conference. Scarborough, Maine: Foundation for Blood Research, 1980.

3. Chwalow AJ, Faden RR, Holtzman NA, et al. [Unpublished results].

4. Andrews LB. Medical genetics: a legal frontier. Chicago: American Bar Foundation, 1987:112.

5. Burke W, Motulsky A. Genetic information may not always be helpful. Am J Hum Genet 1987;41:A194.

6. Holtzman NA, Faden R, Chwalow AJ, Horn SD. Effect of informed parental consent on mothers' knowledge of newborn screening. Pediatrics 1983;72: 807–812. The study also revealed that disparities in knowledge between women of high and low socioeconomic status were overcome by the informing process.

7. Faden RR, Chwalow AJ, Orel-Crosby E, Holtzman NA, Chase GA, Leonard CO. What participants understand about a maternal serum alpha-fetoprotein screening program. Am J Pub Hlth 1985;75:1381–1384.

8. Rothman BK. The tentative pregnancy. New York: Viking, 1986:42.

9. According to one legal commentator, "Removal of blood (without informed consent) is insufficient to state a viable claim for assault and battery unless the blood was used—as in an alcohol test—against the patient's interests in court or in some other way. It would not constitute infliction of emotional distress, since the distress would inevitably occur later, when the child was born. Holder A. Personal communication, August 1987.

10. Schloendorff v. Society of New York Hospital, 1914. Quoted by Rosoff AJ. Informed consent: a guide for health care providers. Rockville, Md.: Aspen, 1981:1.

11. Andrews. Medical genetics:110–111.

12. Faden R, Chwalow AJ, Holtzman NA, Horn SD. A survey to evaluate parental consent as public policy for neonatal screening. Am J Pub Hlth 1982;72:1347–1352.

13. Andrews. Medical genetics:190–197.

14. Holder AR. Medical malpractice law. 2nd ed. New York: John Wiley, 1978:275.

15. Andrews. Medical genetics:199 (italics added).

16. Cited by Andrews. Medical genetics:196,nn.122,124. In these cases the danger was primarily to the partner, not to potential offspring.

17. Holder. Medical malpractice law:276.

18. Andrews. Medical genetics:196. According to Andrews, few other states have yet adopted such policies.

19. President's Commission for the Study of Ethical Problems in Medicine and Biomedical and Behavioral Research. Screening and counseling for genetic conditions: the ethical, social, and legal implications of genetic screening, counseling, and education programs. Washington, D.C.: U.S. Government Printing Office, 1983.

20. Committee for the Study of Inborn Errors of Metabolism (CSIEM). Genetic screening: programs, principles, and research. Washington, D.C.: National Academy of Sciences, 1975:186.

21. Ibid.:187.

22. Andrews. Medical genetics:198.

23. Toon PD, Jones EJ. Serving two masters: a dilemma in general practice. Lancet 1986;1:1196–1198.

24. Rothstein MA. Medical screening of workers. Washington, D.C.: Bureau of National Affairs, 1984:89.

25. Holder. Medical malpractice law:276.

26. Andrews. Medical genetics:205.

27. Ibid.:202.

28. Ibid.:191.

29. President's Commission. Screening and counseling for genetic conditions:42.

30. Shapiro DN, Hutchinson RI. Familial histiocytosis after artificial insemination. N Engl J Med 1981;304:757–759. Other cases in which the donor may have transmitted genetic disease were cited in this report.

31. Garver KL, Holtzman NA, Snyder DL, Marchese SG. Genetic evaluation of prospective semen donors in sperm banking institutions. [Unpublished, 1985].

32. Fisher NL, Plumridge DM, American Society of Human Genetics Social Issues Committee. Adoption laws: the availability of genetic information. Am J Hum Genet 1987;41(suppl):A58.

33. Ethics Committee of the American Fertility Society. Ethical considerations of the new reproductive technologies. Fertil Steril 1986;46(3;suppl):1S–94S.

34. American Association of Tissue Banks. Provisional standards. Addendum 2. Specific standards—Reproductive Council. Rockville, Md.: AATB, September 1984:22–27.

35. Andrews. Medical genetics:171.

36. Kovacs GT, Clayton C, McGarvan P. The attitude of semen donors. Clin Reprod Fertil 1983;2:73–75. See also Rowland R. The social and psychological consequences of secrecy in artificial insemination by donor (AID) programmes. Soc Sci Med 1985;21:391–396.

37. Timmons MC, Rao KW, Sloan CS, et al. Screening of donors for artificial insemination. Fertil Steril 1981;35:451–456.

38. Danks D. Genetic considerations. In: Wood C, Leeton J, Kovacs G, eds. Artificial insemination by donor. Melbourne: Brown, Prior & Anderson, 1980.

39. Fraser FC, Forse RA. On genetic screening of donors for artificial insemination. Am J Med Genet 1981;10:399–405.

40. Kovacs et al. The attitude of semen donors. See also Nicholas MK, Tyler JP. Characteristics, attitudes, and personalities of AI donors. Clin Reprod Fertil 1983;2:47–54.

41. Czeizel A, Szentesi I, Horvath L. Results of genetic screening of donors for artificial insemination. Clin Genet 1983;24:113–116.

42. Employee relations, 1986. Employee Relations Weekly (BNA) 1986;4: 1297,1298.

43. American Council of Life Insurance. Life insurance fact book. Washington, D.C., 1986.

44. Health Insurance Association of America. 1986–1987 source book of health insurance data. Washington, D.C., 1987.

45. Nothing prohibits people with group insurance from taking out additional individual life or health insurance. Such prohibitions ("coordination of benefits") apply to getting reimbursed for a medical care cost from more than one group policy. The only limits on how many different life insurance policies people can purchase is their ability to pay.

46. Corbett JS, vice president and associate general counsel of MIB, Inc. Letter to Dr. Philip Reilly. May 1986.

47. Gibbs JO, Henes C, Kaplan GN. Final report: genetic services benefit study. Chicago: Health Services Foundation, Blue Cross and Blue Shield Association, 1987:47.

48. Committee for the Study of Inborn Errors of Metabolism (CSIEM). Genetic screening: programs, principles, and research. Washington, D.C.: National Academy of Sciences, 1975.

49. American Council of Life Insurance and Health Insurance Association of America. AIDS update. Washington, D.C., September 1987.

50. Andrews LB. State laws and regulations governing newborn screening. Chicago: American Bar Foundation, 1985:16–17.

51. Pear R. States act to provide health care benefits to uninsured people. New York Times, 22 November 1987:1.

52. Rothstein MA. Medical screening of workers. Washington, D.C.: Bureau of National Affairs, 1984.

53. Occupational Safety and Health Administration, 29 C.F.R. 1910.1003(g)(1)(i) (1970).

54. Occupational Safety and Health Administration, Instruction STD 1-23.4 (1980), 1 OSHR ref. file 21:8212.

55. Rothstein MA. Refusing to employ smokers: good public health or bad public policy? Notre Dame Law Rev 1987;62:940–968.

56. Rothstein. Medical screening of workers:171.

57. This is probably illegal, but many handicapped individuals might not know this or, if they did, might be willing to forgo their right in order to gain work. If something did happen, they could file a claim, but their job might not be protected.

58. U.S. Congress, Office of Technology Assessment (OTA). The role of genetic testing in the prevention of occupational disease. Washington, D.C.: U.S. Government Printing Office, 1983; OTA-BA-194.

59. Severo R. Screening of blacks by Du Pont sharpens debate on genetic tests. New York Times, 4 February 1980:1. Du Pont officials said they started screening as a result of requests from black employees.

60. Severo R. Du Pont defends genetic screening. New York Times, 18 October 1981.

61. Uzych L. Genetic testing and exclusionary practices in the workplace. J Pub Hlth Pol 1986;7:37–57.

62. Kark JA, Posey DM, Schumacher HR, Ruehle CJ. Sickle cell trait as a risk factor for sudden death in physical training. N Engl J Med 1987;317:781–787.

63. U.S. Congress, Office of Technology Assessment (OTA). Reproductive health hazards in the workplace. Washington, D.C.: U.S. Government Printing Office, 1985; OTA-BA-267. See also Rothstein. Medical screening of workers.

64. OTA. The role of genetic testing.

65. U.S. Congress, House Committee on Science and Technology. Genetic screening and the handling of high-risk groups in the workplace. Hearings before the Subcommittee on Investigations and Oversight of the Committee on Science and Technology, October 1981. Washington, D.C.: U.S. Government Printing Office, 1981:113.

66. Rothstein M. Personal communication, August 1987.

67. U.S. Chamber of Commerce. Employee benefits. 1985.

68. Medical information may be required if the employee was not actively at work (due, for instance, to sickness) when he or she became eligible for coverage, or if the employee initially elected not to participate. Even then, "open enrollment" periods may permit employees to join the group without providing medical information.

69. The rate paid by employers for group insurance is determined either from costs to the employer in previous years or from a "manual" rate derived from the claims costs of companies whose employees have comparable demographic characteristics. This is known as "experience rating." When the manual rate is used, commercial insurers may grant a rate modification to an eligible group. Firms of intermediate size (10–200 employees) rely more on the actual experience of the group than on the "manual" rate.

70. Medical benefits: employee benefits in medium and large firms, 1985. Med Benefits, 31 August 1986:8–11.

71. This stems from the ruling of the Supreme Court in 1981 (Alessi v. Raybestos-Manhattan, Inc., 451 S. Ct. 504 [1981]) that the federal Employment Retirement Income Security Act (ERISA) preempts the states from regulating health insurance and other benefits offered by employers who are self-insured.

72. Commercial health insurance providers may offer "multiple lives" individual insurance policies to all workers in a small firm, but may limit coverage for some individuals or family members because of their medical history. The firm pays the premiums and absorbs the administrative costs, which are lower than those for policies sold individually.

73. Baram MS. Charting the future course for corporate management of genetic and health risks. In: Milunsky A, Annas GJ, eds. Genetics and the law. III. New York: Plenum, 1985:475–486.

74. Rothstein MA. Legal issues in the medical assessment of physical impairment by third-party physicians. J Leg Med 1984;5:503–548.

75. Ibid.

76. Rothstein. Medical screening of workers:134.

77. Ibid.

78. Ibid.

79. School Board of Nassau Co. v. Arline, 55 U.S.L.W. 4245, 107 S. Ct. 1123 (1987).

80. McGarity TO, Schroeder EP. Risk oriented employment screening. Texas Law Rev 1981;59:999–1076.

81. Ibid.

82. Ibid.

83. Ann. Code of Maryland, art. 100, 95A (1978).

84. Rothstein. Medical screening of workers:124–127. The Wisconsin Supreme Court rejected an employer's exclusion of an epileptic which was based on the 10–30 percent chance that epileptics under medication will still have seizures. The Oregon Supreme Court upheld a Bureau of Labor ruling that a salesperson could not be denied a job because a myocardial infarction 6 years earlier and subsequent sporadic angina failed to indicate a "high probability" of future risk of heart attack.

85. OTA. The role of genetic testing.

86. Ibid.:128. See also Andrews. Medical genetics:205.

87. U.S. Bureau of the Census. Statistical abstract of the United States, 1982–83. Washington, D.C.: U.S. Government Printing Office, 1982:409(table 682).

88. Glass B. Science: endless horizons or golden age? Science 1971;171:23–29.

89. Ibid. Claims that males with the XYY phenotype have criminal or sexually deviant behavior have been disproven (see chapter 5). With recombinant DNA technology, many more than 100 recessive disorders will be detectable.

90. Meister SB, Shepard DS, Zeckhauser R. Cost effectiveness of prenatal screening for neural tube defects. In: Nightingale EO, Meister SB, eds. Prenatal screening, policies, and values: the example of neural tube defect. Cambridge, Mass.: Harvard University, 1987. Measuring the cost per abortion of affected fetuses, as Meister et al. do, permits comparisons only to other technologies in which abortion is also the planned outcome.

91. To make costs that are incurred over different periods of time comparable to each other, cost-benefit analyses discount costs to their current value. For example, the cost of treating someone in the future will be different in dollar value from the cost of treating someone today. No one knows how much costs will change, so the choice of rate used to determine the discount can affect the relationship of benefits to costs; benefits are often farther down the road than costs.

92. Suits in which negligence or poor quality of the laboratory can be proven have been and will continue to be won (see chapter 7). Somewhat more problematic are suits in which false negatives have a biologic basis. If, prior to testing, warning is given that a DNA-based test can fail to give a correct answer because of genetic heterogeneity—and this can then be demonstrated to be the basis for a false negative—the suit might be defensible. It is much harder to prove the biologic basis of a false negative when a continuous variable is measured—for instance, phenylalanine concentration in (gene product) screening for PKU. The high costs of malpractice settlements in cases involving neonatal screening have led to suggestions for limiting the liability of state and private laboratories. (States as well as hospitals and physicians have been sued.) Such limits would put a cap on this component of costs, but would certainly not assure better quality. See Andrews LB, ed. Legal liability and quality assurance in newborn screening. Chicago: American Bar Foundation, 1985.

93. Severe reactions and death have resulted from unnecessarily treating in-

fants who, as a result of neonatal screening, were wrongly diagnosed as having PKU. See Holtzman NA. Dietary treatment of inborn errors of metabolism. Ann Rev Med 1970;21:335–356.

94. Holtzman NA, Leonard CO, Farfel MR. Issues in antenatal and neonatal screening and surveillance for hereditary and congenital disorders. Ann Rev Pub Hlth 1981;2:219–251. See also Meister et al. Cost effectiveness of prenatal screening; and Ostrowsky JT, Lippman A, Scriver CR. Cost-benefit analysis of a thalassemia disease prevention program. Am J Pub Hlth 1985;75:732–736.

95. Chapple JC, Dale R, Evans BG. The new genetics: will it pay its way? Lancet 1987;1:1189–1192.

96. It is not so clear that neonatal screening for maple syrup urine disease or galactosemia would result in a cost savings if they were the only diseases for which screening was done. The frequency of both is considerably less than that of PKU, the course without treatment often leads to death rather than long-term disability, and treatment is not always started in time to prevent irreversible damage. Were it not for the fact that the specimen is being collected anyway, and that the screening laboratory is already established, screening for these conditions would not be justified economically.

97. See, for instance, CSIEM, Genetic screening:203–205.

98. Holtzman NA. [Unpublished estimates].

99. Ostrowsky et al. Cost-benefit analysis of a thalassemia disease prevention program.

100. Berwick DM, Cretin S, Keeler E. Cholesterol, children, and heart disease: an analysis of alternatives. New York: Oxford University Press, 1980.

101. Dickson D. The new politics of science. New York: Pantheon, 1984.

102. Pauling L. Our hope for the future. In: Fishbein M, ed. Birth defects. Philadelphia: J. B. Lippincott, 1963.

103. Shaw M. Conditional prospective rights of the fetus. J Leg Med 1984;5:63–116.

104. Morrison RD. Implications of prenatal diagnosis for the quality of, and right to, human life: society as standard. In: Hilton B, Callahan D, Harris M, Condliffe P, Berkley B, eds. Ethical issues in human genetics. New York: Plenum, 1973:201–211.

105. Saxton M. Prenatal screening and discriminatory attitudes about disability. Genewatch [Committee for Responsible Genetics, Boston, Mass.] 1987;4(1):8–10.

106. Motulsky A, Murray J. Will prenatal diagnosis with selective abortion affect society's attitude toward the handicapped? In: Berg K, Tranoy KE, eds. Research ethics. New York: Alan R. Liss, 1983:277–291.

107. Clow CL, Scriver CR. Knowledge about and attitudes toward genetic screening among high school students: the Tay-Sachs experience. Pediatrics 1977;59:86–91. This study did not elicit knowledge on the disease's mode of transmission, the risks of being a carrier, or the risks to one's offspring. Yet the authors concluded that "the level of knowledge about Tay-Sachs disease is high among students." "Awareness" might be a better description of these findings than "knowledge."

108. Scriver CR, Bardanis M, Cartier L, Clow CL, Lancaster GA, Ostrowsky JT. Beta-thalassemia disease prevention: genetic medicine applied. Am J Hum Genet 1984;36:1024–1038.

109. Ibid. The survey was conducted up to two years following screening.

110. Ibid. Abortion was unacceptable to 32 percent of the respondents; 30 percent were uncertain; and no response was obtained from 6 percent.

111. Zeesman S, Clow CL, Cartier L, Scriver CR. A private view of heterozygosity: eight-year follow-up study on carriers of the Tay-Sachs gene detected by high-school screening in Montreal. Am J Med Genet 1984;18:769–778. Fewer than one-third of those involved in the screening replied to the follow-up questionnaire mailed to them.

112. Stamatoyannopoulos G. Problems of screening and counseling in the hemoglobinopathies. In: Motulsky AG, Lenz W, eds. Birth defects. Amsterdam: Excerpta Medica, 1974:268–276.

113. Dandridge v. Williams, 397 U.S. 471 (1970).

114. Andrews. State laws and regulations:1–2. Five of these states make no provision for parental refusal; thirty-one permit it on religious grounds; nine states allow it on any grounds. In Maryland, North Carolina, and the District of Columbia, screening is voluntary.

115. CSIEM, Genetic screening:44–47.

116. Faden RR, Holtzman NA, Chwalow AJ. Parental rights, child welfare, and public health: the case of PKU screening. Am J Pub Hlth 1982;72:1396–1400.

117. President's Commission. Screening and counseling for genetic conditions.

118. CSIEM. Genetic screening:119. See also Reilly P. Genetics, law, and social policy. Cambridge, Mass.: Harvard University Press, 1977:67–68.

119. Reilly. Genetics, law, and social policy:67–68.

120. Ibid.

121. Simon v. Sargent, 346 F. Supp. 277 (D.Mass. 1972), aff'd, 400 U.S. 1020 (1972).

122. Turpin v. Sortini, 31 Cal. 3d 220, 643 P.2d, 182 Cal. Rptr. 337 (1982).

123. Andrews. Medical genetics:148.

124. Ibid.:142–146. Shaw MW. To be or not to be? That is the question. Am J Hum Genet 1984;36:1–9. Coplan J. Wrongful life and wrongful birth: new concepts for the pediatrician. Pediatrics 1985;75:65–72.

125. Andrews. Medical genetics:148.

126. Gleitman v. Cosgrove, 49 N.J. 22, 227 A.2d 689 (1967).

127. Roe v. Wade, 410 U.S. 113 (1973).

128. Kolder VEB, Gallagher J, Parsons MT. Court-ordered obstetrical interventions. N Engl J Med 1987;316:1192–1196.

129. Eisenstadt v. Baird, 405 U.S. 438 (1972).

130. Bowers v. Hardwick, 106 S. Ct. 2841 (1986).

131. I collected that information in the course of a survey of directors of federally supported genetics programs, but it was not included in the published report. See Holtzman NA. The impact of the federal cutback on genetic services. Am J Med Genet 1983;15:352–365.

132. Holtzman NA. Public participation in genetic policy-making: the Maryland Commission on Hereditary Disorders. In: Milunsky A, ed. Genetics and the law. II. New York: Plenum, 1980:247–258.

133. Shawn W. Notes on justification of putting the audience through a difficult evening. Notes accompanying Shawn's play, Aunt Dan and Lemon, April 1986, reproduced by Center Stage, Baltimore, Md., 1987.

134. Ludmerer KM. Genetics and American society. Baltimore: Johns Hopkins

University Press, 1972. See also Kevles DJ. In the name of eugenics. New York: Alfred A. Knopf, 1985.

135. Kevles. In the name of eugenics:183.

136. The first eugenic law limiting procreation in the United States, passed by Indiana in 1907, required the sterilization of institutionalized people who were mentally retarded or had been convicted of a crime whenever this was recommended by a board of experts. See Ludmerer. Genetics and American society:92. After the Supreme Court declared in 1927 that sterilization on eugenic grounds was within the police power of the state (Buck v. Bell, 274 U.S. 200 [1927]), twenty states adopted sterilization laws, and by 1956, 58,000 sterilizations had been performed on eugenic grounds. Although seldom used, not all of the sterilization laws have been repealed. See Reilly. Genetics, law, and social policy:121–148.

137. Hogben L. Science for the citizen. New York: Alfred A. Knopf, 1938:1053. Cited by Ludmerer, Genetics and American society:93.

138. Kevles. In the name of eugenics:93.

139. Hubbard R. Eugenics and prenatal testing. Intl J Hlth Services 1986;16: 227–242.

140. Kevles. In the name of eugenics:116–118. Prior to 1933 and perhaps for a few years thereafter, the German eugenics movement considered Jews members of the Aryan race and did not target them for extermination.

141. Quoted by Kevles. In the name of eugenics:92.

142. Sterilizing women with PKU will reduce retardation in the next generation, but the retardation prevented is not due to PKU but to the intrauterine exposure of the fetus to high concentrations of phenylalanine or its metabolites. (Placing such women on a low-phenylalanine diet from conception through pregnancy might also prevent retardation of the fetus.) Should these retarded individuals reproduce, their offspring would not have the same problem unless the females mated with males who carried the PKU allele. It is doubtful that there are many similar situations in which the offspring of a person with a recessive disorder is at high risk for disability regardless of the genotype of the spouse.

143. For an allele with a carrier frequency of one in twenty, one partner will be a carrier in 5 percent of the matings, but both partners will be carriers in only 0.25 percent of the matings. Matings of affected individuals would account for only .0625 percent of all matings. For a more extensive treatment of this subject and an indication of how slowly the population frequency of alleles for recessive disorders would be reduced by prenatal diagnosis and selective abortion, see Motulsky AG, Fraser FR, Felsenstein J. Public health and long-term genetic implications of intrauterine diagnosis and selective abortion. Birth Defects: Orig Art Ser 1971; 7(5):636–643.

144. Pauling L. Our hope for the future:164–170.

145. Sorenson et al. Reproductive pasts:42 (table 3-12). Only 6.9 percent of counselors thought this to be a "very important" goal. The very important goals to most counselors were "helping people to cope" (82.8 percent) and "removing or lessening guilt or anxiety" (75.2 percent).

146. Wertz D, Fletcher JC. Attitudes of genetic counselors: a multinational survey. Am J Hum Genet. [In press]. The most active counselors were less likely to consider "reduction of carriers" an important goal.

147. Shaw M. Conditional prospective rights of the fetus.

148. Ludmerer. Genetics and American society:96–113.

149. Shawn. Notes on justification of putting the audience through a difficult evening.

150. Finger A. Claiming *all* of our bodies: reproductive rights and disability. In: Arditti R, Duelli Klein R, Minden S, eds. Test tube women: what future for motherhood? London: Pandora Press, 1984:281–297.

151. Quoted, without attribution, by Saxton. Prenatal screening and discriminatory attitudes about disability.

152. Ibid.

153. Ibid.

154. Motulsky, Murray. Will prenatal diagnosis with selective abortion affect society's attitude toward the handicapped? In: Berg, Tranoy, eds. Research ethics:277–291.

155. Ibid.

156. Kass LR. Implication of prenatal diagnosis for the human right to life. In: Hilton et al., eds. Ethical issues in human genetics:185–199.

157. Annas G. Protecting the liberty of pregnant patients. N Engl J Med 1987;316:1213–1214.

158. Fletcher JC. Moral problems and ethical guidance in prenatal diagnosis. In: Milunsky A, ed. Genetic disorders and the fetus. New York: Plenum, 1986:819–859.

159. Later in the same article, Flectcher attenuates his respect for maternal autonomy: "However, unless that dominance of autonomy is at least balanced by needs and interests expressed from beyond the individual and family, many benefits that could be conferred upon society will not be realized. . . . In a system dominated by the interests of autonomy, the interests of the wider community suffer." Still later he makes clear what some of those interests might be: "Two factors can be expected to create pressure for change in the strong emphasis of the guidance on individual and family concerns: The costs of genetic disease to society will continue to rise, and more persons at higher genetic risk will take the risks of reproduction after genetic counseling." Fletcher acknowledges that this might be seen as eugenical. Ibid.

160. Neel JV. Social and scientific priorities in the use of genetic knowledge. In: Hilton et al., eds. Ethical issues in human genetics:353–368.

161. Motulsky A. Impact of genetic manipulation on society and medicine. Science 1983;219:135–140. Motulsky writes: "From a strictly biologic viewpoint, the necessity for humans to wear clothes is a deleterious trait, in that we lost the genes for hariness that protected us against the elements."

162. Ibid.

163. Dobzhansky T. Comments on genetic evolution. Daedalus 1961;90:461–462.

Chapter 9: What Is (Going) to Be Done?

1. Childs B. Genetics for medical students. Am J Hum Genet 1987;41:296–303.

2. Marks J. Personal communication, August 1987.

3. Committee for the Study of Inborn Errors of Metabolism (CSIEM). Genetic screening: programs, principles, and research. Washington, D.C.: National Academy of Sciences, 1975:36.

4. Holtzman NA. [Unpublished data].

5. Cunningham G. Personal communication, January 1984.

6. Tuerck JM, Buist NRM, Skeels MR, Miyahira RS, Beach PG. Computerized surveillance of errors in newborn screening programs. Am J Pub Hlth 1987;77:1528–1531.

7. Ann. Code of Maryland, Art. 100, 95A (1978).

8. Holtzman NA. The impact of the federal cutback on genetic services. Am J Med Genet 1983;15:353–365.

9. CSIEM, Genetic screening:188.

Index